MATH FOR MEDS
DOSAGES AND SOLUTIONS

MATH FOR MEDS

DOSAGES AND SOLUTIONS

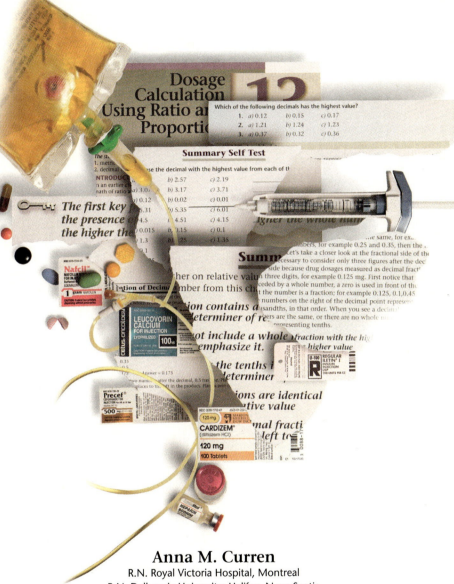

Anna M. Curren

R.N. Royal Victoria Hospital, Montreal

B.N. Dalhousie University, Halifax, Nova Scotia

M.A. California State University, Long Beach, CA

Former Associate Professor of Nursing, Long Beach
City College, Long Beach, CA

Laurie D. Munday

R.N. Los Angeles County U.S.C. Medical Center

B.N. California State University, Los Angeles, CA

M.N., U.C.L.A. Los Angeles, CA

Former Associate Professor of Nursing, San Diego
City College, San Diego, CA

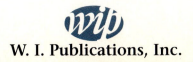

W. I. Publications, Inc.

ACKNOWLEDGMENTS. Hundreds of people have contributed in immeasurable ways to the 7th edition of *Math For Meds* over the past year. They have received our heartfelt thanks as we moved along through each step of the rewriting process. However, some very talented professionals deserve not only thanks but recognition. In particular we wish to thank Rae Richard, RN, BSN, CRNI, Coordinator of the IV Therapy Department, and Jeff Goodban, Pharm. D., Staff Pharmacist, of Scripps Memorial Hospital, La Jolla, Ca., both of whom made our every request for information and assistance a priority. Mark A. Acosta, Pharm. D., Pharmacy Coordinator of Children's Hospital, San Diego, was an invaluable resource on pediatric IV medications. Dr. Shirley Naret, Professor of Nursing, Long Beach City College, Long Beach, Ca. also consulted on the pediatric section. We thank Marlene Murdoch for her timely completion of the Toronto Hospital medication record.

Additional medication records for reproduction in the text were provided by the University of California and Veterans Hospital in San Diego, Ca., and Lionville Systems, Inc. Abbott Laboratories provided photos of their ADD-Vantage® medication system and PCA infusor. IVAC Corporation and McGaw Laboratories loaned equipment for additional photography of IV infusion devices. The following pharmaceutical companies provided labels for reproduction: Abbott, American Cyanamid, Ascot, Astra USA, Ayerst, Beecham, Berlex, Bristol/Apothecon, Bristol Meyers Squibb, Burroughs Wellcome, Cetus Oncology, Ciba-Geighy, Dupont, Eli Lilly/Dista, Elkins-Sinn, Geneva, Glaxo, Hoechst-Roussel, Invenex, Lederle, Lypho Med, Marion Merrell Dow, McNeil, Mead Johnson, Merck, Miles, Nova Nordisk, Parke Davis/Warner-Lambert, Pharmacia, Pfizer/Roerig/Pratt, A.H. Robins, Roxane, Searle, Schering, SmithKline Beecham, E.R. Squibb/Squibb-Marsham, Travenol, Upjohn, Whitby, and Wyeth-Ayerst.

Our final thank you goes to the hundreds of nurse educators continent wide who wrote with suggestions. As always their input was indispensable.

BOOK AND COVER DESIGN
Peter T. Noble Associates, Encinitas, CA

PHOTOGRAPHY
Kim Brun Studios, Inc., San Diego, CA

COMPOSITION AND PAGE MAKEUP
ColorType, San Diego, CA

ELECTRONIC PREPRESS
Northwestern Colorgraphics, Inc., Menasha, WI

PRINTING AND BINDING
Banta Company, Menasha, WI

Printed in the United States of America

Library of Congress catalog card number 76-43259

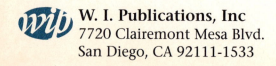

W. I. Publications, Inc
7720 Clairemont Mesa Blvd.
San Diego, CA 92111-1533

PUBLISHER'S NOTICE. The authors have designed this text to assist student nurses to develop professional competence. The authors have taken every reasonable precaution to ensure that the instructional content contained in the text is current and accurate. However, the authors and publisher specifically make no implied or expressed warranties, representations or guarantees of any kind with respect to or responsibility for, any material included in the text. The authors and publisher shall not be liable for any special, consequential or exemplary damages resulting in whole or in part, from the readers use of, or reliance upon, this material.

All instructional information, including but not limited to examples, illustrations, and equations are offered here for the limited purposes of illustrating and explaining general techniques. Still, the facts and circumstances of every case inevitably require variations and unique medical knowledge.

The determination of amounts and proportions and the administration of prescription drugs is the rendering of medical services and no text can assume that responsibility. The responsibility ultimately rests with the individual medical practitioner.

PREFACE

Math For Meds has long been acknowledged for its succinct, thorough and interest maintaining writing style. The seventh edition has not only remained true to the style of previous editions but, with meticulous attention to its instructional intent, improved *Math For Meds* in many ways, some more obvious than others. Using hundreds of instructor submitted suggestions, the entire content has been completely reviewed and, where necessary, revised and expanded. Hundreds of new examples and problems have been added in critical learning areas. Expanded emphasis has been placed on the calculation and administration of intravenous medications, including a unique introductory chapter on IV therapy. In no other clinical area is so much demanded of all levels of nursing personnel, and it is fitting that the scope of the text reflect this. A totally new book design has been utilized which includes an easier to read typeface and full color photographs and illustrations.

As in past editions *Math For Meds* has been written to meet the needs of learners at all curricular levels, and with all levels of ability. The self instructional format has no time constraints, and allows self pacing of instruction. The rapidly changing and increasing nursing responsibilities in medication administration have made assessment of dosage calculations and orders an urgent concern. *Math For Meds* addresses this concern in depth. The focus throughout this edition is on teaching the student how to locate information, how to use information once it is located, and how to assess calculations based on this information. With this emphasis *Math For Meds* provides a wide range of safety for performance based on its teachings.

Since its first edition *Math For Meds* has been the most widely adopted text in its subject area of dosage calculations. It has been and continues to be a trendsetter, often imitated, yet to be equaled. The seventh edition has continued this tradition.

Anna Curren
Laurie Munday

La Jolla, California
October 1994

DEDICATION

For the past eight years we have been both assisted
and consistently challenged by two very talented
graphic designers, who have added much to our
skills and professional life. Through us they have also
made a significant contribution to nursing educa-
tion. In recognition of these contributions we
dedicate this edition of *Math For Meds* to

Louis Neiheisel and Stephen Harrison

DIRECTIONS TO THE STUDENT

Over half a million students have successfully learned dosage calculations from *Math For Meds*, and you can too! You don't have to be a math expert to use this text, all that is required is average ability and a desire to learn. If you have not used your math skills for a number of years you will still have no difficulty, because the refresher math section will quickly bring you up to date. *Math For Meds* lets you move at your own pace through the content, which ranges from easy to thought provoking, and hundreds of examples and problems will keep your learning on track. You will enjoy learning from *Math For Meds*, and here are a few tips to get you started:

1. Have a good supply of paper and pencils ready as you do each chapter. Record your answers to problems here as well as in your text so you won't have to refer back to pages you have completed.

2. As you work your way through *Math For Meds* do exactly as you are instructed to do, and no more.

Programmed learning proceeds in small steps, and jumping ahead can cause confusion.

3. Except for the first few refresher math chapters where you are instructed otherwise, you may use a calculator for all your calculations. Decide which calculator you want to use and set the "F CUT 5/4" setting at 5/4 (this is the rounding off control).

When you have completed your program we recommend that you keep *Math For Meds* as one of your permanent reference texts. You may find yourself needing a refresher in specific calculation skills as a graduate, or you may need the entire text as a refresher if you take time out from the profession at any time. Math does not change very much, and much of *Math For Meds'* content is timeless.

So, provide yourself with pencil, paper, calculator and a distraction free atmosphere as you discover that *Math For Meds* is a fun way to learn!

CONTENTS

ONE

Refresher Math

1

Relative Value, Addition and Subtraction of Decimals

OBJECTIVES

The student will
1. identify the relative value of decimals
2. add decimals
3. subtract decimals

PREREQUISITE

Recognize the abbreviation mg, for milligram, as a drug measure.

INTRODUCTION

In the course of administering medications you will be calculating drug dosages which contain decimals, for example 2.5 mg. The math you will need for these calculations is not difficult, and the first two chapters of this text will provide a complete and easy refresher of everything that you must know about decimals. Let's begin with a review of the relative value of decimals, so that you will be able to recognize which of two or more numbers has the highest (and lowest) value.

Relative Value of Decimals

The easiest way to begin a review of decimal numbers is to visualize them on a scale which has a decimal point at its center. Look for a moment at figure 1.

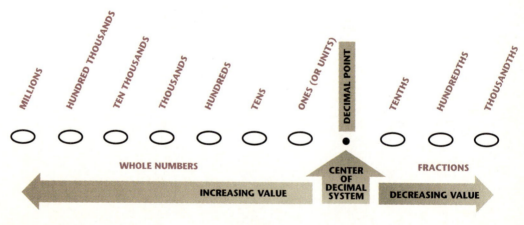

Figure 1

Notice that on the left of the decimal point are the whole numbers, and on the right the fractions. On the whole number (left) side of the scale the measures rise increasingly in value, from ones, to tens, to hundreds, and so on to millions, which is the highest measure you will see in drug dosages. Our monetary system of dollars and cents is a decimal system, and the relative value of the whole numbers is exactly as you now know and use them: the higher the number, the higher the value.

 The first key point in determining relative value of decimals is the presence of whole numbers. The higher the whole number, the higher the value.

EXAMPLE 1 10.1 is higher than 9.1

EXAMPLE 2 3.2 is higher than 2.9

EXAMPLE 3 7.01 is higher than 6.99

Problem

Identify the number with the highest value in each of the following.

1. *a)* 3.5   *b)* 2.7   *c)* 4.2
2. *a)* 6.15   *b)* 5.95   *c)* 4.54
3. *a)* 12.02   *b)* 10.19   *c)* 11.04

ANSWERS   1. c   2. a   3. a

If, however, the whole numbers are the same, for example **10**.2 and **10**.7, or there are no whole numbers, for example **0**.25 and **0**.35, then the fraction will determine the relative value. Let's take a closer look at the fractional side of the scale. Refer to figure 2.

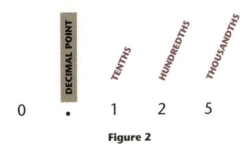

Figure 2

It is necessary to consider only three figures after the decimal point on the fractional side because drug dosages measured as decimal fractions do not contain more than three digits, for example 0.125 mg. First notice that **if a decimal fraction is not preceded by a whole number, a zero is used in front of the decimal point to emphasize that the number is a fraction**; for example **0**.125, **0**.1, **0**.45. Look once again at figure 2. The numbers on the right of the decimal point represent tenths, hundredths, and thousandths, in that order. When you see a decimal fraction in which the whole numbers are the same, or there are no whole numbers, stop and look closely at the number representing the **tenths.**

 The fraction with the highest number representing tenths has the higher value.

EXAMPLE 1 0.3 is higher than 0.2

EXAMPLE 2 0.41 is higher than 0.29

EXAMPLE 3 1.21 is higher than 1.19

Problem

Which of the following decimals has the highest value?

1. *a)* 0.4   *b)* 0.2   *c)* 0.5
2. *a)* 2.73   *b)* 2.61   *c)* 2.87
3. *a)* 0.19   *b)* 0.61   *c)* 0.34

ANSWERS 1. c **2.** c **3.** b

If in decimal fractions the numbers representing the **tenths** are identical, for example, 0.**2**5 and 0.**2**7, then **the number representing the hundredths will determine the relative value.**

 The decimal fraction with the higher number representing hundredths will have the higher value when the tenths are identical.

EXAMPLE 1 0.2**7** is higher than 0.2**5**

EXAMPLE 2 0.1**5** is higher than 0.1 (0.1 is the same as 0.1**0**)

Extra zeros on the end of decimal fractions are omitted because they can cause confusion, although they do not alter the value of the fraction (0.10 is the same as 0.1).

EXAMPLE 3 2.25 is higher than 2.2   (same as 2.20)

EXAMPLE 4 9.77 is higher than 9.75

Problem

Which of the following decimals has the highest value?

1. *a)* 0.12   *b)* 0.15   *c)* 0.17
2. *a)* 1.21   *b)* 1.24   *c)* 1.23
3. *a)* 0.37   *b)* 0.32   *c)* 0.36

ANSWERS 1. c **2.** b **3.** a

Problem

Which decimal fraction has the higher value?

a) 0.125   *b)* 0.25

ANSWER The correct answer is b) 0.25. The decimal fraction which has the higher number representing the **tenths** has the higher value. **2** is higher than **1**; therefore 0.25 has a higher value than 0.125. Medication errors have been made in this **identical** decimal fraction; so remember it well.

 The number of figures on the right of the decimal point is not an indication of relative value. Always look at the figure representing the tenths first, and if these are identical, the hundredths, to determine which is higher.

This completes your introduction to the relative value of decimals. The key points just reviewed will cover all situations in dosage calculations where you will have to recognize high and low values. Therefore, you are now ready to test yourself more extensively on this information.

Problem

Identify the decimal with the highest value in each of the following.

1. *a)* 0.25   *b)* 0.5   *c)* 0.125 _____
2. *a)* 0.4   *b)* 0.45   *c)* 0.5   _____
3. *a)* 7.5   *b)* 6.25   *c)* 4.75   _____
4. *a)* 0.3   *b)* 0.25   *c)* 0.35   _____
5. *a)* 1.125   *b)* 1.75   *c)* 1.5   _____
6. *a)* 4.5   *b)* 4.75   *c)* 4.25   _____
7. *a)* 0.1   *b)* 0.01   *c)* 0.04   _____
8. *a)* 5.75   *b)* 6.25   *c)* 6.5   _____
9. *a)* 0.6   *b)* 0.16   *c)* 0.06   _____
10. *a)* 3.55   *b)* 2.95   *c)* 3.7   _____

ANSWERS   1. b   **2.** c   **3.** a   **4.** c   **5.** b   **6.** b   **7.** a   **8.** c   **9.** a   **10.** c

Addition and Subtraction of Decimals

There are several key points which will make addition and subtraction of decimal fractions easier and safer. Let's look at these.

 When you first write the numbers down, line up the decimal points.

EXAMPLE   To add 0.25 and 0.27

    0.25   0.25
    0.27 is safe   0.27 may be unsafe, it could lead to errors.

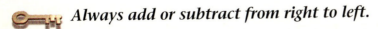 *Always add or subtract from right to left.*

If you found it necessary to write the numbers down, don't confuse yourself by trying to "eyeball" the answer. Also, write any numbers carried, or rewrite those reduced by borrowing if you find this helpful.

EXAMPLE 1 When adding 0.25 and 0.27

$$\begin{array}{r} \overset{1}{0.25} \\ \underline{0.27} \\ 0.52 \end{array}$$
add the 5 and 7 first, then the 2, 2, and
then 1 you carried. Right to left.

EXAMPLE 2 When subtracting 0.63 from 0.71

$$\begin{array}{r} \overset{6\,1}{0.\cancel{7}1} \\ \underline{0.63} \\ 0.08 \end{array}$$
borrow 1 from 7 and rewrite as 6,
write the borrowed 1. Subtract 3 from 11.
Subtract 6 from 6. Work from right to left.

 Add zeros as necessary to make the fractions of equal length.

This does not alter the value of the fractions and it helps prevent confusion and mistakes.

EXAMPLE When subtracting 0.125 from 0.25

$$\begin{array}{l} 0.25 \\ 0.125 \end{array} \quad \text{becomes} \quad \begin{array}{l} 0.250 \\ 0.125 \end{array} \quad \text{Answer} = 0.125$$

If you follow these rules and make them a habit you will automatically reduce calculation errors. The following problems will give you an excellent opportunity to practice them.

Problem

Add the following decimals.

1. $0.25 + 0.5$ = _____
2. $0.1 + 2.25$ = _____
3. $1.7 + 0.75$ = _____
4. $1.4 + 0.02$ = _____
5. $2.3 + 1.45$ = _____

6. $3.7 + 1.05 + 2.2$ = _____
7. $6.42 + 13.3 + 9.55$ = _____
8. $5.57 + 4.03 + 13.02$ = _____
9. $0.33 + 8.41 + 6.09$ = _____
10. $7.44 + 3.04 + 11.31$ = _____

Subtract the following decimals.

11. $1.25 - 1.125$ = _____
12. $3.2 - 0.65$ = _____
13. $2.3 - 1.45$ = _____
14. $0.02 - 0.01$ = _____
15. $5 - 2.5$ = _____

16. $7.33 - 4.04$ = _____
17. $12.45 - 2.07$ = _____
18. $0.07 - 0.035$ = _____
19. $1.175 - 0.23$ = _____
20. $5.75 - 0.95$ = _____

ANSWERS 1. 0.75 **2.** 2.35 **3.** 2.45 **4.** 1.42 **5.** 3.75 **6.** 6.95 **7.** 29.27 **8.** 22.62 **9.** 14.83 **10.** 21.79 **11.** 0.125 **12.** 2.55 **13.** 0.85 **14.** 0.01 **15.** 2.5 **16.** 3.29 **17.** 10.38 **18.** 0.035 **19.** 0.945 **20.** 4.8

Summary

This concludes the refresher on relative value, addition, and subtraction of decimals. The important points to remember from this chapter are:

if the decimal fraction contains a whole number, the value of the whole number is the first determiner of relative value

if the fraction does not include a whole number a zero is placed in front of the decimal point to emphasize it

the number representing the tenths in a decimal fraction is the first determiner of relative value

if the tenths in decimal fractions are identical, the number representing hundredths will determine relative value

when adding or subtracting decimal fractions, first line up the decimal points, then add or subtract from right to left

Summary Self Test

Directions: Choose the decimal with the highest value from each of the following.

1. *a)* 2.45   *b)* 2.57   *c)* 2.19   _____

2. *a)* 3.07   *b)* 3.17   *c)* 3.71   _____

3. *a)* 0.12   *b)* 0.02   *c)* 0.01   _____

4. *a)* 5.31   *b)* 5.35   *c)* 6.01   _____

5. *a)* 4.5   *b)* 4.51   *c)* 4.15   _____

6. *a)* 0.015   *b)* 0.15   *c)* 0.1   _____

7. *a)* 1.3   *b)* 1.25   *c)* 1.35   _____

8. *a)* 0.1   *b)* 0.2   *c)* 0.25   _____

9. *a)* 0.125   *b)* 0.1   *c)* 0.05   _____

10. *a)* 13.7   *b)* 13.5   *c)* 13.25   _____

11. If you have medication tablets whose strength is 0.1 mg, and you must give 0.3 mg, you will need

    a) 1 tablet   *b)* less than 1 tablet   *c)* more than 1 tablet   _____

12. If you have tablets with a strength of 0.25 mg and you must give 0.125 mg you will need

    a) 1 tablet   *b)* less than 1 tablet   *c)* more than 1 tablet   _____

13. If you have an order to give a dosage of 7.5 mg and the tablets have a strength of 3.75 mg you will need

    a) 1 tablet   *b)* less than 1 tablet   *c)* more than 1 tablet   _____

14. If the order is to give 0.5 mg and the tablet strength is 0.5 mg you will give

    a) 1 tablet   *b)* less than 1 tablet   *c)* more than 1 tablet _____

15. The order is to give 0.5 mg and the tablets have a strength of 0.25 mg. You must give

    a) 1 tablet   *b)* less than 1 tablet   *c)* more than 1 tablet _____

Directions: Add the following decimals.

16. 1.31 + 0.4 = _____

17. 0.15 + 0.25 = _____

18. 2.5 + 0.75 = _____

19. 3.2 + 2.17 = _____

20. 1.3 + 1.04 + 0.7 = _____

21. 4.1 + 3.03 + 0.4 = _____

22. 0.5 + 0.5 + 0.5 = _____

23. 5.4 + 2.6 + 0.09 = _____

24. You have just given 2 tablets with a dosage strength of 3.5 mg each. What was the total dosage administered? _____

25. You are to give your patient one tablet labeled 0.5 mg and one labeled 0.25 mg. What is the total dosage of these two tablets? _____

26. If you give two tablets labeled 0.02 mg what total dosage will you administer? _____

27. You are to give one tablet labeled 0.8 mg and two tablets labeled 0.4 mg. What is the total dosage? _____

28. You have two tablets, one is labeled 0.15 mg and the other 0.3 mg. What is the total dosage of these two tablets? _____

Directions: Subtract the following decimals.

29. 4.32 – 3.1 = _____

30. 2.1 – 1.91 = _____

31. 3.7 – 1.93 = _____

32. 5.75 – 4.02 = _____

33. 1.3 – 0.02 = _____

34. 0.2 – 0.07 = _____

35. 3.95 – 0.35 = _____

36. 1.9 – 0.08 = _____

37. Your patient is to receive a dosage of 7.5 mg and you have only one tablet labeled 3.75 mg. How many more milligrams must you give? _____

38. You have a tablet labeled 0.02 mg and your patient is to receive 0.06 mg. many more milligrams do you need? _____

39. The tablet available is labeled 0.5 mg but you must give a dosage of 1.5 mg. How many more milligrams will you need to obtain the correct dosage?

_____

40. Your patient is to receive a dosage of 1.2 mg and you have one tablet labeled 0.6 mg. What additional dosage in milligrams will you need?

_____

41. You must give your patient a dosage of 2.2 mg but have only two tablets labeled 0.55 mg. What additional dosage in milligrams will you need?

_____

Directions: Determine how many tablets will be needed to give the following dosages.

42. Tablets are labeled 0.01 mg. You must give 0.02 mg. _____

43. Tablets are labeled 2.5 mg; you must give 5 mg. _____

44. Tablets are labeled 0.25 mg. Give 0.125 mg. _____

45. Tablets are 0.5 mg. Give 1.5 mg. _____

46. A dosage of 1.8 mg is ordered. Tablets are 0.6 mg. _____

47. Tablets available are 0.04 mg. You are to give 0.02 mg. _____

48. The dosage ordered is 3.5 mg. The tablets available are 1.75 mg.

_____

49. Prepare a dosage of 3.2 mg using tablets with a strength of 1.6 mg.

_____

50. You have tablets labeled 0.25 mg, and a dosage of 0.375 mg is ordered.

_____

ANSWERS   1. b 2. c 3. a 4. c 5. b 6. b 7. c 8. c 9. a 10. a 11. c 12. b 13. c 14. a 15. c
16. 1.71 17. 0.4 18. 3.25 19. 5.37 20. 3.04 21. 7.53 22. 1.5 23. 8.09 24. 7 mg 25. 0.75 mg
26. 0.04 mg 27. 1.6 mg 28. 0.45 mg 29. 1.22 30. 0.19 31. 1.77 32. 1.73 33. 1.28 34. 0.13 35. 3.6
36. 1.82 37. 3.75 mg 38. 0.04 mg 39. 1 mg 40. 0.6 mg 41. 1.1 mg 42. 2 tab 43. 2 tab 44. 1/2 tab
45. 3 tab 46. 3 tab 47. 1/2 tab 48. 2 tab 49. 2 tab 50. 1 1/2 tab

2

Multiplication and Division of Decimals

OBJECTIVES

The student will

1. define product, numerator and denominator
2. multiply decimal fractions
3. reduce fractions using common denominators
4. divide fractions and express answers to the nearest tenth, and hundredth

INTRODUCTION

Multiplication and division of decimals is a routine part of calculating drug dosages. This is an area where using a calculator may be helpful. For the purpose of understanding and review, however, you may wish to do the following exercises without one. Let's begin with multiplication.

Multiplication of Decimals

The main precaution in multiplication of decimals is the **placement of the decimal point in the answer** (which is called the **product**).

 The decimal point in the product of decimal fractions is placed the same number of places to the left as the total of numbers after the decimal point in the fractions multiplied.

EXAMPLE 1 0.35×0.5

Begin by lining the numbers up on the right, since this is somewhat safer; then disregard the decimals during the actual multiplication.

$$
\begin{array}{r}
0.35 \\
\underline{0.5} \\
175
\end{array}
\qquad \text{Answer} = 0.175
$$

0.35 has two numbers after the decimal, 0.5 has one. Place the decimal point three places to the left in the product. Place a zero (0) in front of the decimal to emphasize it.

EXAMPLE 2
$$\begin{array}{r} 1.4 \\ \underline{0.25} \\ 70 \\ \underline{28} \\ 350 \end{array}$$ Answer = 0.35

1.4 has one number after the decimal, 0.25 has two. Place the decimal point three places to the left in the product, and add a zero in front (0.350). Once the decimal is correctly placed the excess zero is dropped from the end of the fraction, and 0.350 becomes 0.35

 If the product contains insufficient numbers for correct placement of the decimal point, add as many zeros as necessary to the left of the product to correct this.

EXAMPLE 3
$$\begin{array}{r} 0.21 \\ \underline{0.32} \\ 42 \\ \underline{63} \\ 672 \end{array}$$ Answer = 0.0672

In this example 0.21 has two numbers after the decimal, and 0.32 also has two. However, there are only three numbers in the product, so a zero must be added to the left of these numbers to place the decimal point correctly: 672 becomes 0.0672

EXAMPLE 4
$$\begin{array}{r} 0.12 \\ \underline{0.2} \\ 24 \end{array}$$ Answer = 0.024

There are a total of three numbers after the decimal points in 0.12 and 0.2. One zero must be added in the product to place the decimal point correctly: 24 becomes 0.024

Problem

Multiply the following decimal fractions.

1. 0.45 × 0.2 = _____

2. 1.3 × 0.15 = _____

3. 3.5 × 1.2 = _____

4. 2.2 × 1.1 = _____

5. 1.3 × 0.05 = _____

6. 6.25 × 3.2 = _____

7. 0.7 × 0.05 = _____

8. 12.5 × 2.2 = _____

9. 16 × 0.3   = _____

10. 0.4 × 0.17 = _____

11. 2.14 × 0.9 = _____

12. 0.35 × 1.9 = _____

ANSWERS 1. 0.09 **2.** 0.195 **3.** 4.2 **4.** 2.42 **5.** 0.065 **6.** 20 **7.** 0.035 **8.** 27.5 **9.** 4.8 **10.** 0.068 **11.** 1.926 **12.** 0.665

Division of Decimals

Look at this sample division:

$$\frac{0.25}{0.125} = \frac{\text{numerator}}{\text{denominator}}$$

You may recall that the **top number,** 0.25, is called the **numerator,** while the **bottom number,** 0.125, is called the **denominator.** (If you have trouble remembering which is which, think of D, for down, for denominator, the denominator is on the bottom). With this basic terminology reviewed we are now ready to look at two preliminary math steps which are used to simplify the fraction prior to final division. The first step is to eliminate the decimal points completely.

Elimination of Decimal Points

Decimal points can be eliminated from the numbers in a decimal fraction without changing its value.

 To eliminate the decimal points from decimal fractions move them the same number of places to the right in both the numerator and the denominator until they are eliminated in both. Zeros may have to be added to accomplish this.

EXAMPLE 1 $\dfrac{0.25}{0.125}$ becomes $\dfrac{250}{125}$

The decimal point must be moved three places to the right in 0.125 to make it 125. Therefore it must be moved three places in 0.25, which requires the addition of one zero to make it 250.

EXAMPLE 2 $\dfrac{0.3}{0.15}$ becomes $\dfrac{30}{15}$

The decimal point must be moved two places in 0.15 to make it 15. It must be moved two places in 0.3, which requires the addition of one zero to become 30.

EXAMPLE 3 $\dfrac{1.5}{2}$ becomes $\dfrac{15}{20}$

Move the decimal point one place in 1.5 to make it 15; add one zero to 2 to make it 20.

EXAMPLE 4 $\dfrac{4.5}{0.95}$ becomes $\dfrac{450}{95}$

Remember that moving the decimal point does not alter the value of the fraction or the answer you will obtain in the final division. It just makes the numbers easier to work with. Now try some problems on your own.

Problem

Eliminate the decimal points from the following decimal fractions.

1. $\dfrac{17.5}{2}$ = _____

2. $\dfrac{0.5}{25}$ = _____

3. $\dfrac{6.3}{0.6}$ = _____

4. $\dfrac{3.76}{0.4}$ = _____

5. $\dfrac{8.4}{0.7}$ = _____

6. $\dfrac{0.1}{0.05}$ = _____

7. $\dfrac{0.9}{0.03}$ = _____

8. $\dfrac{10.75}{2.5}$ = _____

9. $\dfrac{0.4}{0.04}$ = _____

10. $\dfrac{1.2}{0.4}$ = _____

ANSWERS 1. $\dfrac{175}{20}$ 2. $\dfrac{5}{250}$ 3. $\dfrac{63}{6}$ 4. $\dfrac{376}{40}$ 5. $\dfrac{84}{7}$ 6. $\dfrac{10}{5}$ 7. $\dfrac{90}{3}$ 8. $\dfrac{1075}{250}$ 9. $\dfrac{40}{4}$ 10. $\dfrac{12}{4}$

Reduction of Fractions

Once the decimal points are eliminated the next step is to reduce the numbers as far as possible.

 To reduce fractions divide both numbers by their highest common denominator (the highest number which will divide into both).

The highest common denominator is usually 2, 3, 4, 5, or multiples of these numbers, such as 6, 8, 25, and so on.

EXAMPLE 1 $\dfrac{175}{20}$ The highest common denominator is 5

$$\dfrac{\cancel{175}}{\cancel{20}} = \dfrac{35}{4}$$

EXAMPLE 2 $\dfrac{63}{6}$ The highest common denominator is 3

$$\dfrac{\cancel{63}}{\cancel{6}} = \dfrac{21}{2}$$

EXAMPLE 3 $\dfrac{1075}{250}$ The highest common denominator is 25

$$\dfrac{\cancel{1075}}{\cancel{250}} = \dfrac{43}{10}$$

There is a second way you could have reduced the fraction in example 3, and it is equally as correct. Divide by 5, then 5 again.

$$\frac{1075}{250} = \frac{215}{50} = \frac{43}{10}$$

 If the highest common denominator is difficult to determine, reduce several times by using smaller common denominators.

EXAMPLE 4 $\frac{376}{40} = \frac{47}{5}$ Reduce by 8

or divide by 4, then 2 $\frac{376}{40} = \frac{94}{10} = \frac{47}{5}$

or divide by 2, 2, and 2 $\frac{376}{40} = \frac{188}{20} = \frac{94}{10} = \frac{47}{5}$

Remember that simple numbers are easiest to work with, and the time spent in extra reductions may be well worth the payoff in safety.

Problem

Reduce the following fractions as much as possible in preparation for final division.

1. $\frac{84}{8}$ = _____   6. $\frac{40}{14}$ = _____

2. $\frac{20}{16}$ = _____   7. $\frac{82}{28}$ = _____

3. $\frac{250}{325}$ = _____   8. $\frac{100}{75}$ = _____

4. $\frac{96}{34}$ = _____   9. $\frac{50}{75}$ = _____

5. $\frac{175}{20}$ = _____   10. $\frac{60}{88}$ = _____

ANSWERS   1. $\frac{21}{2}$ 2. $\frac{5}{4}$ 3. $\frac{10}{13}$ 4. $\frac{48}{17}$ 5. $\frac{35}{4}$ 6. $\frac{20}{7}$ 7. $\frac{41}{14}$ 8. $\frac{4}{3}$ 9. $\frac{2}{3}$ 10. $\frac{15}{22}$

Reduction of Numbers Ending in Zero

There is one other type of reduction which, while not solely related to decimal fractions, is best covered at this time. This concerns reductions when both numbers in the fraction end with zeros.

EXAMPLE $\frac{2500}{500}$

 Fractions in which both the numerator and denominator end in a zero or zeros may be reduced by crossing off the same number of zeros in each.

EXAMPLE 1 $\dfrac{800}{250}$

In this fraction the numerator, 800, has two zeros, and the denominator, 250, has one zero. The number of zeros crossed off must be the same in both numerator and denominator, so only one zero can be eliminated from each.

$$\dfrac{80\cancel{0}}{25\cancel{0}} = \dfrac{80}{25}$$

EXAMPLE 2 $\dfrac{24\cancel{00}}{20\cancel{00}} = \dfrac{24}{20}$

Two zeros can be eliminated from the denominator and numerator in this fraction.

EXAMPLE 3 $\dfrac{15\cancel{000}}{30\cancel{000}} = \dfrac{15}{30}$

In this fraction three zeros can be eliminated.

Problem

Reduce the following fractions in preparation for final division.

1. $\dfrac{50}{250}$ = _____

2. $\dfrac{120}{50}$ = _____

3. $\dfrac{2500}{1500}$ = _____

4. $\dfrac{1,000,000}{750,000}$ = _____

5. $\dfrac{800}{150}$ = _____

6. $\dfrac{110}{100}$ = _____

7. $\dfrac{200,000}{150,000}$ = _____

8. $\dfrac{1000}{800}$ = _____

9. $\dfrac{60}{40}$ = _____

10. $\dfrac{150}{200}$ = _____

ANSWERS   1. $\dfrac{1}{5}$ **2.** $\dfrac{12}{5}$ **3.** $\dfrac{5}{3}$ **4.** $\dfrac{4}{3}$ **5.** $\dfrac{16}{3}$ **6.** $\dfrac{11}{10}$ **7.** $\dfrac{4}{3}$ **8.** $\dfrac{5}{4}$ **9.** $\dfrac{3}{2}$ **10.** $\dfrac{3}{4}$

Division of Decimals and Expressing to the Nearest Tenth

When a fraction is reduced as much as possible it is ready for final division. This is done by dividing the numerator by the denominator. Answers are most often rounded off and expressed as decimal numbers to the nearest tenth.

   To express an answer to the nearest tenth the division is carried to hundredths (two places after the decimal). When the number representing hundredths is 5 or larger, the number representing tenths is increased by one.

EXAMPLE 1 $\dfrac{0.35}{0.4}$ $=$ $0.35 \div 0.4$ $=$ 0.87

Answer $=$ **0.9**

The number representing hundredths is 5, so the number representing tenths is increased by one.   8.7 becomes 8.8

EXAMPLE 2 $\dfrac{0.5}{0.3}$ $=$ $0.5 \div 0.3$ $=$ 1.66 $=$ **1.7**

The number representing hundredths, 6, is larger than 5, and 6 becomes 7

EXAMPLE 3 $\dfrac{0.16}{0.3}$ $=$ 0.53 $=$ **0.5**

The number representing hundredths, 3, is less than 5, so the number representing tenths, 5, remains unchanged.

EXAMPLE 4 $\dfrac{0.2}{0.3}$ $=$ 0.66 $=$ **0.7**

EXAMPLE 5 An answer of 1.42 remains 1.4

EXAMPLE 6 An answer of 1.86 becomes 1.9

Problem

Divide the following decimal numbers and express your answers to the nearest tenth.

1. $\dfrac{5.1}{2.3}$ $=$ _____

2. $\dfrac{0.9}{0.7}$ $=$ _____

3. $\dfrac{3.7}{2}$ $=$ _____

4. $\dfrac{6}{1.3}$ $=$ _____

5. $\dfrac{1.5}{2.1}$ $=$ _____

6. $\dfrac{2.7}{1.1}$ $=$ _____

7. $\dfrac{4.2}{5}$ $=$ _____

8. $\dfrac{0.5}{2.5}$ $=$ _____

9. $\dfrac{5.2}{0.91}$ $=$ _____

10. $\dfrac{2.4}{2.7}$ $=$ _____

ANSWERS   1. 2.2   **2.** 1.3   **3.** 1.9   **4.** 4.6   **5.** 0.7   **6.** 2.5   **7.** 0.8   **8.** 0.2   **9.** 5.7   **10.** 0.9

Expressing to the Nearest Hundredth

Some drugs are administered in dosages carried to the nearest hundredth. This is common in pediatric dosages, and in some critical care drugs.

To express an answer to the nearest hundredth the division is carried to thousandths (three places after the decimal point). When the number representing thousandths is 5 or larger, the number representing hundredths is increased by one.

EXAMPLE 1   0.736   becomes   0.74

The number representing thousandths, 6, is larger than 5, so the number representing hundredths, 3, is increased by 1 to become 4

EXAMPLE 2   0.777   becomes   0.78

EXAMPLE 3   0.373   remains   0.37

The number representing thousandths, 3, is less than 5, so the number representing hundredths, 7, remains unchanged.

EXAMPLE 4   0.934   remains   0.93

Problem

Express the following numbers to the nearest hundredth.

1.   0.175 = _____   7.   1.081 = _____

2.   0.344 = _____   8.   1.327 = _____

3.   1.853 = _____   9.   0.739 = _____

4.   0.306 = _____   10.   0.733 = _____

5.   3.015 = _____   11.   2.072 = _____

6.   2.154 = _____   12.   0.089 = _____

ANSWERS   1. 0.18   **2.** 0.34   **3.** 1.85   **4.** 0.31   **5.** 3.02   **6.** 2.15   **7.** 1.08   **8.** 1.33   **9.** 0.74   **10.** 0.73   **11.** 2.07   **12.** 0.09

Summary

This concludes the chapter on multiplication and division of decimals. The important points to remember from this chapter are:

when decimal fractions are multiplied the decimal point is placed the same number of places to the left in the product as the total of numbers after the decimal points in the fractions multiplied

zeros must be placed in front of a product if it contains insufficient numbers for correct placement of the decimal point

to simplify division of decimal fractions the preliminary steps of eliminating the decimal points, and reducing the numbers by common denominators can be used

when fractions are divided answers are expressed as decimal fractions to the nearest tenth, or the nearest hundredth

Summary Self Test

Directions: Multiply the following decimals.

1. $1.49 \times 0.05 =$ _____
2. $0.15 \times 3.04 =$ _____
3. $0.025 \times 3.5 =$ _____
4. $0.55 \times 2.5 =$ _____
5. $1.31 \times 2.07 =$ _____

6. $5.3 \times 1.02 =$ _____
7. $0.35 \times 1.25 =$ _____
8. $4.32 \times 0.05 =$ _____
9. $0.2 \times 0.02 =$ _____
10. $0.4 \times 1.75 =$ _____

11. You are to administer four tablets with a dosage strength of 0.04 mg each, what total dosage are you giving? _____

12. You have given 2½ (2.5) tablets with a strength of 1.25 mg, what total dosage is this? _____

13. The tablets your patient is to receive are labeled 0.1 mg and you are to give 3½ (3.5) tablets. What total dosage is this? _____

14. You gave your patient 3 tablets labeled 0.75 mg each, and he was to receive a total of 2.25 mg; did he receive the correct dosage? _____

15. The tablets available for your patient are labeled 12.5 mg, and you are to give 4½ (4.5) tablets. What total dosage will this be? _____

16. Your patient is to receive a dosage of 4.5 mg. The tablets available are labeled 3.5 mg, and there are 2½ tablets in his medication drawer. Is this a correct dosage? _____

Directions: Divide the following fractions and express your answers to the nearest tenth.

17. $\dfrac{1.3}{0.7} =$ _____

18. $\dfrac{1.9}{3.2} =$ _____

19. $\dfrac{32.5}{9} =$ _____

20. $\dfrac{0.04}{0.1} =$ _____

21. $\dfrac{1.45}{1.2} =$ _____

22. $\dfrac{250}{1000} =$ _____

23. $\dfrac{0.8}{0.09} =$ _____

24. $\dfrac{2,000,000}{1,500,000} =$ _____

25. $\dfrac{4.1}{2.05} =$ _____

26. $\dfrac{7.3}{12} =$ _____

27. $\dfrac{150,000}{120,000}$ = _____

29. $\dfrac{2700}{900}$ = _____

28. $\dfrac{0.15}{0.08}$ = _____

30. $\dfrac{0.25}{0.15}$ = _____

Directions: Divide the following fractions and express your answers to the nearest hundredth.

31. $\dfrac{900}{1700}$ = _____

41. $\dfrac{0.13}{0.25}$ = _____

32. $\dfrac{0.125}{0.3}$ = _____

42. $\dfrac{0.25}{0.7}$ = _____

33. $\dfrac{1450}{1500}$ = _____

43. $\dfrac{3.3}{5.1}$ = _____

34. $\dfrac{65}{175}$ = _____

44. $\dfrac{0.19}{0.7}$ = _____

35. $\dfrac{0.6}{1.35}$ = _____

45. $\dfrac{1.1}{1.3}$ = _____

36. $\dfrac{0.04}{0.12}$ = _____

46. $\dfrac{3}{4.1}$ = _____

37. $\dfrac{750}{10,000}$ = _____

47. $\dfrac{62}{240}$ = _____

38. $\dfrac{0.65}{0.8}$ = _____

48. $\dfrac{280,000}{300,000}$ = _____

39. $\dfrac{3.01}{4.2}$ = _____

49. $\dfrac{115}{255}$ = _____

40. $\dfrac{4.5}{6.1}$ = _____

50. $\dfrac{10}{14.3}$ = _____

3

Math of Common Fractions

OBJECTIVES

The student will

1. identify which of several common fractions has the highest (or lowest) value
2. multiply common fractions
3. divide common fractions

INTRODUCTION

The math involving common fractions covered in this chapter may be necessary if you will be doing calculations in the apothecaries' system, which uses common fractions. The review will cover three essentials: relative value, multiplication, and division. We will start with a review of relative value, so that you will be able to recognize which fractions have the highest (and lowest) value.

Relative Value of Common Fractions

Let's start this review by looking at the common fractions $\frac{1}{2}$ and $\frac{1}{4}$. The numerator in both fractions is 1; the numbers 2 and 4 are the denominators.

 When the numerators are the same the fraction with the lowest denominator has the highest value.

2 is a lower number than 4, so $\frac{1}{2}$ has a higher value than $\frac{1}{4}$. Here is a memory cue to help you remember this rule. Think of an aspirin tablet; $\frac{1}{2}$ an aspirin is larger than $\frac{1}{4}$ of an aspirin. The lower denominator, 2, has the higher value. Figure 3 graphically illustrates this.

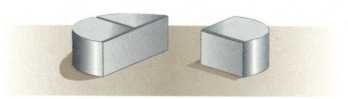

Figure 3

EXAMPLE 1 $\dfrac{1}{3}$ is higher than $\dfrac{1}{8}$ because 3 is a lower denominator than 8

EXAMPLE 2 $\dfrac{1}{100}$ is higher than $\dfrac{1}{150}$

EXAMPLE 3 $\dfrac{1}{150}$ is higher than $\dfrac{1}{200}$

If the denominators are the same, the fraction with the higher numerator will have the higher value.

EXAMPLE 1 $\dfrac{3}{10}$ is higher than $\dfrac{1}{10}$

The denominators, 10, are the same, so the numerator 3, gives the first fraction the highest value.

EXAMPLE 2 $\dfrac{4}{5}$ is higher than $\dfrac{2}{5}$

In drug dosages the numerator is almost always 1, so the relative value is determined by the denominator, for example $\dfrac{1}{4}, \dfrac{1}{100}$

Problem

Identify the fraction with the highest value in each of the following.

1. a) $\dfrac{1}{3}$ b) $\dfrac{1}{6}$ c) $\dfrac{1}{4}$ _____

2. a) $\dfrac{1}{8}$ b) $\dfrac{1}{6}$ c) $\dfrac{1}{4}$ _____

3. a) $\dfrac{1}{4}$ b) $\dfrac{1}{8}$ c) $\dfrac{1}{5}$ _____

4. a) $\dfrac{1}{75}$ b) $\dfrac{1}{50}$ c) $\dfrac{1}{100}$ _____

5. a) $\dfrac{1}{2}$ b) $\dfrac{1}{6}$ c) $\dfrac{1}{4}$ _____

6. a) $\dfrac{1}{200}$ b) $\dfrac{1}{150}$ c) $\dfrac{1}{100}$ _____

7. a) $\dfrac{3}{32}$ b) $\dfrac{4}{32}$ c) $\dfrac{1}{32}$ _____

8. *a)* $\dfrac{1}{10}$ *b)* $\dfrac{1}{15}$ *c)* $\dfrac{1}{5}$ _____

9. *a)* $\dfrac{1}{5}$ *b)* $\dfrac{3}{5}$ *c)* $\dfrac{2}{5}$ _____

10. *a)* $\dfrac{1}{3}$ *b)* $\dfrac{1}{2}$ *c)* $\dfrac{1}{4}$ _____

ANSWERS 1. a **2.** c **3.** a **4.** b **5.** a **6.** c **7.** b **8.** c **9.** b **10.** b

Multiplication of Common Fractions

Multiplication of common fractions will include **proper fractions** in which the **numerator smaller than the denominator,** for example $\dfrac{1}{4}$; and **improper fractions,** in which the **numerator is larger than the denominator,** for example $\dfrac{5}{4}$

Regardless of the type of fraction, multiplication of common fractions in dosage calculations has three steps: reduction of the numbers (if this is possible); multiplication of the remaining numerators, then the remaining denominators; and finally, division of the remaining fraction to express the answer as a decimal number, usually to the nearest tenth. Let's look at some examples.

EXAMPLE 1 $\dfrac{1}{6} \times \dfrac{2}{3}$

$\dfrac{1}{6_3} \times \dfrac{2^1}{3}$ reduce the fractions

$\dfrac{1}{9}$ multiply the remaining numerators ($1 \times 1 = 1$) then the denominators ($3 \times 3 = 9$)

$1 \div 9$ divide the final fraction to two places after the decimal point

0.1   express as a decimal fraction to the nearest tenth

EXAMPLE 2 $\dfrac{7}{50} \times \dfrac{25}{3}$

$\dfrac{7}{50_2} \times \dfrac{25^1}{3}$ reduce; multiply numerators, then denominators

$\dfrac{7}{6}$ divide remaining fraction

$1.16 = \textbf{1.2}$ express answer to nearest tenth

EXAMPLE 3 $\dfrac{1}{8} \times \dfrac{4}{3}$

$$\frac{1}{\cancel{8}_2} \times \frac{\cancel{4}^{1}}{3}$$

$$\frac{1}{6}$$

$$1.66 = \textbf{1.7}$$

 To multiply common fractions reduce the numbers as much as possible; multiply the remaining numerators, then denominators; divide the remaining fraction.

As you can see this math is uncomplicated, and you are now ready for some problems on your own.

Problem

Multiply the following common fractions. Express answers as decimal numbers to the nearest tenth.

1. $\dfrac{1}{8} \times \dfrac{6}{1}$ = _____

2. $\dfrac{3}{5} \times \dfrac{10}{5}$ = _____

3. $\dfrac{2}{7} \times \dfrac{8}{4}$ = _____

4. $\dfrac{1}{50} \times \dfrac{100}{1}$ = _____

5. $\dfrac{1}{3} \times \dfrac{4}{1}$ = _____

6. $\dfrac{2}{9} \times \dfrac{3}{5}$ = _____

7. $\dfrac{1}{6} \times \dfrac{10}{1}$ = _____

8. $\dfrac{7}{12} \times \dfrac{4}{10}$ = _____

9. $\dfrac{7}{8} \times \dfrac{2}{21}$ = _____

10. $\dfrac{1}{5} \times \dfrac{3}{1}$ = _____

ANSWERS 1. 0.8 **2.** 1.2 **3.** 0.6 **4.** 2 **5.** 1.3 **6.** 0.1 **7.** 1.7 **8.** 0.2 **9.** 0.1 **10.** 0.6

Division of Common Fractions

When a dosage calculation involves the division of one common fraction by another it will be written as follows:

$$\frac{\frac{1}{3}}{\frac{1}{6}} \qquad \frac{1}{3} \text{ is a numerator, } \frac{1}{6} \text{ is a denominator}$$

 To divide common fractions the fraction representing the denominator is inverted (turned upside down), and the problem is converted to an equivalent multiplication.

EXAMPLE 1

$$\frac{\frac{1}{3}}{\frac{1}{6}} \quad \text{becomes} \quad \frac{1}{3} \times \frac{6}{1}$$

The denominator, $\frac{1}{6}$, is inverted to become $\frac{6}{1}$, and the problem is converted to a multiplication.

$$\frac{1}{\cancel{3}_1} \times \frac{\cancel{6}^2}{1} = \frac{2}{1} = \mathbf{2}$$

EXAMPLE 2

$$\frac{\frac{1}{150}}{\frac{1}{100}} \quad \text{becomes} \quad \frac{1}{150} \times \frac{100}{1}$$

$$\frac{1}{\cancel{150}_3} \times \frac{\cancel{100}^2}{1}$$

$$\frac{2}{3} = 0.66 = \mathbf{0.7}$$

EXAMPLE 3

$$\frac{\frac{1}{10}}{\frac{1}{8}} \quad \text{becomes} \quad \frac{1}{10} \times \frac{8}{1}$$

$$\frac{1}{\cancel{10}_5} \times \frac{\cancel{8}^4}{1}$$

$$\frac{4}{5} = \mathbf{0.8}$$

Problem

Divide the following common fractions. Express your answers as decimal numbers to the nearest tenth.

1. $\dfrac{\frac{1}{50}}{\frac{1}{60}} = $ _____

4. $\dfrac{\frac{1}{8}}{\frac{1}{4}} = $ _____

2. $\dfrac{\frac{1}{12}}{\frac{1}{4}} = $ _____

5. $\dfrac{\frac{3}{4}}{\frac{1}{2}} = $ _____

3. $\dfrac{\frac{1}{4}}{\frac{1}{6}} = $ _____

6. $\dfrac{\frac{1}{75}}{\frac{1}{150}} = $ _____

7. $\dfrac{\frac{3}{4}}{\frac{2}{3}} = $ _____

9. $\dfrac{\frac{1}{100}}{\frac{1}{50}} = $ _____

8. $\dfrac{\frac{1}{10}}{\frac{1}{6}} = $ _____

10. $\dfrac{\frac{1}{150}}{\frac{1}{200}} = $ _____

ANSWERS 1. 1.2 2. 0.3 3. 1.5 4. 0.5 5. 1.5 6. 2 7. 1.1 8. 0.6 9. 0.5 10. 1.3

Summary

This completes your review of the math of common fractions. The important points to remember from this chapter are:

when the numerators are the same in common fractions the denominator determines relative value

the lower the denominator the higher the value

fractions are multiplied by reducing the numbers as much as possible, multiplying the remaining numerators, then denominators, and dividing the final numerator by the denominator

one common fraction is divided by another by inverting the fraction representing the denominator, thus converting the problem to an equivalent multiplication

answers to division and multiplication are expressed as decimal numbers usually to the nearest tenth

Summary Self Test

Directions: Identify the fraction with the highest value in each of the following.

1. a) $\dfrac{1}{60}$ b) $\dfrac{1}{50}$ c) $\dfrac{1}{70}$ _____

2. a) $\dfrac{1}{12}$ b) $\dfrac{1}{10}$ c) $\dfrac{1}{8}$ _____

3. a) $\dfrac{1}{10}$ b) $\dfrac{4}{10}$ c) $\dfrac{9}{10}$ _____

4. a) $\dfrac{1}{120}$ b) $\dfrac{1}{150}$ c) $\dfrac{1}{175}$ _____

5. a) $\dfrac{1}{4}$ b) $\dfrac{1}{2}$ c) $\dfrac{1}{3}$ _____

6. If you had some tablets whose strength was $\frac{1}{6}$ and you had to give $\frac{1}{4}$, you would need

   a) less than one tablet   b) more than one tablet _____

7. If you had some tablets whose strength was $\frac{1}{100}$, and you needed to give $\frac{1}{150}$, you would need

   a) less than one tablet   b) more than one tablet _____

8. If the tablets available had a strength of $\frac{1}{5}$ and you had to give $\frac{1}{4}$ you would need

   a) less than one tablet   b) more than one tablet _____

9. The order is to give $\frac{1}{10}$ and the tablets available have a strength of $\frac{1}{8}$. You will need

   a) less than one tablet   b) more than one tablet _____

10. You have some tablets labeled $\frac{1}{100}$ and you must give $\frac{1}{200}$. You will need

   a) less than one tablet   b) more than one tablet _____

Directions: Convert the following divisions to multiplications and express your answers as decimal fractions to the nearest tenth.

11. $\dfrac{\frac{1}{2}}{\frac{1}{3}}$ = _____

15. $\dfrac{\frac{1}{100}}{\frac{1}{150}}$ = _____

12. $\dfrac{\frac{1}{4}}{\frac{1}{2}}$ = _____

16. $\dfrac{\frac{1}{10}}{\frac{1}{12}}$ = _____

13. $\dfrac{\frac{1}{4}}{\frac{1}{8}}$ = _____

17. $\dfrac{\frac{1}{200}}{\frac{1}{150}}$ = _____

14. $\dfrac{\frac{1}{50}}{\frac{1}{75}}$ = _____

18. $\dfrac{\frac{1}{3}}{\frac{3}{4}}$ = _____

19. $$\frac{\frac{3}{4}}{\frac{1}{4}} = \underline{\hspace{2cm}}$$

25. $$\frac{\frac{1}{6}}{\frac{1}{4}} = \underline{\hspace{2cm}}$$

20. $$\frac{\frac{1}{8}}{\frac{5}{6}} = \underline{\hspace{2cm}}$$

26. $$\frac{\frac{1}{100}}{\frac{1}{200}} = \underline{\hspace{2cm}}$$

21. $$\frac{\frac{1}{8}}{\frac{1}{2}} = \underline{\hspace{2cm}}$$

27. $$\frac{\frac{1}{300}}{\frac{1}{250}} = \underline{\hspace{2cm}}$$

22. $$\frac{\frac{1}{3}}{\frac{1}{2}} = \underline{\hspace{2cm}}$$

28. $$\frac{\frac{1}{6}}{\frac{1}{5}} = \underline{\hspace{2cm}}$$

23. $$\frac{\frac{2}{3}}{\frac{1}{4}} = \underline{\hspace{2cm}}$$

29. $$\frac{\frac{1}{4}}{\frac{2}{3}} = \underline{\hspace{2cm}}$$

24. $$\frac{\frac{1}{2}}{\frac{1}{6}} = \underline{\hspace{2cm}}$$

30. $$\frac{\frac{1}{80}}{\frac{1}{75}} = \underline{\hspace{2cm}}$$

ANSWERS   1. b   **2.** c   **3.** c   **4.** a   **5.** b   **6.** b   **7.** a   **8.** b   **9.** a   **10.** a   **11.** 1.5   **12.** 0.5   **13.** 2   **14.** 1.5   **15.** 1.5   **16.** 1.2   **17.** 0.8   **18.** 0.4   **19.** 3   **20.** 0.2   **21.** 0.3   **22.** 0.7   **23.** 2.7   **24.** 3   **25.** 0.7   **26.** 2   **27.** 0.8   **28.** 0.8   **29.** 0.4   **30.** 0.9

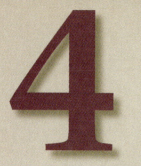

Solving Equations to Determine the Value of X

OBJECTIVES

The student will determine the value of X in equations containing
1. whole numbers
2. decimal numbers
3. common fractions

INTRODUCTION

All the clinical calculations you will be doing will ultimately require that you solve an equation to determine the value of an unknown, represented by X. In the previous three chapters you have reviewed all the basic math you will need to do this. In this chapter we will review step-by-step how these math skills are used together to solve for X. Calculations will involve equations containing whole numbers, decimal numbers, and common fractions, and we will review each of these separately. In this chapter we will concentrate on expressing answers to the nearest tenth, since this is the most common math you will be doing.

Whole Number Equations

The best way to review this material is by actually working with the equations. Follow each step carefully in the following examples.

EXAMPLE 1

$$X = \frac{75}{50} \times 3$$

The only reminder you may need to get started is that 3 is a numerator. If you
wish you can write it as $\frac{3}{1}$

$$X = \frac{75}{50} \times \frac{3}{1}$$

$$\frac{\overset{3}{\cancel{75}}}{\underset{2}{\cancel{50}}} \times \frac{3}{1}$$ reduce 75 and 50 by their highest common denominator, 25

$$\frac{3 \times 3}{2 \times 1}$$ multiply the remaining numerators, $3 \times 3 = 9$; then the remaining denominators, $2 \times 1 = 2$

28

$$\frac{9}{2}$$

divide the numerator 9 by the denominator 2

X = **4.5**

express your answer as a decimal number to the nearest tenth.

EXAMPLE 2 $X = \dfrac{75,000}{300,000} \times 2$

$\dfrac{75,\cancel{000}}{300,\cancel{000}} \times 2$

reduce the zeros by the same number in one numerator and one denominator.

$\dfrac{\cancel{75}^{1}}{\cancel{300}_{4}} \times 2$

reduce 75 and 300 by 75

$\dfrac{1 \times \cancel{2}^{1}}{\cancel{4}_{2}}$

reduce again by 2

$\dfrac{1}{2}$

divide the final fraction

X = **0.5**

express the answer as a decimal fraction to the nearest tenth.

EXAMPLE 3 $X = \dfrac{375}{450} \times 2.5$

It is not uncommon in dosage problems for the second numerator to be a decimal number, as in this equation (2.5). This numerator is usually a small number, and is most easily handled mathematically by keeping it a decimal.

$X = \dfrac{\cancel{375}^{15}}{\cancel{450}_{18}} \times 2.5$ reduce by 25

$\dfrac{15 \times 2.5}{18}$

multiply the remaining numerators (15 × 2.5)

$\dfrac{37.5}{18}$

divide the final fraction

X = 2.08 = **2.1**   express to the nearest tenth

EXAMPLE 4 $X = \dfrac{120}{80} \times 1$

In this example the second numerator is 1. In many dosage problems this is the case, and the math to determine the value of X becomes even simpler.

$X = \dfrac{120}{80} \times 1$ drop the 1 as it has no effect on the equation

$\dfrac{12\cancel{0}}{8\cancel{0}}$

reduce by one zero in the numerator and denominator

$$\frac{\cancel{12}^{3}}{\cancel{8}_{2}}$$ reduce again by 4

$$X = \textbf{1.5}$$ divide the final fraction and express as a decimal number

Problem

Determine the value of X in the following equations. Express your answers to the nearest tenth.

1. $X = \dfrac{350}{400} \times 3 \ =$ _____

2. $X = \dfrac{175}{100} \times 1 \ =$ _____

3. $X = \dfrac{32}{48} \times 1.4 \ =$ _____

4. $X = \dfrac{1000}{1250} \times 2.2 \ =$ _____

5. $X = \dfrac{85}{90} \times 2 \ =$ _____

ANSWERS   1. 2.6   **2.** 1.8   **3.** 0.9   **4.** 1.8   **5.** 1.9

Decimal Fractions

Equations containing decimal fractions are equally as straightforward to handle.

EXAMPLE 1 $X = \dfrac{0.3}{1.65} \times 2.5$

$\dfrac{30}{165} \times 2.5$ eliminate the decimal points from the main fraction by moving two places to the right, and adding a zero to the 3

$\dfrac{\cancel{30}^{6}}{\cancel{165}_{33}} \times 2.5$ reduce the main fraction by dividing by 5

$\dfrac{6 \times 2.5}{33}$ multiply the remaining numerators

$\dfrac{15}{33}$ divide the remaining fraction

$X = 0.45 = \textbf{0.5}$ express to the nearest tenth

EXAMPLE 2 $X = \dfrac{2.5}{1.5} \times 1.2$

$\dfrac{25}{15} \times 1.2$ eliminate the decimal points from the main fraction

$\dfrac{25^5}{15_3} \times 1.2$ reduce by 5 and multiply the remaining numerators

$\dfrac{6}{3}$ divide the remaining fraction

X = **2**

Problem

Solve the following equations to determine the value of X. Express answers to the nearest tenth.

1. $X = \dfrac{2.5}{4} \times 1.1 =$ _____

2. $X = \dfrac{3.1}{2.7} \times 2.2 =$ _____

3. $X = \dfrac{0.05}{1.1} \times 3 \quad =$ _____

4. $X = \dfrac{0.17}{2.2} \times 2.5 =$ _____

5. $X = \dfrac{1.75}{0.95} \times 1.5 =$ _____

ANSWERS   1. 0.7   2. 2.5   3. 0.1   4. 0.2   5. 2.8

Common Fractions

Equations containing common fractions are solved as in the following examples.

EXAMPLE 1

$$X = \dfrac{\dfrac{1}{150}}{\dfrac{1}{200}} \times 2$$

$\dfrac{1}{150} \times \dfrac{200}{1} \times 2$ invert the fraction representing the denominator

$\dfrac{1}{150_3} \times \dfrac{200^4}{1} \times 2$ reduce the numbers by 50

$\dfrac{1}{3} \times \dfrac{4}{1} \times 2$ multiply the remaining numerators (4 × 2) and the remaining denominators (3 × 1)

$\dfrac{8}{3}$ divide the remaining fraction

X = 2.66 = **2.7**   express to the nearest tenth

EXAMPLE 2

$$X = \dfrac{\dfrac{1}{8}}{\dfrac{1}{6}} \times 2$$ invert the fraction representing the denominator

$$\dfrac{1}{\overset{}{8}_4} \times \dfrac{\cancel{6}^3}{1} \times 2$$ reduce the numbers by 2

$$\dfrac{1}{\cancel{4}_2} \times \dfrac{3}{1} \times \cancel{2}^1$$ reduce again by 2

$$\dfrac{3}{2}$$ divide the final fraction

$$X = \mathbf{1.5}$$

Problem

Solve the following equations to determine the value of X. Express answers as decimal numbers to the nearest tenth.

1. $X = \dfrac{\dfrac{1}{150}}{\dfrac{1}{100}} \times 2.1 =$ _____

2. $X = \dfrac{\dfrac{1}{8}}{\dfrac{1}{6}} \times 2.2 =$ _____

3. $X = \dfrac{\dfrac{1}{6}}{\dfrac{1}{4}} \times 1.4 =$ _____

4. $X = \dfrac{\dfrac{1}{3}}{\dfrac{1}{2}} \times 1.2 =$ _____

5. $X = \dfrac{\dfrac{1}{50}}{\dfrac{1}{150}} \times 1.1 =$ _____

ANSWERS   1. 1.4   2. 1.7   **3.** 0.9   4. 0.8   5. 3.3

Summary

This concludes the refresher on solving equations to determine the value of an unknown, X. The important points to remember from this chapter are:

the first step in solving an equation is to reduce the numbers using common denominators

the remaining numerators are then multiplied, and divided by the product of the remaining denominators

answers are expressed as decimal numbers to the nearest tenth (less commonly to the nearest hundredth)

equations are used for calculations which involve whole numbers, decimal numbers, and common fractions

Summary Self Test

Directions: Determine the value of X in the following equations. Express your answers as decimal numbers to the nearest tenth.

1. $X = \dfrac{0.8}{0.65} \times 1.2 =$ _____

2. $X = \dfrac{350}{1000} \times 4.4 =$ _____

3. $X = \dfrac{1.3}{0.95} \times 0.5 =$ _____

4. $X = \dfrac{30}{40} \times 3 =$ _____

5. $X = \dfrac{1,200,000}{800,000} \times 2.7 =$ _____

6. $X = \dfrac{0.35}{1.3} \times 4.5 =$ _____

7. $X = \dfrac{135}{100} \times 2.5 =$ _____

8. $X = \dfrac{0.15}{0.1} \times 1.3 =$ _____

9. $X = \dfrac{320}{150} \times 1 =$ _____

10. $X = \dfrac{0.4}{1.5} \times 2.3 =$ _____

11.   X = $\dfrac{0.08}{0.8}$ × 4   = _____

12.   X = $\dfrac{20}{15}$ × 1.5 = _____

13.   X = $\dfrac{0.003}{0.01}$ × 3   = _____

14.   X = $\dfrac{1500}{500}$ × 0.5 = _____

15.   X = $\dfrac{7.5}{5}$ × 2   = _____

16.   X = $\dfrac{100,000}{80,000}$ × 1.2 = _____

17.   X = $\dfrac{0.3}{0.5}$ × 1.7 = _____

18.   X = $\dfrac{40}{60}$ × 1.2 = _____

19.   X = $\dfrac{0.125}{0.25}$ × 1.5 = _____

20.   X = $\dfrac{0.23}{0.7}$ × 1.1 = _____

21.   X = $\dfrac{300,000}{200,000}$ × 1.7 = _____

22.   X = $\dfrac{1.45}{2.1}$ × 1.5 = _____

23.   X = $\dfrac{0.08}{0.1}$ × 1.1 = _____

24.   X = $\dfrac{0.07}{0.1}$ × 1.4 = _____

25.   X = $\dfrac{\frac{1}{3}}{\frac{1}{5}}$ × 1.1 = _____

26. $X = \dfrac{\frac{1}{200}}{\frac{1}{100}} \times 0.7 =$ _____

27. $X = \dfrac{\frac{3}{4}}{\frac{1}{3}} \times 1 =$ _____

28. $X = \dfrac{\frac{1}{12}}{\frac{1}{8}} \times 1.6 =$ _____

29. $X = \dfrac{\frac{1}{2}}{\frac{1}{4}} \times 1.5 =$ _____

30. $X = \dfrac{\frac{1}{100}}{\frac{1}{150}} \times 1.3 =$ _____

ANSWERS **1.** 1.5 **2.** 1.5 **3.** 0.7 **4.** 2.3 **5.** 4.1 **6.** 1.2 **7.** 3.4 **8.** 2 **9.** 2.1 **10.** 0.6 **11.** 0.4 **12.** 2 **13.** 0.9 **14.** 1.5 **15.** 3 **16.** 1.5 **17.** 1 **18.** 0.8 **19.** 0.8 **20.** 0.4 **21.** 2.6 **22.** 1 **23.** 0.9 **24.** 1 **25.** 1.8 **26.** 0.4 **27.** 2.3 **28.** 1.1 **29.** 3 **30.** 2

5

Introduction to Ratio and Proportion

OBJECTIVES

The student will
1. define ratio
2. define proportion
3. solve simple dosage problems using ratio and proportion

PREREQUISITE

Knowledge of the abbreviations mg (milligram), mL (milliliter), and U (units) as dosage measures.

INTRODUCTION

There are several different ways to calculate drug dosages, but ratio and proportion offers the most logical and safest method of solving any type of dosage or clinical calculation. Once you understand the basic principles of ratio and proportion you will see how simple, yet reliable it is to use. This chapter will review the basics of this method, and give you an opportunity to practice using it to solve a variety of simple dosage problems. Let's begin by reviewing the basic definitions and concepts.

Ratios

A ratio is composed of two numbers which are somehow related to each other. These numbers may be separated by a colon, for example 1:50, or written as a fraction, $\frac{1}{50}$. In this lesson you may use the format you are familiar with.

A ratio can represent any numerical relationship you choose to assign it, but in medications one of the ways it is commonly used is to express the **weight (strength) of a drug in a tablet (tab) or capsule (cap).**

EXAMPLE 1
$$1 \text{ tab} : 50 \text{ mg} \quad \text{or} \quad \frac{1 \text{ tab}}{50 \text{ mg}}$$

This means that 1 tablet contains, or is equal to, 50 mg of drug.
It is equally as correct to reverse the order in which the quantities are written in a ratio. In the previous example the weight of drug can be written first.

$$50 \text{ mg} : 1 \text{ tab} \quad \text{or} \quad \frac{50 \text{ mg}}{1 \text{ tab}}$$

EXAMPLE 2 If 2 cap contain a dosage of 500 mg this could be represented by a ratio as follows:

$$2 \text{ cap} : 500 \text{ mg} \quad \text{or} \quad \frac{2 \text{ cap}}{500 \text{ mg}}$$

EXAMPLE 3 A tab with a strength of 0.25 mg expressed as a ratio is:

$$1 \text{ tab} : 0.25 \text{ mg} \quad \text{or} \quad \frac{1 \text{ tab}}{0.25 \text{ mg}}$$

Another important use of ratios is to express dosages in liquid medications, both oral and injectables. When used for liquid medications a ratio expresses the **weight (strength) of drug in a certain volume of solution.**

EXAMPLE 4 A solution which contains 50 mg of drug in each 1 **mL** would be written as

$$1 \text{ mL} : 50 \text{ mg} \quad \text{or} \quad \frac{1 \text{ mL}}{50 \text{ mg}} \qquad 1 \text{ mL contains 50 mg of drug}$$

EXAMPLE 5 A solution which contains 0.5 mg of drug in 1 mL expressed as a ratio is

$$0.5 \text{ mg} : 1 \text{ mL} \quad \text{or} \quad \frac{0.5 \text{ mg}}{1 \text{ mL}}$$

EXAMPLE 6 A solution which contains 100,000 U in 1.5 mL would be written

$$100,000 \text{ U} : 1.5 \text{ mL} \quad \text{or} \quad \frac{100,000 \text{ U}}{1.5 \text{ mL}}$$

 In review: medication dosage ratios are used to express the amount of drug contained in a tablet or capsule, or in a certain volume of solution.

Problem

Express the following dosages as ratios. Use whichever form of ratio you prefer, either fraction, or separated by a colon. Include the units of measure as well as the numerical value when you write the ratios.

1. An injectable solution which contains 100 mg in each 1.5 mL _____

2. An injectable solution which contains 250 mg in each 0.7 mL _____

3. A tablet which contains 0.4 mg of drug _____

4. Two tablets which contain 450 mg of drug _____

ANSWERS **1.** 1.5 mL : 100 mg; 100 mg : 1.5 mL; $\frac{1.5 \text{ mL}}{100 \text{ mg}}$; $\frac{100 \text{ mg}}{1.5 \text{ mL}}$ **2.** 250 mg : 0.7 mL; 0.7 mL : 250 mg; $\frac{250 \text{ mg}}{0.7 \text{ mL}}$; $\frac{0.7 \text{ mL}}{250 \text{ mg}}$ **3.** 1 tab : 0.4 mg; 0.4 mg : 1 tab; $\frac{1 \text{ tab}}{0.4 \text{ mg}}$; $\frac{0.4 \text{ mg}}{1 \text{ tab}}$ **4.** 2 tab : 450 mg; 450 mg : 2 tab; $\frac{2 \text{ tab}}{450 \text{ mg}}$; $\frac{450 \text{ mg}}{2 \text{ tab}}$. If you did not include the units of measure your answers are incorrect.

To complete the balance of this chapter you will need to choose the style of ratio (and proportion) you prefer to use. If you wish to express ratios as a fraction, for example, $\dfrac{1\ mL}{50\ mg}$, turn now to page 43 under the heading "Ratio and Proportion Expressed as a Fraction." If you prefer ratios separated by a colon continue on this page.

Ratio and Proportion Expressed Using Colons

A proportion is used to show a relationship between two ratios. The ratios can be separated by an equal (=) sign, or by a double colon (: :).

 A true proportion contains two ratios which are equal.

An example of a true proportion would be

1 : 50 = 2 : 100   or   1 : 50 : : 2 : 100

This is a very simple comparison, and by using our previous drug strength examples we can mentally verify that the ratios are equal, and the proportion true.

EXAMPLE 1   1 **tab** : 50 mg = 2 **tab** : 100 mg

If 1 tablet contains 50 mg, 2 tablets will contain 100 mg.

EXAMPLE 2   1 **mL** : 50 mg = 2 **mL** : 100 mg

If 1 mL contains 50 mg, 2 mL will contain 100 mg.

You can also prove mathematically that these ratios are equal, and that the proportion is true. Look again at example 1.

1 tab : 50 mg = 2 tab : 100 mg

The numbers on the **ends** of the proportion (1, 100) are called the **extremes,** while those in the **middle** (50, 2) are called the **means.**

 In a true proportion the product of the means equals the product of the extremes.

If you multiply the means, then the extremes, their products (answers) will be equal.

EXAMPLE 1   1 tab : 50 mg = 2 tab : 100 mg

extremes
1 : 50 = 2 : 100
means

50 × 2 = 100 × 1

100 = 100

The product of the means, 100, equals the product of the extremes, 100. We have now proved mathematically what we previously proved mentally; the ratios are equal, and the proportion is true.

EXAMPLE 2   2 mL : 500 mg = 1 mL : 250 mg

2 : 500 = 1 : 250

500 × 1 = 2 × 250

500 = 500

The product of the means, 500, equals the product of the extremes, 500. This is a true proportion; the ratios are equal.

EXAMPLE 3   1 mL : 10 U = 2 mL : 20 U

10 × 2 = 20

20 = 20

This is a true proportion.

 It is critical in all mathematics involving proportions that the means and extremes not be mixed up, or an incorrect answer will be obtained.

Here is a memory cue that you can use to prevent confusion. Notice that the **means** are in the **middle** of a proportion. Both of these words begin with an **"m"** (**m**eans, **m**iddle). The **extremes** are on the **ends** of the proportion. Both of these words begin with an **"e"** (**e**xtremes, **e**nds). Use these cues as necessary to prevent mix-ups.

Problem

Determine mathematically if the following are true proportions.

1.   34 mg : 2 mL = 51 mg : 3 mL

2.   15 mg : 4 mL = 45 mg : 12 mL

3.   1.3 mL : 46 mg = 0.65 mL : 23 mg

4.   2.3 mL : 150 U = 1.9 mL : 130 U

5.   40 mg : 1.1 mL = 80 mg : 2.2 mL

6.   0.25 mg : 2 mL = 0.5 mg : 4 mL

ANSWERS **1.** True (2 × 51 = 102 and 34 × 3 = 102)   **2.** True (4 × 45 = 180 and 15 × 12 = 180)   **3.** True (1.3 × 23 = 29.9 and 46 × 0.65 = 29.9)   **4.** Not true (2.3 × 130 = 299 and 150 × 1.9 = 285)   **5.** True (40 × 2.2 = 88 and 1.1 × 80 = 88)   **6.** True (0.25 × 4 = 1 and 2 × 0.5 = 1)

Use of Ratio and Proportion in Dosage Calculation

Ratio and proportion is important in dosage calculations because it can be used when only one ratio is known, or complete, and the second is incomplete. For example suppose you have a drug with a dosage strength of 8 mg in 1 mL. This gives you a known or complete ratio of 8 mg : 1 mL. However, the doctor orders a dosage of 10 mg. This is your incomplete ratio, and you will use X to represent the unknown mL which will contain 10 mg.

$$8 \text{ mg} : 1 \text{ mL} \quad = \quad 10 \text{ mg} : X \text{ mL}$$

$$\left(\begin{array}{c} \text{complete ratio} \\ \text{drug strength} \end{array} \right) \qquad \left(\begin{array}{c} \text{incomplete ratio} \\ \text{dosage to give} \end{array} \right)$$

 The major precaution in setting up the proportion is that the ratios must be written in the same sequence of measurement units.

In the above example they are: mg : mL = mg : mL

Next let's look at the math steps used to determine the value of the unknown, X mL. The math will be familiar because it was covered earlier in a refresher math chapter.

EXAMPLE 1 8 mg : 1 mL = 10 mg : X mL	check sequence of measurement units; mg : mL = mg : mL
8 : 1 = 10 : X	drop the measurement units
8X = 10	multiply the means, and the extremes, keeping X on the left of the equation
$X = \dfrac{10}{8}$	divide 10 by the number in front of X
$= \dfrac{\cancel{10}^{5}}{\cancel{8}_{4}}$	reduce the numbers by 2, divide the final fraction
= 1.25 mL	the X in the original proportion was **mL,** so your answer is 1.25 **mL**

To give the ordered dosage of 10 mg you must administer 1.25 mL.

It is routine to check your math twice in dosage calculations. However, it is also necessary to **assess each answer to determine if it seems logical,** and here is where our previous review of relative value of numbers is put to use. Consider the answer you just obtained in example 1.

$$8 \text{ mg} : 1 \text{ mL} = 10 \text{ mg} : X \text{ mL}$$

$$X = 1.25 \text{ mL}$$

If **1 mL** contains **8 mg** you will need a **larger** volume than 1 mL to obtain **10 mg.** The answer you obtained, 1.25 mL, **is** larger, therefore it is logical. This routine check does not guarantee that your math is correct, but it does indicate that you have not mixed up the means and extremes in your calculations. You **can** prove that the proportion is true (and your math correct) by substituting your answer for X in the original proportion.

$$8 \text{ mg} : 1 \text{ mL} = 10 \text{ mg} : \textbf{X mL}$$

$$8 \text{ mg} : 1 \text{ mL} = 10 \text{ mg} : \textbf{1.25 mL}$$

$$10 = 8 \times 1.25$$

$$10 = 10$$

You have now proved mathematically that your answer is correct. However, in most routine calculations it is neither necessary nor practical to mathematically prove each answer you obtain. Dosages such as the 1.25 mL in our example are most often rounded off to the nearest tenth (1.25 = 1.3 mL). Once this is done, the math proofing the answer may contain small discrepancies that could cause confusion.

EXAMPLE 2 The dosage strength available is 25 mg in 1.5 mL. A dosage of 20 mg has been ordered.

$25 \text{ mg} : 1.5 \text{ mL} = 20 \text{ mg} : \text{X mL}$	make sure the units are in the same sequence: mg : mL = mg : mL
$25 : 1.5 = 20 : \text{X}$	drop the measurement units
$25\text{X} = 1.5 \times 20$	multiply the means, and the extremes; keep X on the left
$\dfrac{30}{25}$	divide by the number in front of X
$\dfrac{30^6}{25_5} = 1.2$	reduce by 5, and divide the final fraction
$\text{X} = \textbf{1.2 mL}$	

The dosage ordered, 20 mg, is a smaller amount of drug than the strength available, 25 mg (in 1.5 mL). So your answer should be smaller than 1.5 mL, and it is, 1.2 mL.

EXAMPLE 3 You must give a dosage of 200 mg. The tablets available are labeled 80 mg.

$$80 \text{ mg} : 1 \text{ tab} = 200 \text{ mg} : \text{X tab}$$

$$80\text{X} = 200$$

$$\frac{200^5}{80_2} = \frac{5}{2} = \textbf{2.5 tab}$$

Your original X was tab, so your answer must be tab. 200 mg is a larger dosage than 80 mg, so it must be contained in more than 1 tab. The answer, 2.5 tab, is larger, therefore it is logical.

Problem

Determine the value of **X** in the following proportions. Express your answers to the nearest tenth and include the appropriate unit of measure. Check your answers to determine if they are logical.

1.   12.5 mg : 5 mL = 24 mg : X mL   _____
2.   40 mg : 2.5 mL = 30 mg : X mL   _____
3.   0.6 mg : 0.8 mL = 0.3 mg : X mL _____
4.   36 mg : 2 mL = 24 mg : X mL   _____
5.   78 mg : 0.9 mL = 52 mg : X mL   _____
6.   200 mg : 2 tab = 150 mg : X tab _____
7.   750 mg : 3 mL = 600 mg : X mL   _____
8.   1.5 mg : 1 cap = 4.5 mg : X cap _____
9.   0.5 mg : 1 tab = 0.25 mg : X tab _____
10. 4 mg : 2.7 mL = 3 mg : X mL   _____

ANSWERS   1. 9.6 mL   **2.** 1.9 mL   **3.** 0.4 mL   **4.** 1.3 mL   **5.** 0.6 mL   **6.** 1.5 tab   **7.** 2.4 mL   **8.** 3 cap   **9.** 0.5 tab
10. 2mL   If you did not include the units of measure your answers are incomplete.

As soon as you are comfortable with the math steps in ratio and proportion you can combine several steps at once, and work even more efficiently. You may already have been doing this, but here are a few examples to demonstrate the short cuts.

EXAMPLE 1   300 mg : 1.2 mL = 120 mg : X mL   set up the proportion with the known ratio written first

$$X = \frac{1.2 \times 120}{300}$$ multiply the means, and **immediately** divide by the number in front of X

$$\frac{1.2 \times \cancel{120}^{2}}{\cancel{300}_{5}} = \frac{2.4}{5} = 0.48 = \mathbf{0.5\ mL}$$ reduce (by 60), do final division

EXAMPLE 2   1.5 mg : 0.5 mL = 2 mg : X mL

$$X = \frac{\cancel{0.5}^{1} \times 2}{\cancel{1.5}_{3}} = 0.66 = \mathbf{0.7\ mL}$$

EXAMPLE 3   80 mg : 1 mL = 120 mg : X mL

$$X = \frac{\cancel{120}^{3}}{\cancel{80}_{2}} = \mathbf{1.5\ mL}$$

This completes your introduction to the use of ratio and proportion in solving simple dosage calculations. Turn now to page 48 for the chapter Summary, and Summary Self Test.

Ratio and Proportion Expressed as a Fraction

A proportion is used to show a relationship between two ratios. The ratios can be separated by an equal (=) sign, or by a double colon (: :).

 A true proportion contains two ratios which are equal.

An example of a true proportion would be

$$\frac{1}{50} = \frac{2}{100} \quad \text{or} \quad \frac{1}{50} : : \frac{2}{100}$$

This is a very simple comparison, and by using one of our previous drug strength examples we can mentally verify that the ratios are equal, and the proportion true.

EXAMPLE 1
$$\frac{1\ \textbf{tab}}{50\ \text{mg}} = \frac{2\ \textbf{tab}}{100\ \text{mg}}$$

If 1 tablet contains 50 mg, 2 tablets will contain 100 mg.

EXAMPLE 2
$$\frac{1\ \textbf{mL}}{50\ \text{mg}} = \frac{2\ \textbf{mL}}{100\ \text{mg}}$$

If 1 mL contains 50 mg, 2 mL will contain 100 mg.

You can also prove mathematically that these ratios are equal, and that the proportion is true. Look again at example 1.

$$\frac{1\ \text{tab}}{50\ \text{mg}} = \frac{2\ \text{tab}}{100\ \text{mg}}$$

 In a true proportion the products of cross multiplying will be identical.

To prove a proportion is true cross multiply. The products (answers) you obtain will be identical.

EXAMPLE 1
$$\frac{1\ \text{tab}}{50\ \text{mg}} = \frac{2\ \text{tab}}{100\ \text{mg}}$$

$$\frac{1}{50} \diagdown\!\!\!\!\diagup \frac{2}{100}$$

$$1 \times 100 = 50 \times 2$$

$$100 = 100$$

The products of cross multiplying in this proportion, 100, are the same. We have now proved mathematically what we previously proved mentally; the ratios are equal, and the proportion is true.

EXAMPLE 2

$$\frac{2 \text{ mL}}{500 \text{ mg}} \times \frac{1 \text{ mL}}{250 \text{ mg}}$$

$$2 \times 250 = 500 \times 1$$

$$500 = 500$$

The products of cross multiplying, 500, are identical. This is a true proportion; the ratios are equal.

EXAMPLE 3

$$\frac{1 \text{ mL}}{10 \text{ U}} = \frac{2 \text{ mL}}{20 \text{ U}}$$

$$20 = 20$$

This is a true proportion.

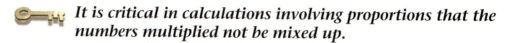 *It is critical in calculations involving proportions that the numbers multiplied not be mixed up.*

If necessary make a habit of drawing an X as in the examples just given to make sure you cross multiply correctly.

Problem

Determine mathematically if the following are true proportions.

1. $\dfrac{34 \text{ mg}}{2 \text{ mL}} = \dfrac{51 \text{ mg}}{3 \text{ mL}}$ _____

2. $\dfrac{15 \text{ mg}}{4 \text{ mL}} = \dfrac{45 \text{ mg}}{12 \text{ mL}}$ _____

3. $\dfrac{1.3 \text{ mL}}{46 \text{ mg}} = \dfrac{0.65 \text{ mL}}{23 \text{ mg}}$ _____

4. $\dfrac{2.3 \text{ mL}}{150 \text{ U}} = \dfrac{1.9 \text{ mL}}{130 \text{ U}}$ _____

5. $\dfrac{40 \text{ mg}}{1.1 \text{ mL}} = \dfrac{80 \text{ mg}}{2.2 \text{ mL}}$ _____

6. $\dfrac{0.25 \text{ mg}}{2 \text{ mL}} = \dfrac{0.5 \text{ mg}}{4 \text{ mL}}$ _____

ANSWERS 1. True (2 × 51 = 102 and 34 × 3 = 102) **2.** True (4 × 45 = 180 and 15 × 12 = 180) **3.** True (1.3 × 23 = 29.9 and 46 × 0.65 = 29.9) **4.** Not true (2.3 × 130 = 299 and 150 × 1.9 = 285) **5.** True (40 × 2.2 = 88 and 1.1 × 80 = 88) **6.** True (0.25 × 4 = 1 and 2 × 0.5 = 1)

Use of Ratio and Proportion in Dosage Calculation

Ratio and proportion is important in dosage calculations because it can be used when only one ratio is known, or complete, and the second is incomplete. For example suppose you have a drug with a dosage strength of 8 mg in 1 mL. This gives you a known or complete ratio of 8 mg in 1 mL. However, the doctor orders a dosage of 10 mg. This is your incomplete ratio, and you will use X to represent the unknown mL which will contain 10 mg.

$$\frac{8 \text{ mg}}{1 \text{ mL}} \quad = \quad \frac{10 \text{ mg}}{\text{X mL}}$$

$$\left(\begin{array}{c}\text{complete ratio} \\ \text{drug strength}\end{array}\right) \quad \left(\begin{array}{c}\text{incomplete ratio} \\ \text{dosage to give}\end{array}\right)$$

 The major precaution in setting up the proportion is that the ratios must be written in the same sequence of measurement units.

In the above example they are.

$$\frac{\text{mg}}{\text{mL}} = \frac{\text{mg}}{\text{mL}}$$

Both **numerators** are **mg,** both **denominators** are **mL.**

Next let's review the steps involved in determining the value of the unknown, X mL. The math will be familiar because it was covered earlier in a refresher math chapter.

EXAMPLE 1 $\dfrac{8 \text{ mg}}{1 \text{ mL}} = \dfrac{10 \text{ mg}}{\text{X mL}}$ set up the proportion to include the measurement units; make sure they are in the same sequence

$\dfrac{8 \text{ mg}}{1 \text{ mL}} \diagup\!\!\!\!\diagdown \dfrac{10 \text{ mg}}{\text{X mL}}$ drop the measurement units as you cross multiply

$8X = 10$ keep X on the left of the equation

$X = \dfrac{\cancel{10}^{5}}{\cancel{8}_{4}}$ divide 10 by the number in front of X; reduce by highest common denominator (2)

$= 1.25$ divide the final fraction to obtain a decimal fraction

$= \mathbf{1.25 \ mL}$ the X in the original proportion was **mL,** so your answer is 1.25 **mL**

To give the ordered dosage you must give 1.25 mL

It is routine to check your math twice in dosage calculations. However, it is also necessary to **assess each answer to determine if it seems logical,** and here is where our previous review of relative value of numbers is put to use. Consider the answer you just obtained in example 1.

$$\frac{8 \text{ mg}}{1 \text{ mL}} = \frac{10 \text{ mg}}{X \text{ mL}}$$

$$X = 1.25 \text{ mL}$$

If **1 mL** contains **8 mg** you will need a **larger** volume than 1 mL to obtain **10 mg.** The answer you obtained, 1.25 mL, **is** larger, therefore it is logical. This routine check does not guarantee that your math is correct, but it does indicate that you did not mix up the units of measure when you set up the proportion and cross multiplied.

You **can** prove that the proportion is true (and your math correct) by substituting your answer for X in the original proportion.

$$\frac{8 \text{ mg}}{1 \text{ mL}} = \frac{10 \text{ mg}}{\textbf{X mL}}$$

$$\frac{8 \text{ mg}}{1 \text{ mL}} = \frac{10 \text{ mg}}{\textbf{1.25 mL}}$$

$$8 \times 1.25 = 10 \times 1$$

$$10 = 10$$

You have now proved mathematically that your answer is correct. However, in most routine calculations it is neither necessary nor practical to mathematically prove each answer you obtain. Dosages such as the 1.25 mL in our example are most often rounded off to the nearest tenth (1.25 = 1.3 mL). Once this is done, the math of proofing the answer may contain small discrepancies that could cause confusion.

EXAMPLE 2 The strength available is 25 mg in 1.5 mL. A dosage of 20 mg has been ordered.

$$\frac{25 \text{ mg}}{1.5 \text{ mL}} = \frac{20 \text{ mg}}{X \text{ mL}}$$ make sure the measurement units are in the correct sequence

$$25X = 1.5 \times 20$$ cross multiply; keep X on left

$$X = \frac{30^6}{25_5}$$ reduce by 5, then divide the final fraction

$$= \textbf{1.2 mL}$$ include the measurement unit in your answer

The dosage ordered, 20 mg, is a smaller amount of drug than the strength available, 25 mg (in 1.5 mL). So your answer should be smaller than 1.5 mL, and it is, 1.2 mL.

EXAMPLE 3 You must give a dosage of 200 mg. The tablets available are labeled 80 mg.

$$\frac{80 \text{ mg}}{1 \text{ tab}} = \frac{200 \text{ mg}}{X \text{ tab}}$$

$$80X = 200$$

$$\frac{200^5}{80_2} = \textbf{2.5 tab}$$

Your original X was tab, so your answer must be tab. 200 mg is a larger dosage than 80 mg, so it must be contained in more than 1 tab. The answer, 2.5 tab, is larger, therefore it is logical.

Problem

Determine the value of X in the following proportions. Express your answers to the nearest tenth and include the appropriate unit of measure. Check your answers to determine if they are logical.

1. $\dfrac{12.5 \text{ mg}}{5 \text{ mL}} = \dfrac{24 \text{ mg}}{X \text{ mL}}$ _____

2. $\dfrac{40 \text{ mg}}{2.5 \text{ mL}} = \dfrac{30 \text{ mg}}{X \text{ mL}}$ _____

3. $\dfrac{0.6 \text{ mg}}{0.8 \text{ mL}} = \dfrac{0.3 \text{ mg}}{X \text{ mL}}$ _____

4. $\dfrac{36 \text{ mg}}{2 \text{ mL}} = \dfrac{24 \text{ mg}}{X \text{ mL}}$ _____

5. $\dfrac{78 \text{ mg}}{0.9 \text{ mL}} = \dfrac{52 \text{ mg}}{X \text{ mL}}$ _____

6. $\dfrac{200 \text{ mg}}{2 \text{ tab}} = \dfrac{150 \text{ mg}}{X \text{ tab}}$ _____

7. $\dfrac{750 \text{ mg}}{3 \text{ mL}} = \dfrac{600 \text{ mg}}{X \text{ mL}}$ _____

8. $\dfrac{1.5 \text{ mg}}{1 \text{ cap}} = \dfrac{4.5 \text{ mg}}{X \text{ cap}}$ _____

9. $\dfrac{0.5 \text{ mg}}{1 \text{ tab}} = \dfrac{0.25 \text{ mg}}{X \text{ tab}}$ _____

10. $\dfrac{4 \text{ mg}}{2.7 \text{ mL}} = \dfrac{3 \text{ mg}}{X \text{ mL}}$ _____

ANSWERS 1. 9.6 mL 2. 1.9 mL 3. 0.4 mL 4. 1.3 mL 5. 0.6 mL 6. 1.5 tab 7. 2.4 mL 8. 3 cap 9. 0.5 tab 10. 2 mL   If you did not include the units of measure your answers are incomplete.

As soon as you are comfortable with the math steps in ratio and proportion you can combine several steps at once, and work even more efficiently. You may already have been doing this, but here are a few examples to demonstrate the short cuts.

EXAMPLE 1 $\qquad \dfrac{300 \text{ mg}}{1.2 \text{ mL}} = \dfrac{120 \text{ mg}}{X \text{ mL}} \qquad$ set up the proportion with the known ratio written first

$$X = \frac{1.2 \times 120}{300}$$

cross multiply, and **immediately** divide by the number in front of X

$$\frac{1.2 \times \cancel{120}^2}{\cancel{300}_5} = \frac{2.4}{5} = 0.48 = \mathbf{0.5\ mL}$$ reduce (by 60), do final division

EXAMPLE 2
$$\frac{1.5\ mg}{0.5\ mL} = \frac{2\ mg}{X\ mL}$$

$$X = \frac{\cancel{0.5}^1 \times 2}{\cancel{1.5}_3} = 0.66 = \mathbf{0.7\ mL}$$

EXAMPLE 3
$$\frac{80\ mg}{1\ mL} = \frac{120\ mg}{X\ mL}$$

$$X = \frac{\cancel{120}^3}{\cancel{80}_2} = \mathbf{1.5\ mL}$$

Summary

This concludes the introductory chapter on ratio and proportion. The important points to remember from this chapter are:

a ratio is composed of two numbers that are somehow related to each other

in medication dosages ratios can be used to express the amount of drug contained in a tablet or capsule, or in a certain volume of solution

a true proportion consists of two ratios which are equal to each other

if one number of a proportion is missing it can be determined mathematically by solving an equation to determine the value of X

when ratio and proportion is used to solve dosage problems the critical first step is to set the ratios up in the same sequence of measurement units

the math of calculations must always be double checked, and the answer must be assessed logically to determine if X is appropriately larger or smaller than the strength available

Summary Self Test

Directions: Determine the value of X in the following proportions. Express answers as decimals to the nearest tenth, and include units of measure in the answer. If you prefer to use the cross multiplication (fraction) method set your problems up using this format. For example #1 would

be written $\dfrac{75\ mg}{5\ mL} = \dfrac{187.5\ mg}{X\ mL}$

1. 75 mg : 5 mL = 187.5 mg : X mL = _____
2. 7500 U : 1.5 mL = 10,000 U : X mL = _____
3. 17 mg : 3 tab = 42.5 mg : X tab = _____
4. 0.25 mg : 0.8 mL = 0.75 mg : X mL = _____
5. 55 mg : 1.1 mL = 165 mg : X mL = _____
6. 14.2 mg : 1.3 mL = 12.1 mg : X mL = _____
7. 250 U : 2.3 mL = 325 U : X mL = _____
8. 40 U : 1 mL = 30 U : X mL = _____
9. 12.5 mg : 1.2 mL = 6.25 mg : X mL = _____
10. 200,000 U : 2.5 mL = 150,000 U : X mL = _____
11. 0.02 mg : 1.2 mL = 0.05 mg : X mL = _____
12. 125 U : 0.8 mL = 100 U : X mL = _____
13. 350 mg : 1.6 mL = 175 mg : X mL = _____
14. 1250 U : 1.4 mL = 625 U : X mL = _____
15. 175 mg : 0.6 mL = 225 mg : X mL = _____
16. 750 mg : 1.5 mL = 1125 mg : X mL = _____
17. 0.7 mg : 1.2 mL = 0.8 mg : X mL = _____
18. 0.04 mg : 0.5 tab = 0.12 mg : X tab = _____
19. 7.5 mg : 3.2 mL = 10 mg : X mL = _____
20. 100,000 U : 2 mL = 75,000 U : X mL = _____
21. 0.1 mg : 0.3 mL = 0.25 mg : X mL = _____
22. 15.7 mg : 2.3 mL = 14.2 mg : X mL = _____
23. 45 mg : 1.2 mL = 35 mg : X mL = _____
24. 275 mg : 2.3 mL = 250 mg : X mL = _____
25. 1.5 mg : 1.4 mL = 0.75 mg : X mL = _____
26. 350 mg : 1 cap = 700 mg : X cap = _____
27. 3.2 mg : 1.5 mL = 1.6 mg : X mL = _____
28. 100 U : 1.2 mL = 75 U : X mL = _____
29. 450 mg : 1.3 mL = 400 mg : X mL = _____
30. 0.1 mg : 1 tab = 0.15 mg : X tab = _____
31. 20 mg : 0.7 mL = 18 mg : X mL = _____
32. 1500 U : 2.2 mL = 1800 U : X mL = _____
33. 75,000 U : 2.1 mL = 60,000 U : X mL = _____
34. 0.05 mg : 1.1 mL = 0.15 mg : X mL = _____
35. 2.5 mg : 1 cap = 7.5 mg : X cap = _____
36. 0.3 mg : 1 tab = 0.45 mg : X tab = _____

37.   150 mg : 2.5 mL = 100 mg : X mL   = _____

38.   80 mg : 1 cap = 160 mg : X cap   = _____

39.   0.2 mg : 1.2 mL = 0.3 mg : X mL   = _____

40.   150 mg : 1 mL = 140 mg : X mL   = _____

41.   1000 U : 1 mL = 1200 U : X mL   = _____

42.   0.4 mg : 0.5 mL = 0.5 mg : X mL   = _____

43.   1.3 mg : 2 mL = 0.7 mg : X mL   = _____

44.   0.25 mg : 1 tab = 0.125 mg : X tab   = _____

45.   1000 U : 2 mL = 750 U : X mL   = _____

46.   0.6 mg : 1.1 mL = 0.5 mg : X mL   = _____

47.   500 U : 1.1 mL = 450 U : X mL   = _____

48.   3.5 mg : 1 tab = 1.75 mg : X tab   = _____

49.   100 mg : 0.8 mL = 130 mg : X mL   = _____

50.   1000 mg : 2.3 mL = 600 mg : X mL   = _____

ANSWERS   **1.** 12.5 mL   **2.** 2 mL   **3.** 7.5 tab   **4.** 2.4 mL   **5.** 3.3 mL   **6.** 1.1 mL   **7.** 3 mL   **8.** 0.8 mL   **9.** 0.6 mL
10. 1.9 mL   **11.** 3 mL   **12.** 0.6 mL   **13.** 0.8 mL   **14.** 0.7 mL   **15.** 0.8 mL   **16.** 2.3 mL   **17.** 1.4 mL   **18.** 1.5 tab
19. 4.3 mL   **20.** 1.5 mL   **21.** 0.8 mL   **22.** 2.1 mL   **23.** 0.9 mL   **24.** 2.1 mL   **25.** 0.7 mL   **26.** 2 cap   **27.** 0.8 mL
28. 0.9 mL   **29.** 1.2 mL   **30.** 1.5 tab   **31.** 0.6 mL   **32.** 2.6 mL   **33.** 1.7 mL   **34.** 3.3 mL   **35.** 3 cap   **36.** 1.5 tab
37. 1.7 mL   **38.** 2 cap   **39.** 1.8 mL   **40.** 0.9 mL   **41.** 1.2 mL   **42.** 0.6 mL   **43.** 1.1 mL   **44.** 0.5 tab   **45.** 1.5 mL
46. 0.9 mL   **47.** 1 mL   **48.** 0.5 tab   **49.** 1 mL   **50.** 1.4 mL

Equivalents in Decimals, Fractions, Ratios and Percents

OBJECTIVES

The student will

1. define ratios as they relate to solutions
2. define percents as they relate to solutions
3. explain the relationship between decimals, common fractions, ratios, and percents
4. express decimals, common fractions, ratios and percents as equivalents of each other

INTRODUCTION

Drug dosage strengths are expressed using a variety of measures. For example you may see 0.25, a decimal; ¼, a common fraction; 1 : 1000, a ratio; and 1%, a percentage. All of these measures can be expressed as equivalents of each other, and the main focus of this chapter is to show you how this is done.

Decimals and common fractions were reviewed in earlier chapters, and now we will define exactly what ratio and percentage strengths mean, and how they are used in dosages. Let's begin with ratio strengths.

Definition of Ratio Strengths

Ratio strengths are used primarily for solutions: drugs in liquid form. An example is 1 : 1000. A ratio represents **parts of solute (drug) per parts of solution.**

EXAMPLE 1   A 1 : 1000 strength solution represents 1 part drug in 1000 parts solution.

EXAMPLE 2   A 1 : 5 strength contains 1 part drug in 5 parts solution.

EXAMPLE 3   A solution which is 1 part drug in 2 parts solution would be written 1 : 2

The more solution the drug is dissolved in the weaker the strength becomes. For example a ratio strength of 1 : 10 (1 part drug to **10** parts solution) is much stronger than a 1 : 100 strength (1 part drug in **100** parts solution).

Ratio strengths are always expressed in their simplest (reduced) forms. For example 2 : 10 would be incorrect, since it can be reduced to 1 : 5.

Dosages expressed using ratio strengths are not common, but you do need to know what they represent.

Problem

Explain what the following ratio strength solutions represent.

    1. 1 : 10 _____

    2. 1 : 1000 _____

    3. 1 : 20 _____

Express the following solution strengths as ratios.

    4. 1 part drug in 200 parts solution _____

    5. 1 part drug in 4 parts solution _____

    6. 1 part drug in 7 parts solution _____

Identify the strongest solution in each of the following.

    7. *a)* 1 : 20   *b)* 1 : 200   *c)* 1 : 2 _____

    8. *a)* 1 : 50   *b)* 1 : 20   *c)* 1 : 100 _____

    9. *a)* 1 : 1000   *b)* 1 : 5000   *c)* 1 : 2000 _____

Reduce the following ratios to their simplest terms.

    10. 10 : 20 _____

    11. 4 : 20 _____

    12. 2 : 200 _____

ANSWERS **1.** 1 part drug (solute) in 10 parts solution **2.** 1 part drug in 1000 parts solution **3.** 1 part drug in 20 parts solution **4.** 1 : 200 **5.** 1 : 4 **6.** 1 : 7 **7.** c **8.** b **9.** a **10.** 1 : 2 **11.** 1 : 5 **12.** 1 : 100

Definition of Percentage Strengths

Percentage strengths are used extensively in intravenous solutions, and somewhat less commonly for a variety of other medications. **Percentage (%) means parts per hundred.**

 A percentage solution represents the number of grams of drug (solute) per 100 mL/cc of solution.

EXAMPLE 1 100 mL of a 1% solution will contain 1 gram of drug or solute

EXAMPLE 2 100 mL of a 2% solution will contain 2 grams of drug or solute

EXAMPLE 3 50 mL of a 1% solution will contain 0.5 grams of drug or solute

EXAMPLE 4 200 mL of a 2% solution will contain 4 grams of drug or solute

Problem

1. How many grams of drug will 100 mL of a 10% solution contain?

   _____

2. How many grams of drug will 50 mL of a 10% solution contain?

   _____

3. How many grams of drug will 200 mL of a 10% solution contain?

   _____

4. A 500 cc IV bag is labeled 5% Dextrose in Water. How many grams of dextrose will it contain? _____

5. A 1000 cc IV bag has a solution strength of 10%. How many grams of solute does this represent? _____

6. An IV of 200 cc 5% Dextrose will contain how many grams of dextrose?

   _____

7. If 350 cc of a 10% Dextrose IV are infused, how many grams will the patient receive? _____

8. An IV of 5% Dextrose is discontinued after only 150 cc have infused. How many grams of dextrose is this? _____

9. A drug is diluted in 100 cc of a 5% Dextrose IV fluid. How many grams of dextrose does this contain? _____

10. A full 1000 cc IV of 5% Dextrose will contain how much dextrose?

    _____

ANSWERS **1.** 10 grams **2.** 5 grams **3.** 20 grams **4.** 25 grams **5.** 100 grams **6.** 10 grams **7.** 35 grams
8. 7.5 grams **9.** 5 grams **10.** 50 grams

 The higher the percentage strength the more drug/solute it contains, and the stronger the solution will be.

For example 2% is stronger than 1%, and 10% is stronger than 5%.

Regardless of the dosage used all drug measures, decimals, common fractions, ratios and percents, can be converted into equivalents of each other. The balance of this chapter will show you how to do this.

Converting Between Ratios and Common Fractions

The easiest of the conversions to do is between ratios and common fractions, because they are essentially the same. Refer to figure 4 and notice how the colon of the ratio (:), and the fraction bar (—) of the common fraction both serve to identify the numerator and denominator of these two measures.

$$7 : 100 \qquad\qquad \frac{7}{100} \quad \text{numerator}$$
$$\text{numerator} \quad \text{denominator} \qquad\qquad\qquad \text{denominator}$$

Figure 4

Conversion from ratio to common fraction, and vice versa, requires just a physical realignment of the numbers.

EXAMPLE 1 $2 : 5 = \dfrac{2}{5}$

EXAMPLE 2 $\dfrac{1}{10} = 1 : 10$

EXAMPLE 3 $\dfrac{1}{5} = 1 : 5$

Problem

Convert the following ratios and common fractions to their equivalents.

	Ratio	Common Fraction
1.	1 : 2	_____
2.	3 : 4	_____
3.	_____	$\dfrac{2}{5}$
4.	_____	$\dfrac{1}{6}$
5.	1 : 8	_____

ANSWERS 1. $\dfrac{1}{2}$ 2. $\dfrac{3}{4}$ 3. 2 : 5 4. 1 : 6 5. $\dfrac{1}{8}$

Changing Ratios, Common Fractions and Decimals to Percent

If it is necessary to express a decimal, ratio or common fraction as a percent, you must simply multiply by 100. **Percent is always obtained by multiplying by 100 and adding the % sign.** Ratios and common fractions are converted by changing ratios to common fractions first, because the physical alignment of the numbers is easier to work with.

EXAMPLE 1 $1:4 = \dfrac{1}{\cancel{4}_1} \times \cancel{100}^{25} = 25\%$

EXAMPLE 2 $2:5 = \dfrac{2}{\cancel{5}_1} \times \cancel{100}^{20} = 40\%$

EXAMPLE 3 $1:6 = \dfrac{1}{6} \times 100 = 16.67 = 16.7\%$ (Round off to the nearest tenth percent)

EXAMPLE 4 $1:100 = \dfrac{1}{100} \times 100 = 1\%$

Notice that **when the denominator is 100,** as in example 4, **the percent equivalent is always the same as the original numerator**

($\dfrac{1}{100} = 1\%$). Therefore if the denominator is 100, the conversion is already

done: the percent equivalent is the same as the numerator.

EXAMPLE 5 $3:100 = \dfrac{3}{\cancel{100}_1} \times \cancel{100}^1 = 3\%$

Problem

Express the following ratios as common fractions, then as percentage equivalents.

Ratio	Common Fraction	%
1. 3 : 4	_____	_____
2. 1 : 8	_____	_____
3. 1 : 1000	_____	_____
4. 3 : 10	_____	_____
5. 0.9 : 100	_____	_____

ANSWERS 1. $\frac{3}{4}$, 75% **2.** $\frac{1}{8}$, 12.5% **3.** $\frac{1}{1000}$, 0.1% **4.** $\frac{3}{10}$, 30% **5.** $\frac{0.9}{100}$, 0.9%

    To convert a decimal to a percent it is also necessary to multiply by 100. However, in decimal numbers this is done by simply moving the decimal point. **The number of places the decimal point is moved is the same as the number of zeros in the multiplier.** For 100, this is 2 places. **When you multiply, the quantity must get larger, so the decimal point is moved two places to the right.** Zeros may need to be eliminated or added to accomplish this.

	Decimal	Percent	
EXAMPLE 1	0.02	2%	

Move the decimal point in 0.02 two places to the right making it 2. One zero is eliminated.

	Decimal	Percent	
EXAMPLE 2	0.001	0.1%	Two zeros are dropped
EXAMPLE 3	0.3	30%	One zero is added

Problem

Convert the following decimals to percents.

1. 0.4   = _____
2. 0.05 = _____
3. 0.25 = _____
4. 0.004 = _____
5. 0.15 = _____

6. 0.03 = _____
7. 0.5   = _____
8. 0.04 = _____
9. 0.17 = _____
10. 0.005 = _____

ANSWERS 1. 40% **2.** 5% **3.** 25% **4.** 0.4% **5.** 15% **6.** 3% **7.** 50% **8.** 4% **9.** 17% **10.** 0.5%

 All multiplications (and divisions) by units of 10 (10, 100, 1000) can be done by moving the decimal point. The number of places the decimal point is moved is always the same as the number of zeros in the multiplier (or divider).

For 10, this is one place; for 100 it is two places; for 1000 it is three places.

Converting Percent to Decimals, Common Fractions, and Ratios

Percent can easily be converted back to the other three measures. To do this you must **divide by 100.**

  Percent is converted to a **decimal** by moving the decimal point **two** places to the **left.** Because you are dividing the quantity will get **smaller.**

	Percent	**Decimal**
EXAMPLE 1	7%	0.07
EXAMPLE 2	25%	0.25
EXAMPLE 3	0.1%	0.001
EXAMPLE 4	0.02%	0.0002

Problem

Change the following percents to decimal equivalents.

1. 20%   = _____
2. 0.5% = _____
3. 2.5% = _____
4. 0.08% = _____
5. 4%   = _____

6. 0.9% = _____
7. 3%   = _____
8. 1.4% = _____
9. 2.3% = _____
10. 5%   = _____

ANSWERS 1. 0.2 **2.** 0.005 **3.** 0.025 **4.** 0.0008 **5.** 0.04 **6.** 0.009 **7.** 0.03 **8.** 0.014 **9.** 0.023 **10.** 0.05

To convert from **percent to common fractions and ratios** make the common fraction conversion first.

		Common Fraction	Ratio
EXAMPLE 1	3%	$\dfrac{3}{100}$	3 : 100
EXAMPLE 2	1%	$\dfrac{1}{100}$	1 : 100
EXAMPLE 3	2%	$\dfrac{2}{100}$	2 : 100

$\dfrac{2}{100}$ should be reduced to its lowest terms $\dfrac{1}{50}$, 1 : 50

		Common Fraction	Ratio
EXAMPLE 4	25%	$\dfrac{25}{100}$	25 : 100
	reduce to lowest terms	$\dfrac{1}{4}$	1 : 4
EXAMPLE 5	0.9%	$\dfrac{0.9}{100}$	0.9 : 100

The 0.9 can also be expressed as a whole number by eliminating the decimal point.

$\dfrac{0.9}{100}$ becomes $\dfrac{9}{1000}$ and 9 : 1000

		Common Fraction	Ratio
EXAMPLE 6	0.01%	$\dfrac{0.01}{100}$	0.01 : 100
	becomes	$\dfrac{1}{10,000}$	1 : 10,000

Problem

Express the following percents as common fractions and ratios. Reduce the equivalents to their lowest terms, and **express decimal fraction strengths as whole numbers.**

	Percent	Common Fraction	Ratio
1.	4%	_____	_____
2.	10%	_____	_____
3.	2.5%	_____	_____
4.	0.5%	_____	_____
5.	0.02%	_____	_____
6.	5%	_____	_____
7.	0.3%	_____	_____

8. 0.05% _____ _____

9. 30% _____ _____

10. 7% _____ _____

ANSWERS 1. $\frac{1}{25}$, 1 : 25 2. $\frac{1}{10}$, 1 : 10 3. $\frac{1}{40}$, 1 : 40 4. $\frac{1}{200}$, 1 : 200 5. $\frac{1}{5,000}$, 1 : 5,000 6. $\frac{1}{20}$, 1 : 20
7. $\frac{3}{1000}$ 3 : 1000 8. $\frac{1}{2000}$, 1 : 2000 9. $\frac{3}{10}$, 3 : 10 10. $\frac{7}{100}$, 7 : 100

Changing Decimals to Common Fractions and Ratios

To change a decimal fraction to a common fraction or ratio you must first recognize that **a decimal fraction has an unwritten denominator of 10, or a multiple of 10 (100, 1000). Identify the denominator by looking at the position of the decimal point.**

EXAMPLE 1 **One number** after the decimal identifies **tenths.**

$$0.3 \text{ becomes } \frac{3}{10} \qquad 3 : 10$$

EXAMPLE 2 **Two numbers** after the decimal identifies **hundredths.**

$$0.01 = \frac{1}{100} \qquad 1 : 100$$

EXAMPLE 3 **Three numbers** after the decimal point identifies **thousandths.**

$$0.015 = \frac{15}{1000} \qquad 15 : 1000$$

This fraction/ratio would be reduced to its lowest terms, and expressed as

$$\frac{3}{200} \qquad 3 : 200$$

Problem

Change the following decimal fractions to their common fraction and ratio equivalents. Reduce to lowest terms.

Decimal Fraction	Common Fraction	Ratio
1. 0.9	_____	_____
2. 0.75	_____	_____
3. 0.01	_____	_____
4. 0.45	_____	_____
5. 0.003	_____	_____
6. 0.5	_____	_____
7. 0.04	_____	_____

8.   0.2   _____   _____

9.   0.33   _____   _____

10. 0.03   _____   _____

ANSWERS 1. $\frac{9}{10}$, 9 : 10 2. $\frac{3}{4}$, 3 : 4 3. $\frac{1}{100}$, 1 : 100 4. $\frac{9}{20}$, 9 : 20 5. $\frac{3}{1000}$, 3 : 1000 6. $\frac{1}{2}$, 1 : 2 7. $\frac{1}{25}$, 1 : 25 8. $\frac{1}{5}$, 1 : 5 9. $\frac{33}{100}$, 33 : 100 10. $\frac{3}{100}$, 3 : 100

Changing Ratios and Common Fractions to Decimal Equivalents

The last equivalent to be discussed, changing ratios and common fractions to decimals, is one you have already practiced. **To change a ratio or common fraction to a decimal divide the numerator by the denominator.**

	Ratio	Common Fraction	Decimal Fraction
EXAMPLE 1	2 : 5	$\frac{2}{5}$	$2 \div 5 = 0.4$
EXAMPLE 2	3 : 4	$\frac{3}{4}$	$3 \div 4 = 0.75$
EXAMPLE 3	2 : 3	$\frac{2}{3}$	$2 \div 3 = 0.666 = 0.67$

Problem

Convert the following ratios to common fractions, then to decimal fractions. Round to the nearest hundredth.

	Ratio	Common Fraction	Decimal Fraction
1.	1 : 5	_____	_____
2.	1 : 6	_____	_____
3.	1 : 50	_____	_____
4.	1 : 20	_____	_____
5.	1 : 15	_____	_____
6.	3 : 7	_____	_____
7.	4 : 5	_____	_____
8.	1 : 4	_____	_____
9.	3 : 5	_____	_____
10.	1 : 100	_____	_____

ANSWERS 1. $\frac{1}{5}$, 0.2 2. $\frac{1}{6}$, 0.17 3. $\frac{1}{50}$, 0.02 4. $\frac{1}{20}$, 0.05 5. $\frac{1}{15}$, 0.07 6. $\frac{3}{7}$, 0.43 7. $\frac{4}{5}$, 0.8 8. $\frac{1}{4}$, 0.25 9. $\frac{3}{5}$, 0.6 10. $\frac{1}{100}$, 0.01

Summary

This concludes the chapter on equivalents in drug measures. The important points to remember are:

dosages may be expressed as ratios, percents, common fractions, or decimal fractions

all of these measures can be expressed as equivalents of each other

ratios and common fractions are essentially the same, with only the colon or fraction bar making them look different

to change a percent to any other equivalent divide by 100

to change any other equivalent to a percent multiply by 100

to change a common fraction or ratio to a decimal fraction divide the numerator by the denominator

to reverse this calculation, and express a decimal fraction as a common fraction or ratio, write the appropriate denominator beneath the decimal fraction and reduce to simplest terms

Summary Self Test

Directions: Express each of the following measures as their three mathematic equivalents. Reduce to simplest terms where appropriate.

	Percent	Ratio	Common Fraction	Decimal
1.	0.01%			
2.		1 : 2000		
3.		1 : 25		
4.				0.02
5.	10%			
6.			$\frac{1}{3}$	
7.			$\frac{1}{150}$	
8.				0.15
9.				0.03
10.	0.45%			
11.			$\frac{1}{4}$	
12.		1 : 100		
13.				0.06
14.	2.5%			

15. 20% _____ _____ _____

16. _____ _____ $\frac{1}{2}$ _____

17. _____ _____ _____ 0.9

18. _____ 1 : 200 _____ _____

19. _____ 1 : 15 _____ _____

20. _____ _____ $\frac{3}{50}$ _____

ANSWERS

Percent	Ratio	Common Fraction	Decimal Fraction
1. 0.01%	1 : 10,000	$\frac{1}{10,000}$	0.0001
2. 0.05%	1 : 2000	$\frac{1}{2,000}$	0.0005
3. 4%	1 : 25	$\frac{1}{25}$	0.04
4. 2%	1 : 50	$\frac{1}{50}$	0.02
5. 10%	1 : 10	$\frac{1}{10}$	0.1
6. 33.3%	1 : 3	$\frac{1}{3}$	0.33
7. 0.67%	1 : 150	$\frac{1}{150}$	0.0067
8. 15%	3 : 20	$\frac{3}{20}$	0.15
9. 3%	3 : 100	$\frac{3}{100}$	0.03
10. 0.45%	9 : 2000	$\frac{9}{2000}$	0.0045
11. 25%	1 : 4	$\frac{1}{4}$	0.25
12. 1%	1 : 100	$\frac{1}{100}$	0.01
13. 6%	3 : 50	$\frac{3}{50}$	0.06
14. 2.5%	1 : 40	$\frac{1}{40}$	0.025
15. 20%	1 : 5	$\frac{1}{5}$	0.2
16. 50%	1 : 2	$\frac{1}{2}$	0.5
17. 90%	9 : 10	$\frac{9}{10}$	0.9
18. 0.5%	1 : 200	$\frac{1}{200}$	0.005
19. 6.7%	1 : 15	$\frac{1}{15}$	0.067
20. 6%	3 : 50	$\frac{3}{50}$	0.06

SECTION

TWO

Systems of Drug Measure

7

Metric International (SI) System

OBJECTIVES

The student will

1. list the commonly used units of measure in the metric system
2. distinguish between the official abbreviations and variations in common use
3. express metric weights and volumes using correct notation rules
4. convert metric weights and volumes within the system

INTRODUCTION

The major system of weights and measures used in medicine is the metric/international/SI (from the French **S**ystème **I**nternational). The metric system was invented in France in 1875, and takes its name from the **meter,** a length roughly equivalent to a yard, from which all other units of measure in the system are derived. The strength of the metric system lies in its simplicity, since all units of measure differ from each other in powers of ten (10). Conversions between units in the system are accomplished by simply moving a decimal point.

While it is not necessary for you to know the entire metric system to administer medications safely, you must understand its basic structure, and become familiar with the units of measure you will be using.

Basic Units of Metric Measure

Three types of metric measures are in common use, those for **length, volume** (or capacity), and **weight.** The **basic units** or beginning points of these three measures are

length _____ meter   volume _____ liter   weight _____ gram

You must memorize these basic units: do so now if you do not already know them. In addition to these basic units there are both larger and smaller units of measure for length, volume, and weight. Let's compare this concept with something familiar. The pound is a unit of weight that we use every day. A smaller unit of measure is the ounce, a larger, the ton. **However, all are units measuring weight.**

In the same way there are smaller and larger units than the basic meter, liter, and gram. However, in the metric system there is one very important advantage: **all other units, whether larger or smaller than the basic units, have the name of the**

64

basic unit incorporated in them. So there is never need for doubt when you see a unit of measure just what it is measuring. **Meter-length, liter-volume, gram-weight.**

Problem

Identify the following metric measures with their appropriate category of weight, length, or volume.

1. milligram   _____
2. centimeter   _____
3. milliliter   _____
4. millimeter   _____
5. kilogram   _____
6. microgram   _____

ANSWERS   **1.** weight   **2.** length   **3.** volume   **4.** length   **5.** weight   **6.** weight

Metric Prefixes

The prefixes used in combination with the names of the basic units identify the larger and smaller units of measure. The same prefixes are used with all three measures. Therefore there is a kilo**meter,** kilo**gram,** and a kilo**liter.** Prefixes also change the value of each of the basic units by the same amount. For example the prefix "kilo" identifies a unit of measure which is larger than, or multiplies the basic unit by 1000. Therefore,

> 1 kilometer = 1000 meters
> 1 kilogram = 1000 grams
> 1 kiloliter = 1000 liters

Kilo is the only prefix you will be using which identifies a measure **larger** than the basic unit. Kilograms are frequently used as a measure for body weight, especially for infants and children.

You will see only three measures **smaller** than the basic unit in common use. The prefixes for these are:

> centi—as in centimeter
> milli—as in milligram
> micro—as in microgram

Therefore, you will actually be working with only four prefixes; kilo, which identifies a larger unit of measure than the basics, and centi, milli, and micro, which identify smaller units than the basics.

Metric Abbreviations

In actual use the units of measure are abbreviated. **The basic units are abbreviated to their first initial, and printed in small letters, with the exception of liter, which is capitalized.**

> gram is g   liter is L   meter is m

The abbreviations for the prefixes used in combination with the basic units are all printed using small letters.

kilo —— k —— as in kilogram —— kg
centi —— c —— as in centimeter —— cm
milli —— m —— as in milligram —— mg
micro —— mc —— as in microgram —— mcg

Micro has an additional abbreviation, the symbol μ, which is used in combination with the basic unit, as in microgram, **μg.**

While you will see the symbol μg on drug labels for microgram, you should be aware that it has an inherent safety risk. When hand printed it is very easy for microgram (*ug*) to be mistaken for milligram (*mg*). These units differ from each other in value by 1000 (1 mg = 1000 mcg), and misreading these dosages could be critical.

To assure safety when transcribing orders by hand always use the abbreviation mc to designate micro rather than its symbol: Example mcg.

In combination liter remains capitalized. Therefore milliliter is mL, and kiloliter kL.

Problem

Print the abbreviations for the following metric units.

1. microgram _____
2. liter _____
3. kilogram _____
4. milliliter _____
5. centimeter _____
6. milligram _____
7. meter _____
8. kiloliter _____
9. millimeter _____
10. gram _____

ANSWERS 1. mcg 2. L 3. kg 4. mL 5. cm 6. mg 7. m 8. kL 9. mm 10. g

Variations of SI/Metric Abbreviations

Although the metric system was invented in 1875 it was not until 1960, nearly 100 years later, that a standard system of abbreviations, the **International System of Units,** was adopted. Therefore a variety of unofficial abbreviations are still in use. Most of the variations were designed to prevent confusion with the much older apothecaries' system, which was in common use at that time in drug dosages. The major difference is that gram was abbreviated **Gm,** in an effort to differentiate it from the apothecaries' grain, **gr.** This of course led to milligram and microgram being abbreviated **mgm,** and **mcgm.** Liter was routinely abbreviated small **l,** and milliliter, **ml.** While you may see these abbreviations used do not fall into the habit of using them yourself. They are officially obsolete.

Metric Notation Rules

The easiest way to learn the rules of metric notations, in which a unit of measure is expressed with a quantity, is to memorize some prototypes (examples) which incorporate all the rules. Then if you get confused, you can stop and think and remember the correct way to write them. For the metric system the notations for one-half, one, and one and one-half milliliters will incorporate all the rules you must know.

Prototype Notations: **0.5 mL   1 mL   1.5 mL**

RULE: **The quantity is written in Arabic numerals, 1,2,3,4, etc.**

example: 0.5   1   1.5

RULE: **The numerals representing the quantity are placed in front of the abbreviations.**

example: 0.5 mL   1 mL   1.5 mL   (not mL 0.5, etc.)

RULE: **A full space is used between the numeral and abbreviation.**

example: 0.5 mL   1 mL   1.5 mL   (not 0.5mL, etc.)

RULE: **Fractional parts of a unit are expressed as decimal fractions.**

example: 0.5 mL   1.5 mL   (not $\frac{1}{2}$ mL, $1\frac{1}{2}$ mL)

RULE: **A zero is placed in front of the decimal when it is not preceded by a whole number to emphasize the decimal point.**

example: 0.5 mL   (not .5 mL)

RULE: **Unnecessary zeros are omitted so they cannot be misread and lead to medication errors.**

example: 0.5 mL   1 mL   1.5 mL   (not 0.50 mL, 1.0 mL, 1.50 mL)

So once again, as examples of the rules of metric notations, memorize the prototypes 0.5 mL—1 mL—1.5 mL. Just refer back to these in your memory if you get confused and you will be able to write them correctly.

Problem

Write the following metric measures using official abbreviations and notation rules.

1. two grams .... _____
2. five hundred milliliters..................................... _____
3. five-tenths of a liter .... _____
4. two-tenths of a milligram................................. _____
5. five-hundredths of a gram............................... _____
6. two and five-tenths kilograms .... _____
7. one hundred micrograms................................. _____

8.   two and three-tenths milliliters .... _____

9.   seven-tenths of a milliliter .... _____

10. three-tenths of a milligram .... _____

11. two and four-tenths liters................................ _____

12. seventeen and five-tenths kilograms .... _____

13. nine-hundredths of a milligram....................... _____

14. ten and two-tenths micrograms....................... _____

15. four-hundredths of a gram .... _____

ANSWERS   1. 2 g   2. 500 mL   3. 0.5 L   4. 0.2 mg   5. 0.05 g   6. 2.5 kg   7. 100 mcg   8. 2.3 mL   9. 0.7 mL
10. 0.3 mg   11. 2.4 L   12. 17.5 kg   13. 0.09 mg   14. 10.2 mcg   15. 0.04 g

Conversion Between Metric/SI Units

When you administer medications you will routinely be converting units of measure within the metric system, for example g to mg, and mg to mcg. Learning the relative value of the units you will be working with is the first prerequisite to accurate conversions. There are only four metric **weights** commonly used in medicine. From **highest** to **lowest** value these are:

kg   = kilogram
g   = gram
mg   = milligram
mcg = microgram

Only two units of **volume** are frequently used. From **highest** to **lowest** value these are:

L   = liter
mL   = milliliter

Each of these units differs in value from the next by 1000

1 kg = 1000 g
1 g = 1000 mg
1 mg = 1000 mcg

1 L   = 1000 mL (1000 cc)

 The abbreviations for milliliter (mL) and cubic centimeter (cc) are used interchangeably. A cc is actually the amount of physical space that a 1 mL volume occupies, but the two measures are considered identical.

Once again, from highest to lowest value the units are, for weight: kg—g—mg—mcg; for volume: L—mL (cc). Each unit differs in value from the next by 1000, and **all conversions will be between touching units of measure,** for example g to mg, mg to mcg, L to mL.

Problem

Indicate if the following statements are true or false.

1. T F 1000 cc = 1000 L
2. T F 1000 mg = 1 g
3. T F 1000 mL = 1000 cc
4. T F 1000 mg = 1 mcg
5. T F 1000 mcg = 1 g
6. T F 1 kg = 1000 g
7. T F 1 mg = 1000 g
8. T F 1000 mcg = 1 mg
9. T F 1000 mL = 1 L
10. T F 3 cc = 3 mL

ANSWERS 1.F 2.T 3.T 4.F 5.F 6.T 7.F 8.T 9.T 10.T

Since the metric system is a decimal system, **conversions between the units are simply a matter of moving the decimal point.** Also because each unit of measure in common use differs from the next by 1000, if you know one conversion you know them all.

How far do you move the decimal point? Each of the units differs from the next by 1000. There are three zeros in 1000, **move the decimal point three places.**

Which way do you move the decimal point? If you are converting **down** the scale to a **smaller** unit of measure, for example g to mg, the quantity must get **larger,** so move the decimal three places to the **right.**

EXAMPLE 1 0.5 g = _____ mg

You are converting down the scale. Move the decimal point three places to the right. To do this you have to add two zeros. Your answer, 500 mg, is a larger number because you moved down the scale (0.5 g = 500 mg).

EXAMPLE 2 2.5 L = _____ mL

Converting down, L to mL, move the decimal point three places to the right. Your answer will be a larger quantity (2.5 L = 2500 mL).

Problem

Convert the following metric measures

1. 7 mg = _____ mcg
2. 1.7 L = _____ mL
3. 3.2 g = _____ mg
4. 0.03 kg = _____ g
5. 0.4 mg = _____ mcg
6. 1.5 mg = _____ mcg
7. 0.7 g = _____ mg
8. 0.3 L = _____ mL
9. 7 kg = _____ g
10. 0.01 mg = _____ mcg

ANSWERS 1. 7000 mcg 2. 1700 mL 3. 3200 mg 4. 30 g 5. 400 mcg 6. 1500 mcg 7. 700 mg 8. 300 mL 9. 7000 g 10. 10 mcg

In metric conversions up the scale, from smaller to larger units of measure, the quantity will get smaller, for example mL to L. The decimal point moves **three places to the left.**

EXAMPLE 1   200 mL = _____ L

You are converting up the scale. Move the decimal point three places left. The quantity becomes smaller 200 mL = 0.2 L (remember the safety feature of adding a zero in front of the decimal).

EXAMPLE 2   500 mcg = _____ mg

Move the decimal point three places to the left. The quantity becomes smaller. 500 mcg = 0.5 mg.

Problem

Convert the following metric measures.

1.   3500 mL   = _____ L
2.   520 mg   = _____ g
3.   1800 mcg = _____ mg
4.   750 cc   = _____ L
5.   150 mg   = _____ g

6.   250 mcg = _____ mg
7.   1200 mg = _____ g
8.   600 mL = _____ L
9.   100 mg = _____ g
10.   950 mcg = _____ mg

ANSWERS   **1.** 3.5 L   **2.** 0.52 g   **3.** 1.8 mg   **4.** 0.75 L   **5.** 0.15 g   **6.** 0.25 mg   **7.** 1.2 g   **8.** 0.6 L   **9.** 0.1 g
10. 0.95 mg

Summary

This concludes your refresher on the metric system. The important points to remember from this chapter are:

the meter, liter, and gram are the basic units of metric measures

larger and smaller units than the basics are identified by the use of prefixes

the only larger unit you will be seeing is the kilo, whose prefix is k

the only smaller units you will be seeing are milli—m, micro—mc, and centi—c

each prefix changes the value of the basic unit by the same amount

converting from one unit to another within the system is accomplished by moving the decimal point

when you convert down the scale to smaller units of measure the quantity will get larger

when you convert up the scale to larger units of measure the quantity will get smaller

Summary Self Test

1. List the basic units of measure of the metric system and indicate what type of measure they are used for.

   _____   _____

   _____   _____

   _____   _____

2. Which of the following are official metric/SI abbreviations?

   a) L

   b) g

   c) kL

   d) mgm

   e) mg

   f) kg

   g) ml

   h) G   _____

Directions: Express the following measures using official metric abbreviations and notation rules.

3. six-hundredths of a milligram   _____

4. three hundred and ten milliliters _____

5. three-tenths of a kilogram   _____

6. four-tenths of a cubic centimeter _____

7. one and five-tenths grams   _____

8. one-hundredths of a gram   _____

9. four thousand milliliters   _____

10. one and two-tenths milligrams   _____

11. List the four commonly used units of weight and the two of volume, from highest to lowest value.

    _____   _____

    _____   _____

    _____

    _____

Directions: Convert the following metric measures.

12. 160 mg   = _____ g

13. 10 kg   = _____ g

14. 1500 μg = _____ mg

15. 750 mg   = _____ g

16. 200 mL   = _____ L

17. 0.3 g   = _____ mg

18. 0.05 g   = _____ mg

19. 0.15 g   = _____ mg

20. 1.2 L   = _____ mL

21. 15 mL   = _____ cc

22. 2 mg   = _____ mcg

23. 900 mcg = _____ mg

24. 2.1 L   = _____ mL

25. 475 mL   = _____ L

26. 0.9 cc   = _____ mL

27. 300 mg   = _____ g

28. 2.5 mg   = _____ mcg

29. 1 kL   = _____ L

30. 3 L   = _____ cc

31. 10 cc   = _____ mL

32. 0.7 mg   = _____ mcg

33. 4 g   = _____ mg

34. 1000 mL = _____ L

35. 2.5 mL   = _____ cc

36. 1000 mg = _____ g

37. 0.2 mg   = _____ mcg

38. 2000 g   = _____ kg

39. 1.4 g   = _____ mg

40. 2.5 L   = _____ cc

ANSWERS 1. gram-weight; liter-volume; meter-length **2.** a, b, c, e, f **3.** 0.06 mg **4.** 310 mL **5.** 0.3 kg **6.** 0.4 cc **7.** 1.5 g **8.** 0.01 g **9.** 4000 mL **10.** 1.2 mg **11.** kg, g, mg, mcg; L, mL **12.** 0.16 g **13.** 10,000 g **14.** 1.5 mg **15.** 0.75 g **16.** 0.2 L **17.** 300 mg **18.** 50 mg **19.** 150 mg **20.** 1200 mL **21.** 15 cc **22.** 2000 mcg **23.** 0.9 mg **24.** 2100 mL **25.** 0.475 L **26.** 0.9 mL **27.** 0.3 g **28.** 2500 mcg **29.** 1000 L **30.** 3000 cc **31.** 10 mL **32.** 700 mcg **33.** 4000 mg **34.** 1 L **35.** 2.5 cc **36.** 1 g **37.** 200 mcg **38.** 2 kg **39.** 1400 mg **40.** 2500 cc

Apothecary and Household Systems

OBJECTIVES

The student will

1. list the symbols, abbreviations, and notation rules for apothecary and household measures
2. convert apothecary and household measures to metric equivalents
3. explain why discrepancies exist in such conversions

INTRODUCTION

The apothecaries' and household are the oldest of the drug measurement systems. Apothecary measures are not frequently used, but you may occasionally see them on drug labels and doctors orders. Household measures are still in use, especially for patients being cared for at home, and in children's dosages. It is important that you be able to recognize the symbols of measures in these systems, and if necessary convert the dosages to metric units of measure.

Apothecary and Household Measures

There are only four apothecary units for which you must memorize the abbreviations and symbols. Take a minute to learn them now and practice printing them before moving ahead in the lesson.

WEIGHT	VOLUME
grain gr	minim m min
	dram ℈ dr
	ounce ℥ oz

You may initially have difficulty remembering the difference between the symbols for dram and ounce. So let's take a minute to clarify these. **An ounce equals 30 mL,** or a full medication cup in case it's easier for you to relate to that. It is the larger of the two measures and the symbol is likewise larger, having an extra loop on top. In fact it almost looks like oz written carelessly ℥ . **A dram equals 4 mL.** It just covers the bottom of a medication cup and is therefore very small compared with an ounce. Its symbol is also smaller ℈ . It is important not to confuse these symbols because the large difference in measures, 30 mL for ounce as opposed to 4 mL for dram could make errors very serious.

Once again: ounce = ℥ = 30 mL

dram = ℨ = 4 mL

A **minim** is approximately equal in size to a **drop,** so it is a very small measure.

1 minim = m or min = 1 drop

Three **household** measures still in common use are

tablespoon — T or tbs   teaspoon — t or tsp   drop — gtt

Memorize these if you are not already familiar with them. Be careful not to confuse the single letter abbreviations for table and teaspoon. A tablespoon is larger (15 mL) and is printed with a capital T; the teaspoon, which is smaller (5 mL), is printed with a small t.

Once again: tablespoon = T or tbs = 15 mL

teaspoon = t or tsp = 5 mL

Problem

Write the symbols and/or abbreviations for the following measures.

1.   minim   _____   _____
2.   teaspoon   _____   _____
3.   ounce   _____   _____
4.   grain   _____
5.   dram   _____   _____
6.   drop   _____
7.   tablespoon   _____   _____

ANSWERS 1. min, m **2.** t, tsp **3.** ℥ , oz **4.** gr **5.** ℨ , dr **6.** gtt **7.** T, tbs

Apothecary and Household Notations

The best overall description of **apothecary notations** is that they are the exact opposite of metric notations.

RULE: **The symbol is placed in front of the quantity.**

example: gr 7½   gr ¹/₁₅₀   (not 7½ gr, ¹/₁₅₀ gr)

RULE: **Fractions are expressed as common fractions in Arabic numerals.**

example: gr ¼   gr ¹/₁₅₀

RULE: **Larger quantities may be written in Roman *or* Arabic numerals.**

example: Roman: gr $\overset{..}{VII}$ Arabic: gr 7

Need a refresher in Roman numerals? Here's how they are used in dosages (1–10)

$$\dot{\overline{I}} \quad \ddot{\overline{II}} \quad \dddot{\overline{III}} \quad \dot{\overline{IV}} \quad \overline{V} \quad \dot{\overline{VI}} \quad \ddot{\overline{VII}} \quad \dddot{\overline{VIII}} \quad \dot{\overline{IX}} \quad \overline{X}$$

You should also know 20, $\overline{XX}$ and 30, $\overline{XXX}$ since these are occasionally used. Note that it is the usual practice when writing Roman numerals to **draw a line over the digits, and to dot the number 1 (one) each time as a safeguard against errors.** For example, a hastily written 5 ($\overline{V}$) could be mistaken for 2 ($\overline{II}$), but not if each numeral 1 has a dot ($\ddot{\overline{II}}$).

RULE: **The symbol ss may be used for ¹/₂**

example gr $\dot{\overline{I}}ss$ gr $\ddot{\overline{VII}}ss$

If you find memorizing prototypes helpful here are two notations which incorporate all the above rules:

gr 1¹/₂   gr $\ddot{\overline{VII}}ss$

There are no standard notation rules for **household measures,** so be prepared to see quite a variety in use, for example 1 T, gtt 2, $\overline{II}$ tsp, etc.

Problem

Express the following measures using the abbreviations/symbols and notation rules just discussed.

1. nine and one-half grains .... _____
2. five minims... _____
3. one two-hundredths of a grain .... _____
4. four ounces .... _____
5. one-sixteenth of a grain .... _____
6. one hundred fiftieth of a grain.......................... _____
7. twenty grains .... _____
8. one and one-half grains..................................... _____
9. four drams.. _____
10. three and a half grains....................................... _____
11. two tablespoons.. _____
12. six teaspoons.. _____
13. four drops... _____
14. one-quarter grain .... _____
15. one and a half ounces.. _____

ANSWERS   1. gr $\dot{\overline{IX}}ss$ **2.** m $\overline{V}$, min 5   **3.** gr ¹/₂₀₀   **4.** ℥ $\overline{IV}$, oz 4   **5.** gr ¹/₁₆   **6.** gr ¹/₁₅₀   **7.** gr $\overline{XX}$ **8.** gr $\dot{\overline{I}}ss$
9. ℥ $\overline{IV}$, dr 4   **10.** gr $\dddot{\overline{III}}ss$ **11.** 2 T, 2 tbs, etc.   **12.** 6 t, 6 tsp, etc.   **13.** 4 gtt, gtt $\overline{IV}$, etc.   **14.** gr ¹/₄
15. ℥ $\dot{\overline{I}}ss$; 1¹/₂ oz, etc.

Problem

Write the Roman numerals for the following numbers.

1. seven   _____

2. thirty   _____

3. four   _____

4. one   _____

5. nine   _____

6. twenty   _____

7. two   _____

8. five   _____

9. eight   _____

10. six   _____

ANSWERS 1. V̄IĪ   2. X̄X̄X̄   3. ĪV̇   4. İ   5. İX   6. X̄X̄   7. İİ   8. V̇   9. V̈IIï   10. V̇İ

Apothecary/Household/Metric Conversions

Drug labels which contain apothecary units of measure will also contain metric equivalents, so you can match up dosages ordered with the appropriate measurement system. However when an **order is written in apothecary** measures and the **label contains only metric,** conversion will be necessary. For example, a doctor may order gr ⅙, but the label reads 15 mg. If you do conversions infrequently the safest way to proceed is to refer to a conversion/equivalents table or chart. All hospitals and doctors offices will have one available. Let's begin by looking at a typical conversion/equivalents table. Refer to figure 5, and notice that the equivalents for **liquid** measures are on the left, and for **weight** on the right.

APOTHECARY/HOUSEHOLD/METRIC EQUIVALENTS			
Liquid		**Weight**	

oz	mL	min	mL	gr	mg	gr	mg
1 = 30		45 = 3		15 = 1000		1/4 = 15	
½ = 15		30 = 2		10 = 600		1/6 = 10	
		15 = 1		7½ = 500		1/8 = 8	
dr mL		12 = 0.75		5 = 300		1/10 = 6	
2½ = 10		10 = 0.6		4 = 250		1/15 = 4	
2 = 8		8 = 0.5		3 = 200		1/20 = 3	
1¼ = 5		5 = 0.3		2½ = 150		1/30 = 2	
1 = 4		4 = 0.25		2 = 120		1/40 = 1.5	
		3 = 0.2		1½ = 100		1/60 = 1	
1 min = 1 gtt		1½ = 0.1		1 = 60		1/100 = 0.6	
1 T = 15 mL		1 = 0.06		3/4 = 45		1/120 = 0.5	
1 t = 5 mL		¾ = 0.05		1/2 = 30		1/150 = 0.4	
		½ = 0.03		1/3 = 20		1/200 = 0.3	
						1/250 = 0.25	

Figure 5

The numbers on this conversion table, as on most conversion tables, are small and close together. This contributes to the most common error in the use of conversion tables, which is to misread from one column to another. For example, if you are converting gr 1/8 to mg, it is not impossible to incorrectly read one line above the correct equivalent, 10 mg, or one line below, 6 mg. To eliminate this possibility **always use a guide to read from one column to the other.** Use any straight edge available and you will see immediately that gr 1/8 is equivalent to 8 mg. Very simple, very safe.

Problem

Use the conversion table in figure 5 to determine the following equivalent measures.

1. gr 1/4 = _____ mg	9. 300 mg = gr _____
2. 30 mL = oz _____	10. 15 mg = gr _____
3. 100 mg = gr _____	11. gr 1/100 = _____ mg
4. gr 1/6 = _____ mg	12. 0.4 mg = gr _____
5. 60 mg = gr _____	13. 2 min = _____ gtt
6. 4 mL = dr _____	14. 30 mg = gr _____
7. gr 7 1/2 = _____ mg	15. 10 mL = _____ t
8. oz 1/2 = _____ mL	16. 2 T = _____ mL

ANSWERS   1. 15 mg   **2.** 1 oz   **3.** gr 1 1/2   **4.** 10 mg   **5.** gr 1   **6.** dr 1   **7.** 500 mg   **8.** 15 mL   **9.** gr 5   **10.** gr 1/4   **11.** 0.6 mg   **12.** gr 1/150   **13.** 2 gtt   **14.** gr 1/2   **15.** 2 t   **16.** 30 mL

The Apothecary/Metric Conversion Clock

Another way to remember some common conversions is to visualize an "apothecary/metric clock." Because 60 mg equal gr 1, and there are 60 minutes in one hour, mg can be used to represent minutes, and fractions of the hour to represent gr. Refer to Figure 6 to see how this works for conversions.

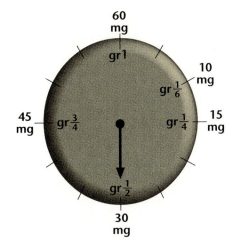

Figure 6

As you can see on this "clock" 60 mg (representing 60 min) equals gr 1 (1 hour). It then follows that 30 mg equals gr 1/2, 10 mg = gr 1/6 and so on. Two hours (gr 2) = 120 mg, and gr 5 = 300 mg. One additional equivalent to remember which does not correspond exactly to the clock is gr 15, which equals 1000 mg (1 gram).

A few moments ago you also learned that 1 oz = 30 mL, 1 dr = 4 mL, 1 T = 15 mL, 1 tsp = 5 mL. Use these equivalents now in the following problems.

Problem

Convert the following to equivalent measures.

1. gr ¾ = _____ mg
2. gr ¼ = _____ mg
3. ½ oz = _____ mL
4. gr 15 = _____ mg
5. 8 mL = dr _____

6. 300 mg = gr _____
7. gr ⅙ = _____ mg
8. 10 mL = _____ t
9. dr İ = _____ mL
10. 2 T = _____ mL

ANSWERS 1. 45 mg **2.** 15 mg **3.** 15 mL **4.** 1000 mg **5.** dr 2 **6.** gr 5 **7.** 10 mg **8.** 2 t **9.** 4 mL **10.** 30 mL

Discrepancies in Equivalents

There is an inconsistency in conversions that you need to be aware of. The conversion table you used is in fact a table of **equivalent,** not **exact** measures. To illustrate this read the dosage strengths which are circled on the labels in figures 7 and 8.

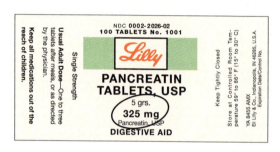

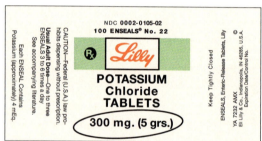

Figure 7   **Figure 8**

As you can see the label in figure 7 indicates that 5 gr equals 325 mg, while the label in figure 8 states that 300 mg equals 5 gr. Which is correct? In fact they both are, and you need to understand why.

The table of equivalents tells you that gr 1 equals 60 mg. In actual fact it equals approximately 64 mg. However, the tendency is to round off the numbers, so you are more likely to see 60 mg than 64 mg. But you may well see both. You will also see gr ½ listed as 30 mg, and 32 mg. And you have just discovered that gr 5 is equivalent to 300 mg, and 325 mg. You may also see it recorded as 324 mg.

The point being reinforced here is that conversions are **equivalent** not **equal** measures. The discrepancy results from the fact that the apothecaries' system is so inaccurate. The original gr was defined as the weight of a grain of wheat, which will give you some idea what an obsolete system of measure the apothecaries' is. So, don't be surprised when you see small discrepancies, they do exist. The important thing is that you **question all inconsistencies you are unfamiliar with,** and keep in mind that the **smaller the dosage the more significant the discrepancy will be.** For example, the difference between 300 and 325 mg may be slight in terms of drug action; the difference between 0.3 and 0.4 mg is enormous, since the drug potency is obviously so much greater. **Never guess at equivalents, take the time to be absolutely certain.**

Calculating Equivalents Mathematically

You can also calculate equivalents mathematically using ratio and proportion. All you will need to know is one equivalent.

EXAMPLE 1   You must convert gr $\frac{1}{6}$ to mg. You know that gr 1 = 60 mg. This is the complete or known ratio, so always write it first. Then add the incomplete ratio, making sure it is written in the same sequence of measurement units, gr : mg

$$\text{gr } 1 : 60 \text{ mg} = \text{gr } \frac{1}{6} : X \text{ mg} \qquad \text{or} \qquad \frac{\text{gr } 1}{60 \text{ mg}} = \frac{\text{gr } \frac{1}{6}}{X \text{ mg}}$$

$$X = 60 \times \frac{1}{6} = \textbf{10 mg} \qquad\qquad X = 60 \times \frac{1}{6} = \textbf{10 mg}$$

EXAMPLE 2   You must convert gr $\frac{1}{150}$ to mg.

$$\text{gr } 1 : 60 \text{ mg} = \text{gr } \frac{1}{150} : X \text{ mg} \qquad \text{or} \qquad \frac{\text{gr } 1}{60 \text{ mg}} = \frac{\text{gr } \frac{1}{150}}{X \text{ mg}}$$

$$X = 60 \times \frac{1}{150} = \textbf{0.4 mg} \qquad\qquad X = 60 \times \frac{1}{150} = \textbf{0.4 mg}$$

Problem

Use ratio and proportion to determine metric equivalents for the following apothecary measures. Round answers to the nearest tenth.

1. gr $\frac{1}{4}$ = _____ mg   3. gr $\frac{1}{100}$ = _____ mg

2. gr $\frac{1}{200}$ = _____ mg   4. gr $\frac{1}{8}$ = _____ mg

ANSWERS   1. 15 mg   **2.** 0.3 mg   **3.** 0.6 mg   **4.** 8 mg

Apothecary Dosage Calculations

You have already practiced the math needed to solve dosage problems containing common fractions. Use whichever format of ratio and proportion you chose earlier.

EXAMPLE 1   A dosage of gr $\frac{1}{2}$ is contained in 2 mL. gr $\frac{1}{8}$ has been ordered.

$$\text{gr } \frac{1}{2} : 2 \text{ mL} = \text{gr } \frac{1}{8} : X \text{ mL} \qquad \text{or} \qquad \frac{\text{gr } \frac{1}{2}}{2 \text{ mL}} = \frac{\text{gr } \frac{1}{8}}{X \text{ mL}}$$

$$\frac{1}{2} X = 2 \times \frac{1}{8} \qquad\qquad\qquad \frac{1}{2} X = 2 \times \frac{1}{8}$$

$$= \frac{2 \times \frac{1}{8}}{\frac{1}{2}} \qquad\qquad\qquad\qquad = \frac{2 \times \frac{1}{8}}{\frac{1}{2}}$$

$$= 2 \times \frac{1}{8} \times \frac{2}{1}$$

$$= \cancel{2}^1 \times \frac{1}{\cancel{8}_{\cancel{4}_2}} \times \cancel{2}^1$$

$$= \frac{1}{2} = \textbf{0.5 mL}$$

$$= 2 \times \frac{1}{8} \times \frac{2}{1}$$

$$= \cancel{2}^1 \times \frac{1}{\cancel{8}_{\cancel{4}_2}} \times \cancel{2}^1$$

$$= \frac{1}{2} = \textbf{0.5 mL}$$

Check your answer: gr ⅛ is less than gr ½ and the quantity should be smaller than 2 mL, which it is, **0.5 mL**

Several steps can be combined to make the calculation even simpler.

EXAMPLE 2 A dosage strength of gr ¼ in 1.5 mL is available, gr ½ is ordered.

$$\text{gr} \frac{1}{4} : 1.5 \text{ mL} = \text{gr} \frac{1}{2} : X \text{ mL} \quad \text{or} \quad \frac{\text{gr} \frac{1}{4}}{1.5 \text{ mL}} = \frac{\text{gr} \frac{1}{2}}{X \text{ mL}}$$

$$\frac{1}{4} X = 1.5 \times \frac{1}{2}$$
multiply the means and extremes, or cross multiply, keeping X on the left.

$$1.5 \times \frac{1}{\cancel{2}_1} \times \frac{\cancel{4}^2}{1}$$
immediately invert the fraction with X, ¼, to an equivalent multiplication, ⁴/₁. Reduce and do final division to obtain answer.

$$X = \textbf{3 mL}$$
express answer with unit of measure, mL

Your answer should be larger than 1.5 mL because gr ½ is a larger quantity than gr ¼, and it is (3 mL).

EXAMPLE 3 A dosage strength of gr ¹/₁₅₀ in 2 mL is available. Give gr ¹/₁₀₀

$$\text{gr} \frac{1}{150} : 2 \text{ mL} = \text{gr} \frac{1}{100} : X \text{ mL} \quad \text{or} \quad \frac{\text{gr} \frac{1}{150}}{2 \text{ mL}} = \frac{\text{gr} \frac{1}{100}}{X \text{ mL}}$$

$$\frac{1}{150} X = 2 \times \frac{1}{100}$$

$$\cancel{2}^1 \times \frac{1}{\cancel{100}_2} \times \frac{\cancel{150}^3}{1} = \textbf{3 mL}$$

$$\frac{1}{150} X = 2 \times \frac{1}{100}$$

$$\cancel{2}^1 \times \frac{1}{\cancel{100}_2} \times \frac{\cancel{150}^3}{1} = \textbf{3 mL}$$

gr ¹/₁₀₀ is a larger quantity than gr ¹/₁₅₀ and the answer, 3 mL, is also larger (than 2 mL), so it is logical.

Problem

Determine the value of X in the following proportions. If you prefer to use the cross multiplication (fraction) ratio and proportion format set the problems up using this method. Express answers to the nearest tenth.

1. gr ½ : 1 mL = gr ⅛ : X mL _____

2. gr 1/75 : 4 mL = gr 1/100 : X mL _____

3. gr ¼ : 1.6 mL = gr ⅛ : X mL _____

4. gr ⅕ : 1.8 mL = gr ¼ : X mL _____

5. gr 1/100 : 1.3 mL = gr 1/150 : X mL _____

ANSWERS   1. 0.3 mL   **2.** 3 mL   **3.** 0.8 mL   **4.** 2.3 mL   **5.** 0.9 mL

Summary

This concludes your introduction to the apothecaries' and household systems of measure. The important points to remember from this chapter are:

the four apothecary measures sometimes used are the grain, minim, dram, and ounce

the symbol is placed in front of the quantity in apothecary notations; and both Arabic and Roman numerals may be used

the three household measures still in use are the tablespoon, teaspoon, and drop

there are no standard notation rules for household measures

conversions between metric and apothecary/household measures are equivalent not equal measures

a conversion table is the safest way to determine metric, apothecary, and household equivalents

the apothecary/metric conversion clock is a handy memory cue for simple apothecary/metric conversions

equivalents can also be calculated mathematically using ratio and proportion

dosage calculations within the apothecaries' system are also done using ratio and proportion

Summary Self Test

Directions: What unit of measure do the following symbols/abbreviations identify?

1. ℥ _____   7. t _____
2. oz _____   8. min _____
3. m _____   9. T _____
4. dr _____   10. gr _____
5. gtt _____   11. tsp _____
6. ℥ _____   12. tbs _____

Directions: Write the dosages identified by the following notations.

13. ℥ $\overset{\cdot}{\text{IV}}$ _____   18. 3 gtt _____

14. $\overset{\cdot\cdot}{\text{II}}$ T _____   19. gr $\overset{\cdot\cdot}{\text{VII}}$ss _____

15. gr $\overset{\cdot\cdot\cdot}{\text{III}}$ss _____   20. oz 3 _____

16. ℥ $\overset{\cdot}{\text{I}}$ _____   21. dr $\overset{\cdot}{\text{I}}$ _____

17. $\overset{\cdot\cdot}{\text{II}}$ tsp _____   22. gr $^1/_{100}$ _____

Directions: Convert the following to the equivalent measures specified. You may use the equivalents you have memorized from the apothecary/metric clock, the equivalents table on page xx or ratio and proportion for this section.

23. 3 T   = _____ mL   32. 500 mg = gr _____

24. gr $^1/_2$ = _____ mg   33. gr $^1/_2$ = _____ mg

25. 1 mL   = min _____   34. gr $^1/_{150}$ = _____ mg

26. 15 mL   = _____ tbs   35. ℥ $\overline{\text{ss}}$ = _____ mL

27. ℥ $\overset{\cdot\cdot}{\text{II}}$ = _____ mL   36. 1 min   = _____ gtt

28. gr $\overset{\cdot}{\text{I}}$ = _____ mg   37. 1 t   = _____ mL

29. gr 5   = _____ mg   38. 1 oz   = _____ mL

30. 1 g   = gr _____   39. 1 tbs   = _____ mL

31. 4 tsp   = _____ mL   40. gr $^1/_4$ = _____ mg

Directions: Determine the value of X in the following dosage problems. Express answers to the nearest tenth.

41. The strength available is gr $^1/_{10}$ in 1.8 mL. The order is to give gr $^1/_{12}$.

42. A dosage of gr $^1/_3$ has been ordered. The dosage strength available is gr $^1/_4$ in 1.4 mL.

43. The label reads gr $^1/_6$ in 2 mL. You must give gr $^1/_{10}$.

44. The order is to administer gr $^1/_{75}$. The label reads gr $^1/_{50}$ in 1.1 mL.

45. A dosage strength of gr $^1/_{200}$ in 1.4 mL is available. You must give gr $^1/_{150}$.

46. Give gr $^1/_3$ from an available dosage strength of gr $^1/_4$ in 1.8 mL.

ANSWERS 1. dram 2. ounce 3. minim 4. dram 5. drop 6. ounce 7. teaspoon 8. minim 9. tablespoon 10. grain 11. teaspoon 12. tablespoon 13. 4 drams 14. 2 tablespoons 15. 3½ grains 16. 1 ounce 17. 2 teaspoons 18. 3 drops 19. 7½ grains 20. 3 ounces 21. 1 dram 22. ¹/₁₀₀ grain 23. 45 mL 24. 30 mg 25. min 15 26. 1 tbs 27. 8 mL 28. 60 mg 29. 300 mg 30. gr 15 31. 20 mL 32. gr 7½ 33. 30 mg 34. 0.4 mg 35. 15 mL 36. 1 gtt 37. 5 mL 38. 30 mL 39. 15 mL 40. 15 mg 41. 1.5 mL 42. 1.9 mL 43. 1.2 mL 44. 0.7 mL 45. 1.9 mL 46. 2.4 mL

SECTION THREE

Reading Medication Labels and Syringe Calibrations

9

Reading Oral Medication Labels

OBJECTIVES

The student will

1. identify scored tablets, unscored tablets, and capsules
2. read drug labels to identify trade and generic names
3. locate dosage strengths and calculate simple dosages
4. measure oral solutions using a medicine cup

INTRODUCTION

Medication labels contain a variety of information, which ranges from simple to complex. In this chapter you will be introduced to labels of oral medications which are generally the least complicated. With this instruction you will be able to locate drugs and calculate simple dosages without confusion, as well as understand the more complicated labels presented in later chapters.

We will begin with labels for solid drug preparations. These include tablets; scored tablets (which contain an indented marking to make breakage for partial dosages possible); enteric coated tablets (which delay absorption until the drug reaches the small intestine); capsules (powdered or oily drugs in a gelatin cover); and sustained or controlled release capsules (action spread over a prolonged period of time, for example 12 hours). See illustrations in figure 9.

Reading Tablet and Capsule Labels

The most common type of label you will see in the hospital setting is the **unit dosage label,** in which each tablet or capsule is packaged separately.

EXAMPLE 1 Look at the Lanoxin label in figure 10, which is a unit dosage label. The first thing to notice is that this drug has two names. The first, Lanoxin, is its **trade name,** which is identified by the ® registration symbol. Trade names are usually capitalized and printed first on the label. The name in smaller print, digoxin, is the **generic or official name** of the drug. Each drug has only one official name, but may have several trade names, each for the exclusive use of the company which manufactures it. It is important to remember, however, that most labels do contain **both** names, because drugs may be ordered by either name depending on hospital policy or physician preference. You will frequently need to cross check trade and generic names for accurate drug identification.

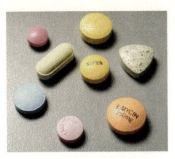
Tablets

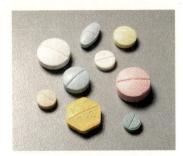
Scored Tablets

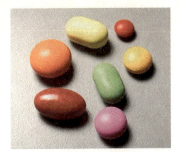
Enteric Coated Tablets

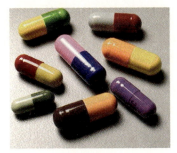
Capsules

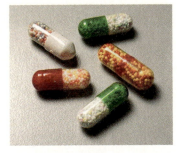
Controlled Release Capsules

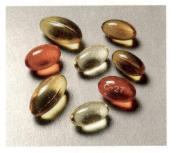
Gelatin Capsules

Figure 9

Next on the label is the **dosage strength,** 250 mcg (written with its SI symbol, μg) or 0.25 mg. The dosage is often representative of the **average dosage strength, the dosage given to the average patient at one time.** This label also identifies the manufacturer of this drug, Burroughs Wellcome Co.

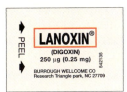

Figure 10

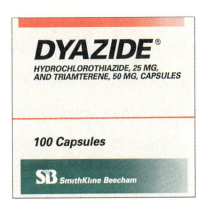

Figure 11

EXAMPLE 2 The Dyazide® label in figure 11 is **not** a unit dosage label. Notice the "100 Capsules" labeling near the center, which indicates that this package contains 100 capsules. All multiple tablet/capsule packages will list the actual number of drugs they contain, and this must not be confused with the dosage strength. **The dosage strength will have units of measure incorporated with it.** Dyazide actually contains two drugs: hydrochlorothiazide 25 mg, and triamterene 50 mg. These are the generic names, and **each has the dosage**

incorporated with the name. It is not uncommon for tablets or capsules to contain more than one drug, and when this is the case dosages are usually ordered by trade name, in this case Dyazide, and number of capsules to be administered.

Tablets and capsules which contain more than one drug are ordered by trade name and number of tablets or capsules to be given, rather than by dosage.

EXAMPLE 3 The label in figure 12 bears only one name, phenobarbital, which is actually the generic name of the drug. This labeling is common with drugs which have been in use for many years. The official (generic) name was so well established that drug manufacturers did not try to promote their own trade names. Also notice that immediately after the drug name are the initials **U.S.P.** This is the abbreviation for **U**nited **S**tates **P**harmacopeia, one of the two official national listings of drugs. The other is the **N**ational **F**ormulary, **N.F.** You will see U.S.P. and N.F. on drug labels, and must not confuse this with other initials which identify additional drugs, or specific action of drugs in a preparation.

Next, notice that this label gives the dosage strength of phenobarbital in both metric and apothecaries' units of measure, 15 mg and gr 1/4. Finally, on the right of the label, printed sideways, are the letters "EXP". This represents

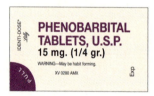

Figure 12

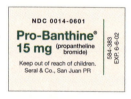

Figure 13

"expiration"; the last date when the drug should be used. Make a habit of checking the expiration dates on labels.

Problem

Refer to the label in figure 13 and answer the following questions about this drug.

1. What is the generic name? _____

2. What is the trade name? _____

3. What is the dosage strength? _____

4. What is the expiration date? _____

ANSWERS **1.** propantheline bromide **2.** Pro-Banthine® **3.** 15 mg **4.** 6-6-02 (2002)

Problem

Refer to the label in figure 14 and answer the following questions about this drug.

1. What is the generic name? _____

2. What is the trade name? _____

3. What is the dosage strength? _____

4. What is the expiration date? _____

ANSWERS 1. ampicillin trihydate **2.** Principen® **3.** 500 mg (If you said the dosage strength was 500 you were only half right. Dosage strengths must always be expressed with a unit of measure, in this case mg, 500 mg) **4.** expires 4-2-01 (2001)

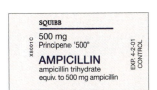

Figure 14

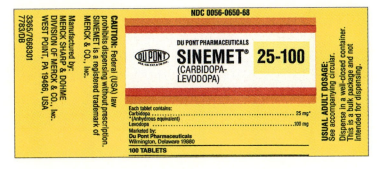

Figure 15

While most drugs are available in the unit dosage format, you will see packages or bottles containing multiple capsules or tablets. The labels are larger, and contain more information. Refer to the Sinemet® label in figure 15.

Sinemet® is another example of a combined drug tablet. The generic names of the drugs it contains are carbidopa and levodopa. These are listed on the label in several places: directly under the trade name, then with the **amount** of each drug in the fine print at the bottom of the label. Also notice the yellow box to the right of the trade name, which contains the numbers 25–100. This again is the amount of carbidopa–25 mg, and levodopa–100 mg. Contrast this with the Sinemet labels in figures 16 and 17.

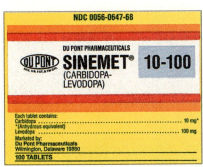

Figure 16

Figure 17

In figure 16 the dosage strengths are different. A blue box to the right of the trade name identifies the strengths of carbidopa and levodopa as 10 mg and 100 mg, actually a lower dosage. And finally, figure 17 is a label for Sinemet **CR,** a **c**ontrolled **r**elease or sustained release tablet, with yet another dosage strength (in the pink box) of 50–200, carbidopa 50 mg, levadopa 200 mg.

Extra initials after a drug name identify additional drugs in the preparation, or a special drug action.

Unlike the previous combined drug tablet discussed, an order for Sinemet **must** include the dosage, since it is available in several strengths.

Calculating Simple Dosages

When the time comes for you to administer medications you will have to read a medication record or Kardex to prepare the dosage. This will tell you the name and amount of drug to be given, but **it will not tell you how many tablets or capsules contain this dosage.** This you must calculate yourself. However, this is not difficult. Most tablets/capsules are prepared in average dosage strengths, and most orders will involve giving one half to three tablets (or one to three capsules, since capsules cannot be broken in half). **Learn to question orders for more than three tablets or capsules.** Although a few drugs require multiple tablets, most do not, and an unusual number could be a warning of an error in prescribing, transcribing, or your calculations.

 Regardless of the source of an error, if you give a wrong drug or dosage you are legally responsible for it.

Let's look at some sample orders and do some actual dosage calculations. Assume that both tablets in our problems are scored and can be broken in half.

Problem

Refer to the Thorazine® label in figure 18 and answer the following questions.

1. What is the dosage strength? _____
2. If you have an order for 100 mg give _____
3. If you have an order for 150 mg give _____
4. If 300 mg are ordered give _____
5. What is the generic name of this drug? _____
6. What is the total number of tablets in this package? _____

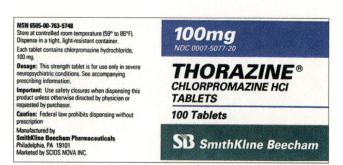

Figure 18

ANSWERS **1.** 100 mg **2.** 1 tab **3.** 1½ tab **4.** 3 tabs **5.** chlorpromazine HCl **6.** 100 tab

Problem

Refer to Cardizem® label in figure 19 and answer the following questions.

1. What is the dosage strength? _____
2. If 15 mg is ordered give _____
3. If 60 mg is ordered give _____
4. If 30 mg is ordered give _____
5. What is the generic name of this drug? _____
6. What is the total number of tablets in this package? _____

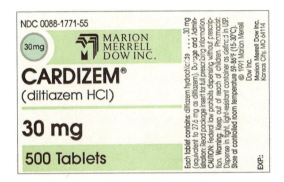

Figure 19

ANSWERS   **1.** 30 mg   **2.** ½ tab   **3.** 2 tab   **4.** 1 tab   **5.** diltiazem HCl   **6.** 500 tablets

It is not uncommon to have a drug **ordered** in one unit of metric measure, for example mg, and discover that it is **labeled** in another measure, for example g. It will then be necessary to **convert the units to calculate the dosage.** This is not difficult because conversions will always be between touching units of measure: g and mg, or mg and mcg. Converting is a matter of moving the decimal point three places.

EXAMPLE 1   Refer to the Tigan label in figure 20. A dosage of 0.25 g has been ordered. The label reads 250 mg. Convert the g to mg and you can mentally verify that these dosages are identical. Give 1 capsule.

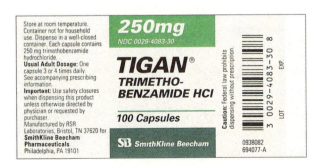

Figure 20

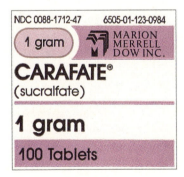

Figure 21

EXAMPLE 2   Refer to the Carafate label in figure 21. Carafate 2000 mg is ordered. The label reads 1 gram. You must give 2 tablets. (1 tab = 1000 mg, so 2000 mg requires 2 tab).

Problem

Locate the appropriate labels for the following dosages, and indicate how many tablets or capsules are needed to give them.

1.   Achromycin V 1 g _____ cap

2.   Catapres 100 mcg _____ tab

3.   Tagamet 0.8 g _____ tab

4.   Ceclor 0.5 g _____ cap

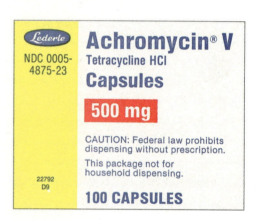

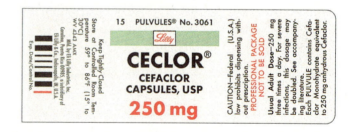

ANSWERS   1. 2 cap   **2.** 1 tab   **3.** 1 tab   **4.** 2 cap

Problem

Locate the appropriate labels for the following drug orders and indicate the number of tablets/capsules which will be required to administer the dosages ordered. Assume that all tablets are scored. Notice that both generic and trade names are used for the orders, and a label may be used in more than one problem.

1. isosorbide dinitrate 80 mg _____ tab

2. sulfasalazine 0.5 g _____ tab

3. sulfasalazine 1 g _____ tab

4. hydrochlorothiazide 25 mg _____ tab

5. chlordiazepoxide HCl 50 mg _____ cap

6. Stelazine® 7.5 mg _____ tab

7. Minipress® 2 mg _____ cap

8. phenytoin Na 90 mg _____ cap

9. diphenhydramine HCl 100 mg _____ cap

10. allopurinal 450 mg _____ tab

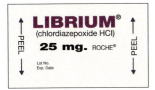
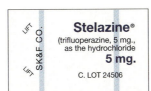
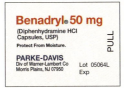

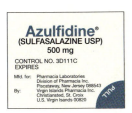
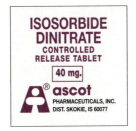
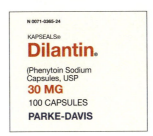

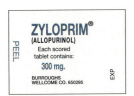
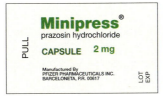
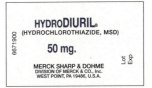

ANSWERS **1.** 2 tab **2.** 1 tab **3.** 2 tab **4.** ½ tab **5.** 2 cap **6.** 1½ tab **7.** 1 cap **8.** 3 cap **9.** 2 cap
10. 1½ tab

Reading Oral Solution Labels

In liquid drug preparations the weight of the drug is contained in a certain **volume of solution,** most frequently mL or cc's. Let's review dosages in some solid and liquid drug preparations to illustrate the difference.

EXAMPLE 1 **Solid:** 250 mg in **1 tablet**   **Liquid:** 250 mg in **5 mL**

EXAMPLE 2 **Solid:** 100 mg in **1 capsule**   **Liquid:** 100 mg in **10 mL**

Solution strength can also be expressed in ounces, drams, teaspoons or tablespoons, but these measures are less common. Let's look at some solution labels so that you can become familiar with them.

EXAMPLE 3 Refer to the Tegopen® label in figure 22. The information it contains will be familiar. Tegopen® is the trade name, cloxacillin sodium is the generic or official name. The **dosage strength is 125 mg per 5 mL.**

As with solid drugs the medication record will tell you the dosage of the drug to be administered, but rarely will it specify the volume which contains this dosage.

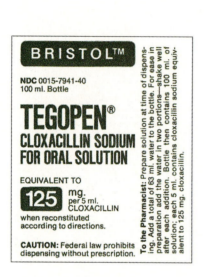

Figure 22

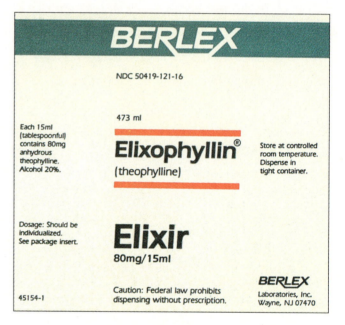

Figure 23

Problem

Refer to the cloxacillin label in figure 22 again, and calculate the following dosages.

1.   The order is for cloxacillin Na soln. 125 mg. Give _____

2.   The order is for Tegopen soln. 0.25 g. Give _____

> **ANSWERS   1.** 5 mL   **2.** 10 mL   If you did not express your answers as mL they are incorrect. Numbers have no meaning unless they are expressed with a unit of measure, in this case mL.

Problem

Refer to the Elixophyllin® label in figure 23, and calculate the following dosages.

1.   The order is for theophylline soln. 160 mg. Give _____

2.   The order is for Elixophyllin soln. 40 mg. Give _____

3.   Theophyllin soln. 80 mg has been ordered. Give _____

> **ANSWERS   1.** 30 mL   **2.** 7.5 mL   **3.** 15 mL   Your answers are incorrect unless they include mL as the unit of measure.

Problem

Refer to the solution labels in figures 24 and 25 and calculate the following dosages.

1. Prozac soln. 10 mg _____

2. cefaclor susp. 187 mg _____

3. Ceclor susp. 374 mg _____

4. fluoxetine HCl soln. 30 mg _____

5. Prozac soln. 40 mg _____

6. fluoxetine HCl soln. 20 mg _____

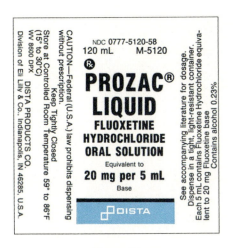

Figure 24

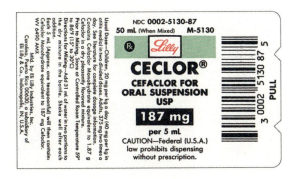

Figure 25

ANSWERS **1.** 2.5 mL **2.** 5 mL **3.** 10 mL **4.** 7.5 mL **5.** 10 mL **6.** 5 mL

Measurement of Oral Solutions

Oral solutions can be measured using a **calibrated medicine cup** such as the one shown in figure 26. Notice that it contains calibrations in mL (cc), tbs, tsp, dr, and oz. To pour accurately hold the cup at eye level, then line up the measure you need and pour.

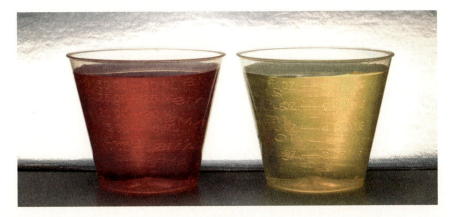

Figure 26

Solutions can also be measured using specially calibrated **oral syringes** such as those illustrated in figures 27 and 28. Oral syringes have safety features built into their design to prevent their being mistaken for hypodermic syringes. One of these features is color, as illustrated in figure 27 (hypodermic syringes are not colored, although their packaging and needle covers may be, to aid in identification). A second feature is the syringe tip, which is a different size and shape, and is often off center (termed **eccentric**). Figure 28 illustrates an eccentric oral syringe tip.

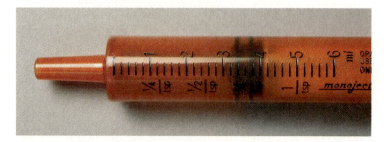

Figure 27

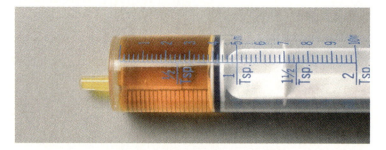

Figure 28

Hypodermic syringes (without a needle) can also be used to measure and administer oral dosages. The main concern with correct syringe identification is that oral syringes, which are **not sterile,** not be confused and used for hypodermic medications, which **are** sterile. This mistake has been made, in spite of the fact that hypodermic needles do not fit correctly on oral syringes. The precaution, therefore, does need to be stressed.

Oral solutions may also be ordered as drops (gtt), and when this is the case the dropper is usually attached to the bottle stopper. It is also common for medicine droppers to be calibrated, for example in mL, or by actual dosage, 125 mg, 250 mg, etc.

Summary

This concludes the chapter on reading oral medication labels. The following are important points to remember:

most labels contain both generic and trade names

dosages are clearly printed on the label, except for preparations containing multiple drugs, which will list the name and dosage of all ingredients

multiple dosage medications will be ordered by trade name and number of tablets/capsules to be given

the letters U.S.P. (United States Pharmacopeia) and N.F. (National Formulary) on drug labels identify their official generic listings

additional letters which follow a drug name are used to identify additional drugs in the preparation, or a special action of the drug

most dosages of oral medications will involve giving one half to three tablets (1–3 capsules, which cannot be broken in half)

check drug expiration dates before use

drug expiration dates are printed on each label

oral solution dosages are measured in cc's, oz, tsp, tbs, or gtt

for accurate measurement oral solutions are poured at eye level when a medicine cup is used

liquid medications may be measured and administered with an oral syringe, or hypodermic syringe (without the needle)

care must be taken not to use oral syringes for hypodermic medication preparation as these are not sterile

---

Summary Self Test

Directions: Locate the appropriate label for each of the following drug orders, and indicate the number of tablets/capsules or mL/cc which will be required to administer them. Assume that all tablets are scored, and can be broken in half.

PART I

1. Glucotrol 15 mg _____

2. ciprofloxacin HCl 0.5 g _____

3. Verapamil HCl 240 mg _____

4. Trental 200 mg _____

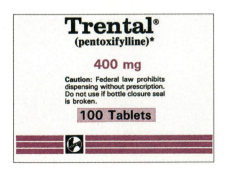

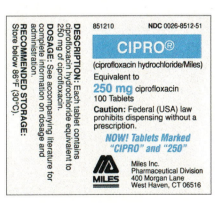

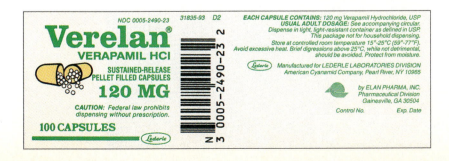

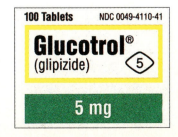

PART II

5. Theo-24 200 mg _____

6. amoxicillin susp 250 mg _____

7. Coumadin 4 mg _____

8. Calan SR 240 mg _____

9. Myambutol 300 mg _____

10. phenobarbital 30 mg _____

11. ZIAC 5 mg _____

12. lithium 600 mg _____

13. terfenadine 90 mg _____

14. captopril 12.5 mg _____

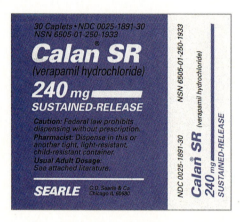

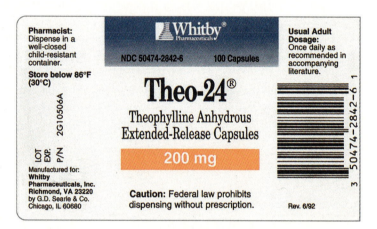

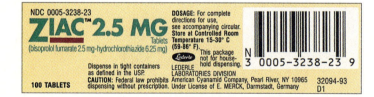

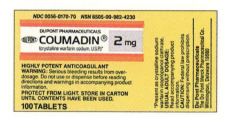

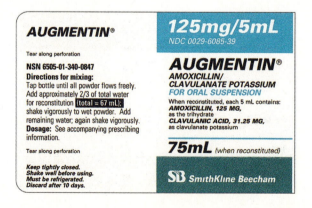

NDC 0068-0723-61   6505-01-220-8416

(60 mg)

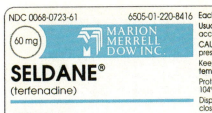

Each tablet contains: terfenadine..................60 mg

Usual Adult Dose: One tablet twice daily. See accompanying product information.

CAUTION: Federal law prohibits dispensing without prescription.

Keep tightly closed. Store at controlled room temperature 59-86°F (15-30°C).

Protect from exposure to temperatures above 104°F (40°C) and moisture.

Dispense in tight container with child-resistant closure.

©1991 Marion Merrell Dow Inc.

Merrell Dow Pharmaceuticals Inc.
Subsidiary of Marion Merrell Dow Inc.
Kansas City, MO 64114

SELDANE®
(terfenadine)

60 mg

100 Tablets

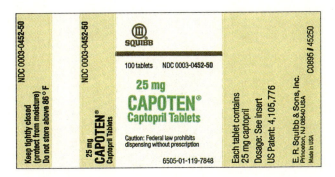

NDC 0003-0452-50

NDC 0003-0452-50

100 tablets   NDC 0003-0452-50

25 mg
CAPOTEN®
Captopril Tablets

Caution: Federal law prohibits dispensing without prescription

6505-01-119-7848

Keep tightly closed (protect from moisture) Do not store above 86° F

25 mg **CAPOTEN®** Captopril Tablets

Each tablet contains 25 mg captopril

Dosage: See insert

US Patent: 4,105,776

E. R. Squibb & Sons, Inc. Princeton, NJ 08540 USA Made in USA

C0895 *I* 45250

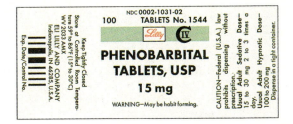

Exp. Date/Control No.

Keep Tightly Closed Store at Controlled Room Temperature 59° to 86°F (15° to 30°C)

ELI LILLY AND COMPANY Indianapolis, IN 46285, U.S.A. WV 2033 AMX

NDC 0002-1031-02

100   **TABLETS No. 1544**

PHENOBARBITAL
TABLETS, USP

15 mg

WARNING—May be habit forming.

CAUTION—Federal (U.S.A.) law prohibits dispensing without prescription.

Usual Adult Sedative Dose—15 to 30 mg 2 to 3 times a day.

Usual Adult Hypnotic Dose—100 to 200 mg

Dispense in a tight container.

NSN 6505-00-482-8058

Store at controlled room temperature (59° to 86°F). Dispense in a tight container. Each capsule contains lithium carbonate, 300 mg.

Usual Dosage: 1 or 2 capsules t.i.d. See accompanying prescribing information.

Important: Use safety closures when dispensing this product unless otherwise directed by physician or requested by purchaser.

Caution: Federal law prohibits dispensing without prescription.

Manufactured by
SmithKline Beecham Pharmaceuticals
Philadelphia, PA 19101
Marketed by SCIOS NOVA INC.

300mg
NDC 0007-4007-20

ESKALITH®
LITHIUM CARBONATE
CAPSULES

100 Capsules

SB SmithKline Beecham

Lederle

NDC 0005-5015-23

20451-92 D12

6505-00-403-7645

Myambutol®
Ethambutol Hydrochloride
Tablets 100 mg

CAUTION: Federal law prohibits dispensing without prescription. This package not for household dispensing.

100 TABLETS

Store at Controlled Room Temperature 15-30°C (59-86°F).

Control No.

N 3   0005-5015-23   4   Exp. Date

AVERAGE ADULT DAILY DOSAGE: 15 mg/kg or 25 mg/kg once every 24 hours. See accompanying circular.
Dispense in well-closed containers as defined in the USP.
LEDERLE LABORATORIES DIVISION American Cyanamid Company, Pearl River, NY 10965

PART III

15. acetaminophen 650 mg _____
16. Aldactone® 75 mg _____
17. meclizine HCl 50 mg _____
18. Reglan® 15 mg _____
19. propranolol HCl 30 mg _____
20. metroprolol tartrate 0.15 g _____
21. nifedipine 10 mg _____
22. furosemide 10 mg _____
23. Lasix® 30 mg _____
24. dexamethasone 3 mg _____
25. Tenormin® 150 mg _____
26. terbutaline 2.5 mg _____
27. Procan SR® 0.75 g _____
28. Synthroid® 225 mcg _____
29. Diabeta® 5 mg _____

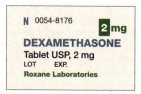
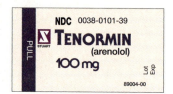
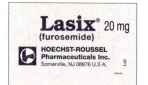
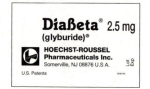
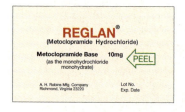
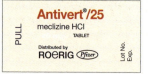
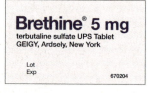
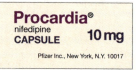
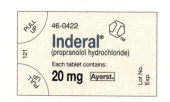
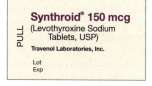
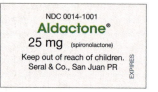
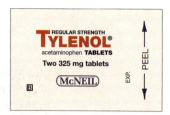
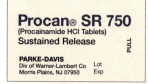
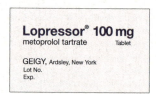

PART IV

30. erythromycin susp 0.25 g _____

31. Percocet 2 tabs _____

32. Flagyl 0.75 g _____

33. piroxicam 40 mg _____

34. cimetidine 200 mg _____

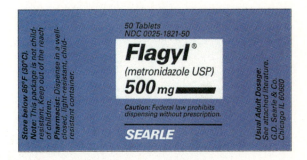

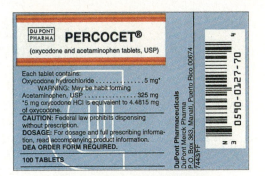

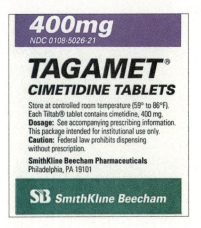

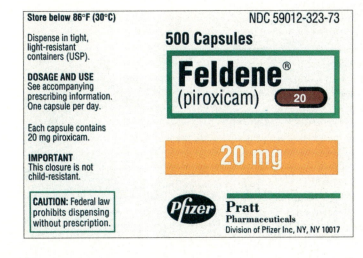

PART V

35. cefaclor oral susp 0.5 g _____

36. spironolactone 100 mg _____

37. Trimox 0.5 g _____

38. Augmentin 0.75 g _____

39. Proventil syrup 4 mg _____

40. ritodrine HCl 15 mg _____

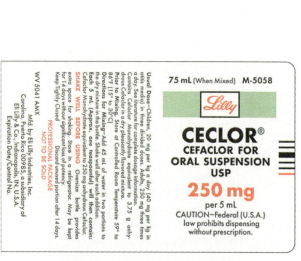

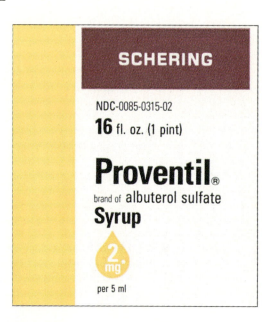

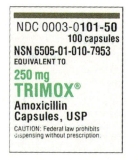

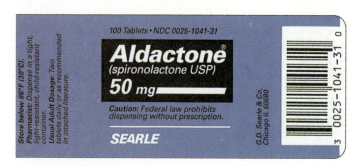

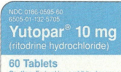

ANSWERS 1. 3 tab **2.** 2 tab **3.** 2 tab **4.** ¹/₂ tab **5.** 1 cap **6.** 10 mL **7.** 2 tab **8.** 1 cap **9.** 3 tab **10.** 2 tab **11.** 2 tab **12.** 2 cap **13.** 1¹/₂ tab **14.** ¹/₂ tab **15.** 2 tab **16.** 3 tab **17.** 2 tab **18.** 1¹/₂ tab **19.** 1¹/₂ tab **20.** 1¹/₂ tab **21.** 1 cap **22.** ¹/₂ tab **23.** 1¹/₂ tab **24.** 1¹/₂ tab **25.** 1¹/₂ tab **26.** ¹/₂ tab **27.** 1 tab **28.** 1¹/₂ tab **29.** 2 tab **30.** 10 mL **31.** 2 tab **32.** 1¹/₂ tab **33.** 2 cap **34.** ¹/₂ tab **35.** 10 mL **36.** 2 tab **37.** 2 cap **38.** 1¹/₂ tab **39.** 10 mL **40.** 1¹/₂ tab

Hypodermic Syringe Measurement

10

OBJECTIVES

The student will measure parenteral solutions using
1. a standard 3 cc syringe
2. a tuberculin syringe
3. Tubex® and Carpuject® cartridges
4. 5, 6, 10 and 12 cc syringes
5. a 20 cc syringe

INTRODUCTION

A variety of hypodermic syringes are in common use. They have different capacities (3 cc, 6 cc, 20 cc, etc.) and different calibrations. **All are calibrated in cc's,** but the smaller capacity syringes are further divided into tenths, or two-tenths, or hundredths of a cc. The objective of this chapter is to teach you how to read syringe calibrations, so that you will be comfortable with **any** type of syringe you may encounter.

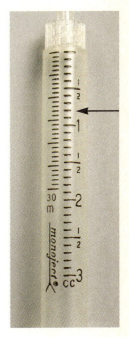

Figure 29

Standard 3 cc Syringe

The most commonly used hypodermic syringe is the 3 cc size illustrated in figure 29. Look at the calibrations on the right side, for metric (cc) measures. **The first thing to notice about any syringe is exactly how many calibrations there are in each 1 cc.** On this 3 cc syringe there are ten calibrations in each cc, which indicates that the syringe is calibrated in tenths. Larger calibrations identify the 0, ½ (0.5), and full cc measures. The shorter calibrations between these identify the tenths. For example the arrow in figure 29 identifies 0.8 cc.

Problem

Use decimal numbers, for example 2.2 cc, to identify the measurements indicated by the arrows on the standard 3 cc syringes in figure 30.

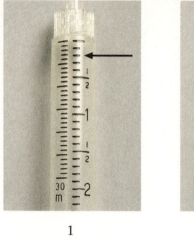 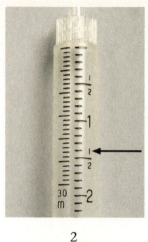 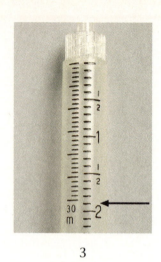

| 1 | 2 | 3 |

Figure 30

1. _____   2. _____   3. _____

Did you have difficulty with 0.2 cc calibration in problem 1? Remember that **the first long calibration on all syringes is zero.** It is slightly longer than the 0.1 cc and subsequent one tenth calibrations. Be careful not to mistakenly count it as 0.1 cc.

You have just been looking at photos of syringe barrels only. Next look at the assembled syringes in figure 31. Notice that the black suction tip of the plunger has two widened areas in contact with the barrel, which look like two distinct rings. **Calibrations are read from the front, or top ring.** Do not become confused by the second, bottom ring, or by the raised middle section of the suction tip.

Problem

What dosages are measured by the three assembled syringes in figure 31.

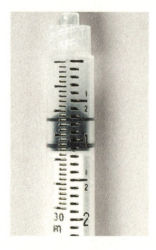 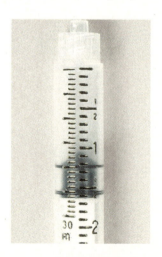 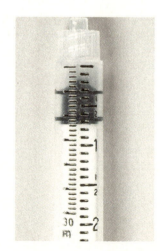

Figure 31

1. _____   2. _____   3. _____

Refer back to figure 29 and look at the small calibrations on the left of the barrel. This is the minim (m) scale of the apothecaries' system. These calibrations measure a total of 30 m, with larger calibrations identifying each 5 m increment, for example 5, 10, etc. Only the 30 m calibration is numbered. This scale is infrequently used, but you should be aware that the syringe contains it.

Problem

Draw an arrow or shade in the following syringe barrels to indicate the required dosages. Have your instructor double check your accuracy.

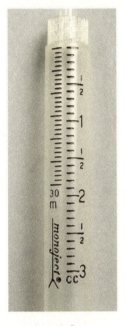 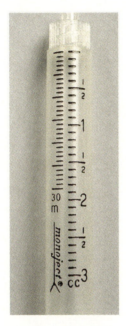 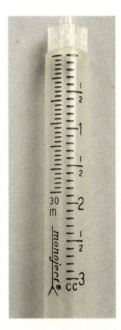

1.   1.3 cc   2.   2.4 cc   3.   0.9 cc

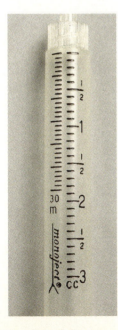 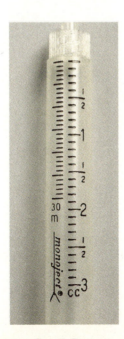 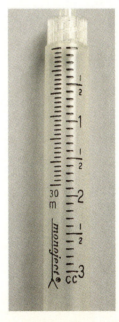

4.   2.5 cc   5.   1.7 cc   6.   2.1 cc

Problem

Identify the dosages measured on the following 3 cc syringes.

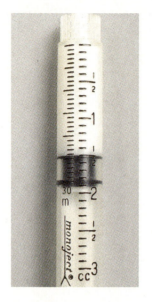

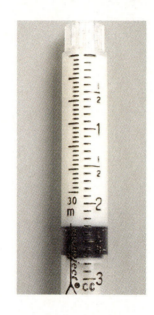

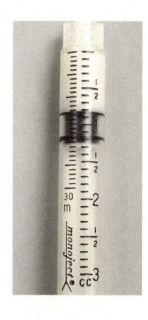

1. _____

2. _____

3. _____

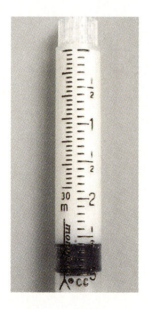

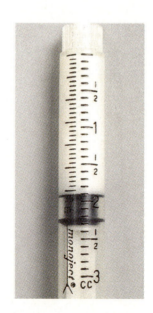

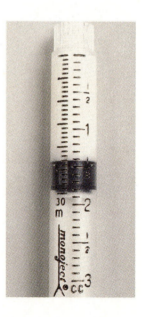

4. _____

5. _____

6. _____

Tuberculin Syringe

When dosages of **small volumes** are necessary they are measured in **hundredths,** rather than tenths, for example 0.27 cc, and 0.64 cc. Pediatric dosages usually require measurement in hundredths, as does heparin. A special 1 cc syringe calibrated in hundredths, called the tuberculin (TB), is used for these measurements. Refer to figure 32.

Once again first notice there is a 30 m scale on the left of the barrel. Then take a close look at the metric scale on the right. As you can see the calibrations are very small and close together. This mandates particular care and an unhurried approach when dosages are measured using this syringe. Notice that the total capacity of the syringe is 1.00 (1 cc), and that longer calibrations identify zero, and each successive .05 cc. Also notice that only alternate tenths are numbered: .20, .40, .60 etc., and that the actual calibration which identifies these falls between the 2 and 0, the 4 and 0, and so on. The shorter calibrations measure hundredths. Spend some time examining the calibrations to be sure you understand them. For example, the syringe in figure 32 measures 0.63 cc.

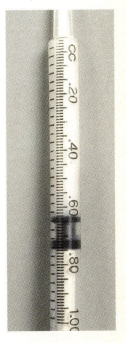

Figure 32

Problem

Identify the measurements on the following tuberculin syringes.

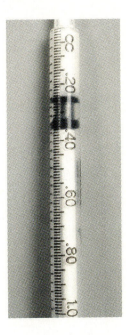 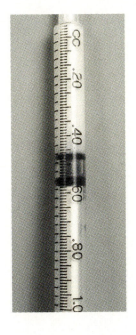 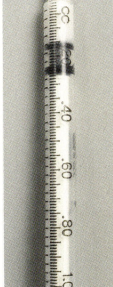

1. _____ 2. _____ 3. _____

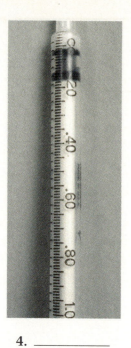

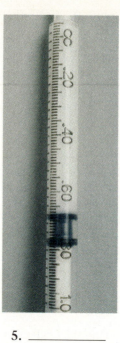

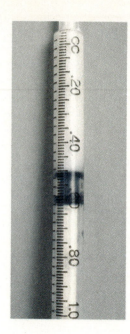

4. _____

5. _____

6. _____

ANSWERS 1. 0.24 cc 2. 0.46 cc 3. 0.15 cc 4. 0.06 cc 5. 0.67 cc 6. 0.50 cc

Problem

Draw an arrow or shade in the barrel to identify the dosages indicated on the following TB syringes. Have your instructor check your answers.

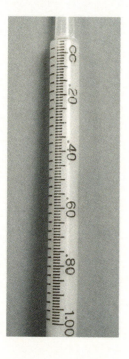

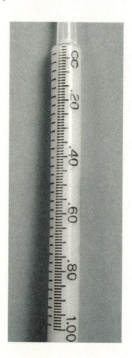

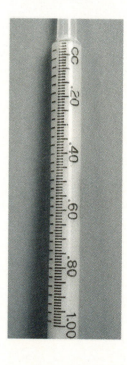

1. 0.28 cc

2. 0.61 cc

3. 0.45 cc

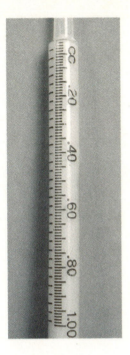
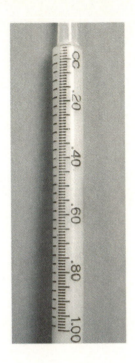
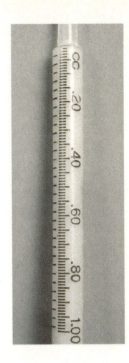

4. 0.12 cc   5. 0.97 cc   6. 0.70 cc

Tubex® and Carpuject® Cartridges

Tubex® and Carpuject® are the trade names of the two most widely used **injection cartridges.** These cartridges come **pre-filled** with sterile medication and are **clearly labeled to identify both drug and dosage.** The cartridges are designed to slip into **plastic injectors,** which provide the plunger for the actual injection. Refer to the Tubex® cartridge in figure 33, and the Carpuject® cartridge in figure 34.

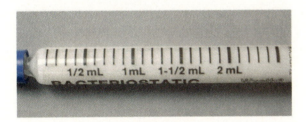

Figure 33

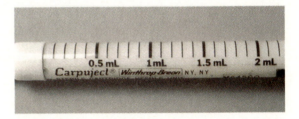

Figure 34

Both cartridges have a volume of 2.5 mL. They are calibrated in tenths, and each 0.5 (½) mL has a heavier calibration, which is also numbered. The cartridges are routinely overfilled with 0.1 mL to 0.2 mL of medication to allow for manipulation of the syringe to expel air from the needle prior to injection. The cartridges are designed with sufficient capacity to allow for addition of a second drug when combined dosages are ordered.

Problem

Identify the dosages measured on the following cartridges.

1. _____

2. _____

3. _____

4. _____

5. _____

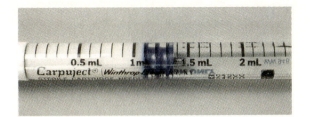

6. _____

Problem

Shade in the cartridges to indicate the following dosages. Have your instructor double check your answers.

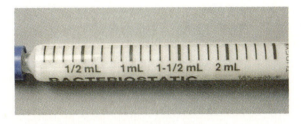

1.   2.5 mL

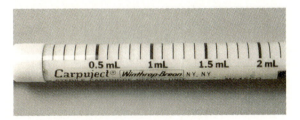

2.   1.4 mL

3.   The cartridge is pre-filled with 1 mL of medication, and you are adding 0.8 mL of a second drug.

Total Volume _____

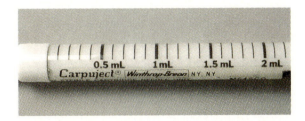

4. The cartridge contains 0.8 mL, and you must add an additional 0.8 mL.

Total Volume _____

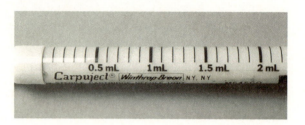

5. The cartridge contains 1.5 mL, and you are to add another 1 mL.

Total Volume _____

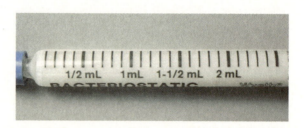

6. The cartridge contains 1 mL, and you must add an additional 1.2 mL.

Total Volume _____

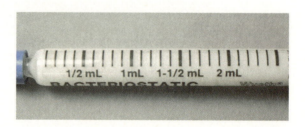

ANSWERS   3. 1.8 mL   **4.** 1.6 mL   **5.** 2.5 mL   **6.** 2.2 mL

5, 6, 10, and 12 cc Syringes

When volumes larger than 3 cc are required a 5, 6, 10 or 12 cc syringe may be used. Refer to figure 35 and examine the calibrations between each numbered cc to determine how these syringes are calibrated.

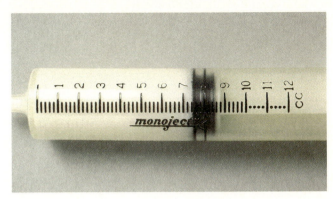

Figure 35

As you have discovered the calibrations divide each cc of these syringes into **five,** so that **each shorter calibration actually measures two tenths, 0.2 cc.** The 6 cc syringe on the left measures 4.6 cc, and the 12 cc syringe on the right measures 7.4 cc. These syringes are most often used to measure whole rather than fractional cc's, but in your practice readings we will include a full range of measurements.

Problem

What dosages are measured on the following syringes?

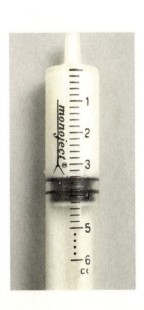

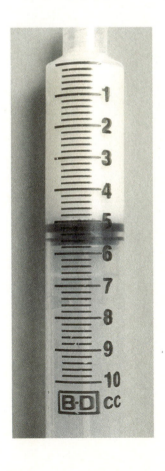

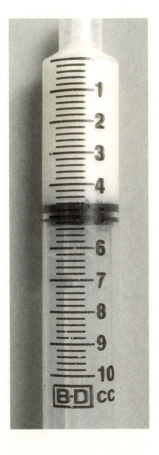

1. _____   2. _____   3. _____

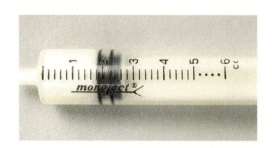 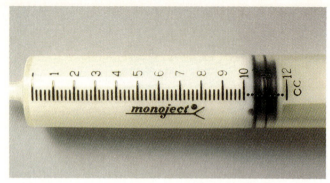

4. _____   5. _____

ANSWERS   1. 3.4 cc   **2.** 5 cc   **3.** 4.6 cc   **4.** 1.8 cc   **5.** 10.4 cc

Problem

Measure the dosages indicated on the following syringes. Have an instructor double check your accuracy.

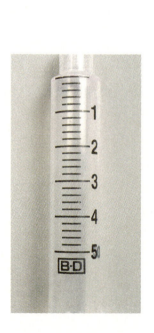 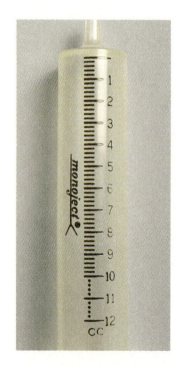 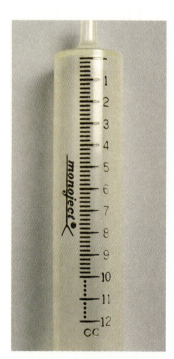

1.   1.4 cc   2.   3.2 cc   3.   6.8 cc

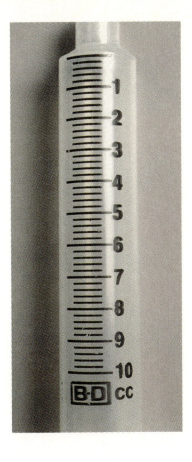

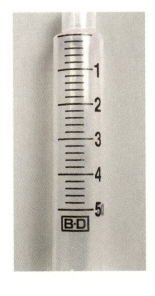

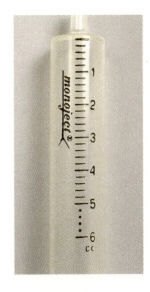

4. 9.4 cc

5. 3 cc

6. 5.6 cc

Syringes 20 cc and Larger

Examine the 20 cc syringe in figure 36 and determine how it is calibrated.

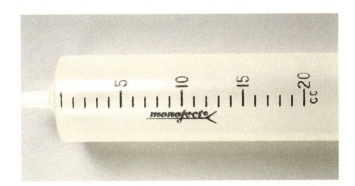

Figure 36

As you can see this syringe is calibrated in **1 cc increments,** with larger calibrations identifying the 0, 5, 10, 15 and 20 cc volumes. Syringes with a 50 cc capacity are also calibrated in full cc measures. These syringes are used only for measurement of large volumes.

Problem

What dosages are measured on the following 20 cc syringes?

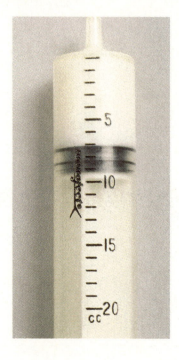 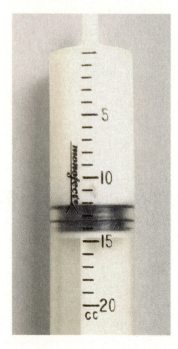 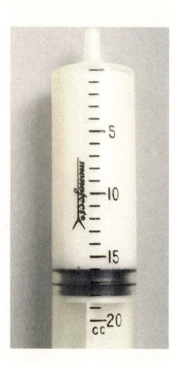

1. _____   2. _____   3. _____

Problem

Shade in or draw arrows on the following syringe barrels to identify the volumes listed. Have your answers checked by your instructor.

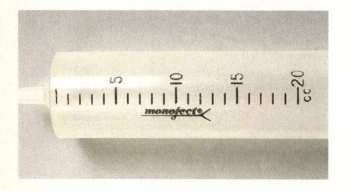 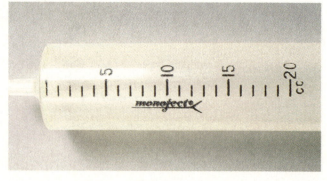

1.   11 cc   2.   18 cc

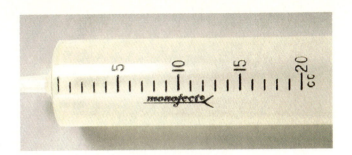

3. 9 cc

Summary

This concludes your introduction to syringe calibrations. The important points to remember from this chapter are:

3 cc syringes are calibrated in tenths

TB syringes are calibrated in hundredths

5, 6, 10 and 12 cc syringes are calibrated in fifths

syringes larger than 12 cc are calibrated in full cc measures

the first long calibration on all syringes indicates zero

pre-filled cartridges such as the Tubex® and Carpuject® are overfilled with 0.1 to 0.2 mL of medication to allow for air expulsion from the needle

pre-filled cartridges are sufficiently large to allow for the addition of a second compatible drug

all syringe calibrations must be read from the top, or front ring of the plunger's suction cup

Summary Self Test

Directions: Identify the dosages measured on the following syringes and cartridges.

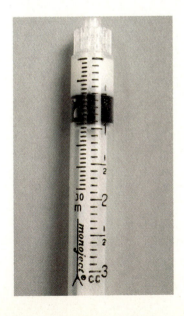

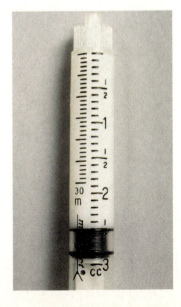

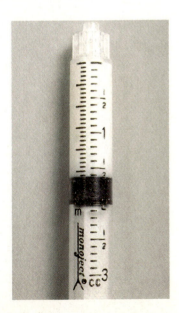

1. _____   2. _____   3. _____

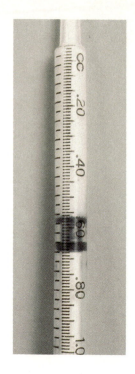

4. _____

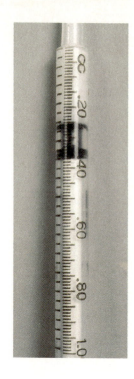

5. _____

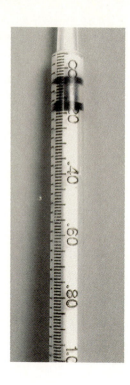

6. _____

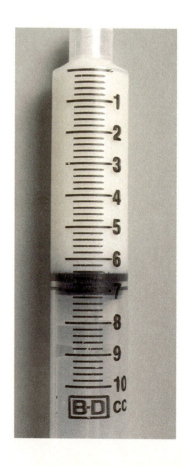

7. _____

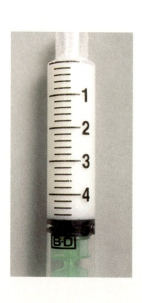

8. _____

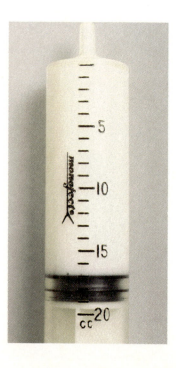

9. _____

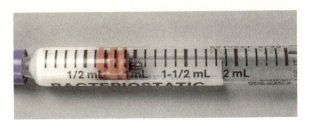

10. _____

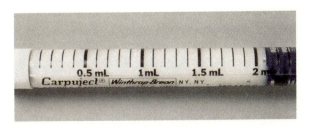

11. _____

Directions: Draw arrows or shade the barrels on the following syringes/cartridges to measure the indicated dosages. Have your answers checked by your instructor.

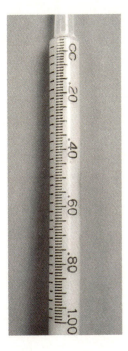

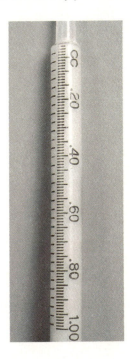

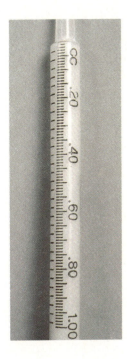

12. 0.52 cc   **13.** 0.31 cc   **14.** 0.94 cc

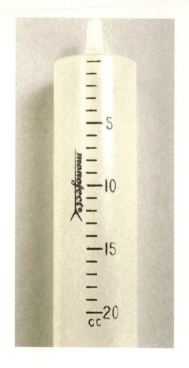

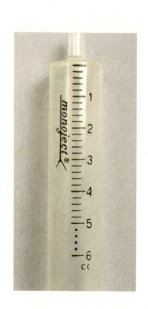

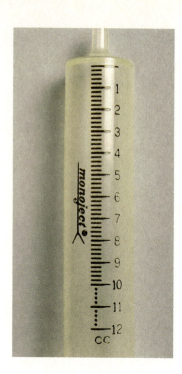

15. 13 cc

16. 1.2 cc

17. 7.6 cc

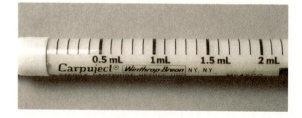

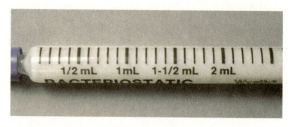

18. 1.1 mL

19. 0.7 mL

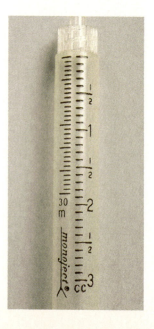

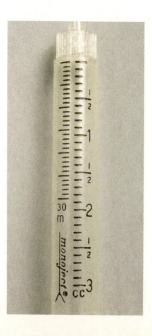

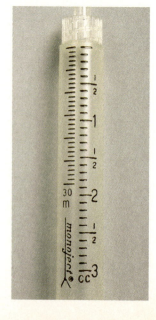

20. 1.7 cc

21. 2.2 cc

22. 0.9 cc

Reading Parenteral Medication Labels

OBJECTIVES

The student will

1. read parenteral solution labels and identify dosage strengths
2. identify milliequivalents and International Units as drug dosage measurements
3. measure parenteral dosages in metric, milliequivalent, unit, percentage, and ratio strengths using a 3 cc syringe

INTRODUCTION

Parenteral medications are administered by injection, the intravenous (IV), intramuscular (IM), and subcutaneous (s.c.) being the most frequently used routes. The labels of oral and parenteral solutions are very similar, but the volume of the average parenteral dosage is much smaller. Intramuscular and subcutaneous solutions in particular are manufactured so that the **average adult dosage will be contained in a volume of between 1 and 3 mL.** Volumes larger than 3 mL are difficult for a single injection site to absorb, while dosages contained in a volume of less than 1 mL may require the use of a tuberculin syringe to prepare accurately. The 1-3 mL volume can be used as a guideline for accuracy of calculations in IM and s.c. dosages. Excessively larger or smaller volumes would need to be questioned, and calculations rechecked.

Intravenous medication administration is usually a two step procedure: the dosage is prepared first, then may be further diluted in IV fluids prior to administration. In this chapter we will be concerned only with the first step of IV drug preparation, which is accurate measurement of the prescribed dosage.

Parenteral drugs are packaged in a variety of single use glass ampules, single and multiple use rubber stoppered vials and increasingly, in pre-measured syringes and cartridges. See figure 37.

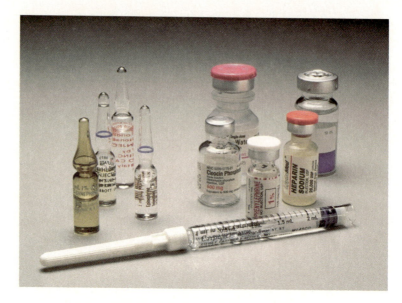

Figure 37

Ampules, vials, and pre-filled cartridge

Reading Solution Labels

We will begin by looking at parenteral solution labels on which the dosages are expressed in metric, percentage and ratio strengths, since these measures are now familiar to you.

EXAMPLE 1 Refer to the Vistaril® label in figure 38. The immediate difference you will notice between this and oral solution labels is the **size.** Ampules and vials are small and their labels are small, which requires that they be **read with particular care.** The information, however, is similar to oral labels. Vistaril® is the trade name of the drug, hydroxyzine hydrochloride is the generic name. The dosage strength is 50 mg per mL (in red rectangular area). The total vial contents are 10 mL (in black, upper left). Calculating dosages is not usually complicated. For example if a dosage of Vistaril® 100 mg is ordered you would give 2 mL, if 50 mg are ordered give 1 mL, for 25 mg give 0.5 mL.

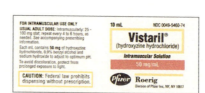

Figure 38

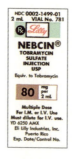

Figure 39

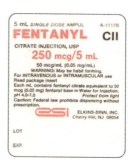

Figure 40

EXAMPLE 2 The Nebcin® (tobramycin) label in figure 39 has a dosage strength of 80 mg per 2 mL. To prepare an 80 mg dosage you would draw up 2 mL; 40 mg requires 1 mL; and 60 mg would be 1.5 mL.

EXAMPLE 3 The fentanyl citrate solution in figure 40 has a dosage strength of 250 mcg/5 mL. To prepare a 0.25 mg (250 mcg) dosage you will need 5 mL; for a 0.125 mg dosage 2.5 mL. Once again these simple dosages can be calculated mentally.

Problem

Refer to the Garamycin® label in figure 41 and answer the following questions.

1. What is the total volume of this vial? _____

2. What is the dosage strength? _____

3. If gentamicin 80 mg were ordered how many mL would this be? _____

4. If gentamicin 60 mg were ordered how many mL would this be? _____

5. How many mL would you need to prepare a 20 mg dosage? _____

ANSWERS 1. 20 mL   2. 40 mg/mL   3. 2 mL   4. 1.5 mL   5. 0.5 mL

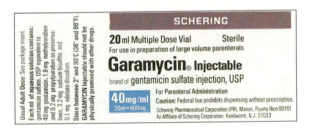

Figure 41

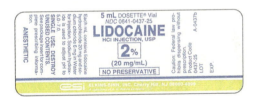

Figure 42

Percentage and Ratio Solutions

Drugs labeled as **percentage solutions** often express the drug strength in **metric measures in addition to percentage strength.** Refer to the lidocaine label in figure 42. Notice that this is a 2% solution, and the vial which contains it has a total volume of 5 mL. Also notice that the dosage strength is listed in metric measures: 20 mg/mL. Lidocaine is most often ordered in mg, for example 20 mg requires 1 mL, 10 mg would require 0.5 mL, and 30 mg would require 1.5 mL. However, lidocaine is also used as a local anesthetic and a doctor may request for example, that you prepare 3 mL of 2% lidocaine, which requires no calculation at all, but simply locating the correct percentage strength, and drawing up 3 mL.

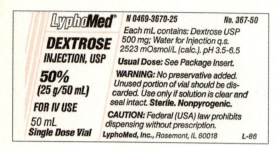

Figure 43

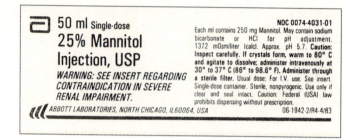

Figure 44

Problem

Refer to the dextrose label in figure 43 and answer the following questions.

1. What is the percentage strength of this dextrose solution? _____

2. How many mL does the vial contain? _____

3. If you are asked to prepare 20 mL of a 50% dextrose solution how much will you draw up in the syringe? _____

4. The dosage also appears on this label in metric measures. What is the metric dosage strength of this solution? _____

5. If you are asked to prepare 25 g of dextrose from this vial what volume will you draw up? _____

Refer to the Mannitol label in figure 44 and answer the following questions.

6. What is the percentage strength of this solution? _____

7. How many mL does this preparation contain? _____

8. What is the metric dosage strength of this solution? _____

9. If you were asked to prepare a 1 g dosage what volume would this require? _____

ANSWERS   1. 50%   2. 50 mL   3. 20 mL   4. 25 g/50 mL   5. 50 mL   6. 25%   7. 50 mL   8. 250 mg/mL   9. 4 mL

Parenteral medications expressed in **ratio strengths** are not common, and **when they are ordered it will be by number of cc/mL.** Labels may also contain metric weights.

Problem

Refer to the epinephrine label in figure 45 and answer the following questions.

1. What is the ratio strength of this solution? _____

2. What volume is this contained in? _____

3. What is the metric dosage strength of this solution? _____

<table>
<tr><td>
1 mL ampule

epinephrine HCl

1 : 1000

contains 1 mg epinephrine as
the hydrochloride in each 1 mL
</td></tr>
</table>

Figure 45

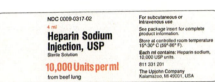

Figure 46

Solutions Measured in Units (U)

A number of drugs are measured in **International Units.** Insulin, penicillin and heparin are examples of drugs commonly measured in units. A unit measures a drug in terms of its action, not its physical weight. Units may be abbreviated **U,** and are expressed using Arabic numerals with the abbreviation following, for example 2,000 U, or 1,000,000 U.

Problem

Refer to the heparin label in figure 46 and answer the following questions.

1. What is the total volume of this vial? _____

2. What is the dosage strength? _____

3. If a volume of 1.5 mL is prepared how many units will this be? _____

4. How many mL will you need to prepare a dosage of 55,000 U? _____

5. If 0.25 mL of this medication is prepared what dosage will this be? _____

Refer to the oxytocin label in figure 47 and answer the following questions.

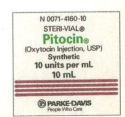

6. What is the dosage strength of this solution? _____

7. If a dosage of 10 U is ordered what volume will you need? _____

Figure 47

8. If a dosage of 5 U is ordered what volume will you prepare? _____

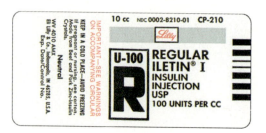

Figure 48

Refer to the insulin label in figure 48 and answer the following questions.

9. What is the dosage strength of this insulin? _____

10. If 50 U of regular insulin was ordered how many cc would this require? _____

ANSWERS **1.** 4 mL **2.** 10,000 U/mL **3.** 15,000 U **4.** 5.5 mL **5.** 2500 U **6.** 10 U per mL **7.** 1 mL **8.** 0.5 mL **9.** 100 U per cc **10.** 0.5 cc

Solutions Measured as Milliequivalents (mEq)

Milliequivalents (mEq) is an expression of the number of grams of a drug contained in 1 mL of a normal solution. This is a definition which will be quite understandable to a pharmacist, but you need not memorize it. Refer to the calcium gluconate label in figure 49 and notice that this solution has a dosage strength of 0.465 mEq/mL. If a dosage of 0.465 mEq were ordered you would draw up 1 mL in the syringe.

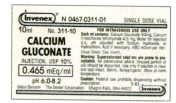

Figure 49

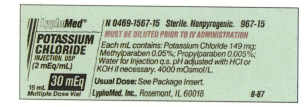

Figure 50

Problem

Refer to the potassium chloride label in figure 50 and answer the following questions.

1. What is the total volume and total dosage strength of this vial? _____

2. What is the dosage in mEq per mL? _____

3. If you are asked to prepare 30 mEq for addition to an IV what volume would you draw up? _____

Refer to the potassium chloride label in figure 51, and answer the following dosage questions. Notice that this label lists the strength of potassium chloride in mg as well as mEq. All of the questions can be answered by careful reading of the label.

4. What is the strength of this solution in mEq per mL? _____

5. If you were asked to prepare 40 mEq for addition to an IV solution what volume would you draw up in the syringe? _____

6. What is the strength of this solution expressed in mg per mL? _____

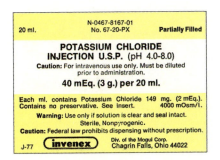

Figure 51

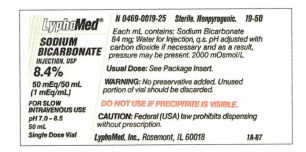

Figure 52

Refer to the sodium bicarbonate label in figure 52. Notice that this solution lists the drug strength in mEq, percentage, and mg. Read the label very carefully and locate the answers to the following questions.

7. What is the dosage strength expressed in mEq/mL? _____

8. What is the total volume of the vial, and how many mEq does this volume contain? _____

9. What is the strength per mL expressed as mg? _____

10. If you were asked to prepare 10 mL of an 8.4% sodium bicarbonate solution, what volume would you draw up in a syringe? _____

ANSWERS 1. 15 mL/30 mEq **2.** 2 mEq/mL **3.** 15 mL **4.** 2 mEq/mL **5.** 20 mL **6.** 149 mg **7.** 1 mEq/mL
8. 50 mL/50 mEq **9.** 84 mg/mL **10.** 10 mL

Summary

This concludes the introduction to parenteral solution labels. The important points to remember from this chapter are:

> *the most commonly used parenteral administration routes are IV, IM, and s.c.*

> *the labels of most parenteral solutions are quite small and must be read with particular care*

> *the average IM and s.c. dosage will be contained in a volume of between 1 and 3 mL. This volume can be used as a guideline to accuracy of calculations*

> *IV medication preparation is usually a two step procedure: measurement of the dosage, then dilution according to manufacturers recommendations or doctors order*

> *parenteral drugs may be measured in metric, ratio, percentage, unit or mEq dosages*

> *if dosages are ordered by percentage or ratio strength they are usually specified in cc/mL to be administered*

> *most IM and s.c. dosages are prepared using a 3 cc or 1 cc tuberculin syringe*

Summary Self Test

Directions: Read the parenteral drug labels provided to measure the following dosages. Then indicate on the syringe provided exactly how much solution you will draw up to obtain these dosages. Have your answers checked by your instructor to be sure you have measured the dosages correctly.

Dosage Ordered	mL/cc Needed
1. Depo-Provera® 0.2 g	_____

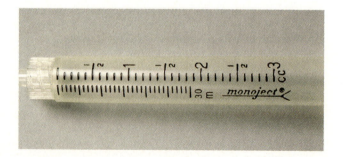

NDC 0009-0248-02
5 ml Vial
Depo-Provera®
Sterile Aqueous Suspension
sterile medroxyprogesterone
acetate suspension, USP
100 mg per ml

For intramuscular use only
See package insert for complete product information.
Shake vigorously immediately before each use.
Store at controlled room temperature 15°-30° C (59°-86° F)
811 851 201
The Upjohn Company
Kalamazoo, Michigan 49001, USA

2. furosemide 10 mg _____

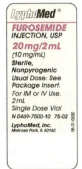

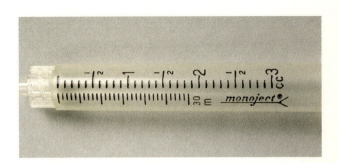

3. heparin 2,500 U _____

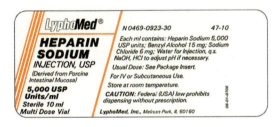

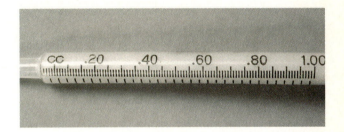

4. Cleocin® 0.9 g _____

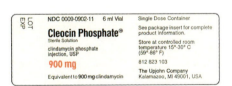

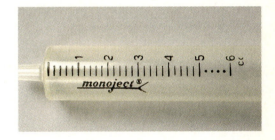

5. atropine 0.2 mg _____

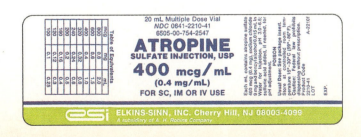

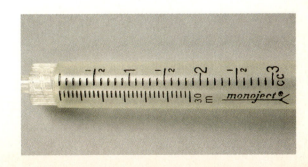

6. hydroxyzine HCl 25 mg _____

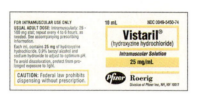

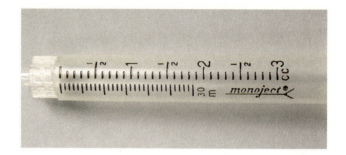

7. Robinul® 100 mcg _____

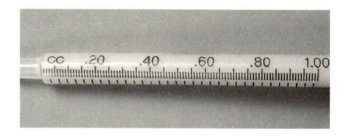

8. Tigan® 200 mg _____

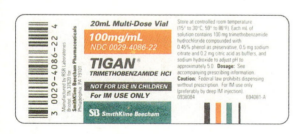

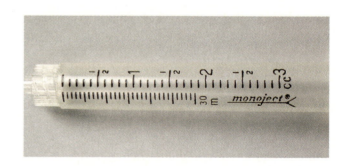

9. aminophylline 0.25 g _____

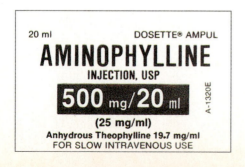

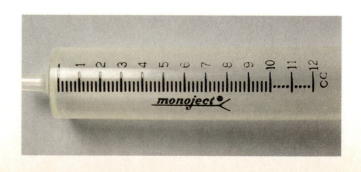

10. cyanocobalamin 1000 mcg _____

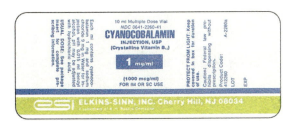

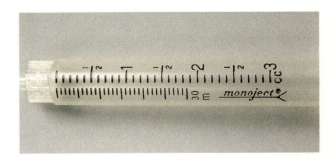

11. Yutopar 0.15 g _____

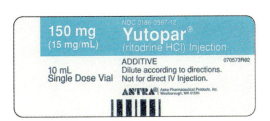

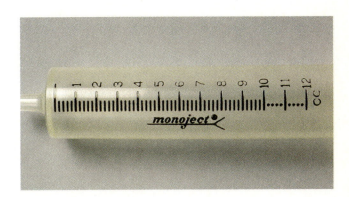

12. amikacin 100 mg _____

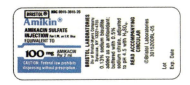

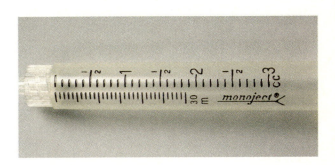

13. Zantac 75 mg _____

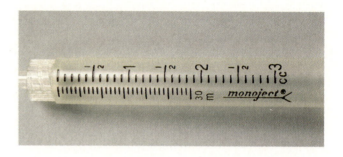

NDC 0173-0363-39

Glaxo

Zantac®
(ranitidine hydrochloride)
Injection

25 mg/ml
Sterile
10-ml Multi-dose Vial

Caution: Federal law prohibits dispensing without
prescription.
Each ml contains ranitidine 25 mg (as the hydrochloride)
in a buffered aqueous solution with phenol 5 mg as
preservative.
Usual Adult Dosage: 50 mg (2 ml) every 6 to 8 hours.
For IV or IM injection or IV infusion.
See package insert for full prescribing information.
Store below 30°C (86°F). Protect from light.
Glaxo Inc., Research Triangle Park, NC 27709
Manufactured in England   10/87

14. calcium gluconate 0.93 mEq _____

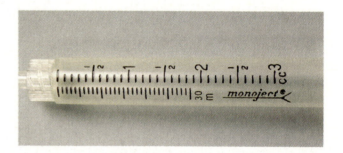

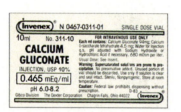

Invenex N 0467-0311-01   SINGLE DOSE VIAL
10ml   No. 311-10
CALCIUM GLUCONATE
INJECTION, USP 10%
0.465 mEq/ml
pH 6.0-8.2
Gibco Division   The Dexter Corporation   Chagrin Falls, Ohio 44022   **Invenex**

15. diazepam 7.5 mg _____

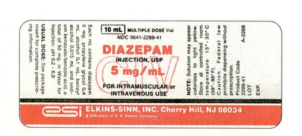

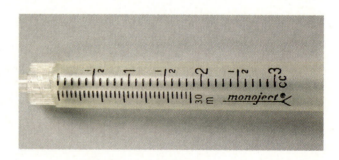

10 mL MULTIPLE DOSE Vial
NDC 0641-2289-41
DIAZEPAM
INJECTION, USP
5 mg/mL
FOR INTRAMUSCULAR or
INTRAVENOUS USE
esi **ELKINS-SINN, INC. Cherry Hill, NJ 08034**

16. heparin 1000 U _____

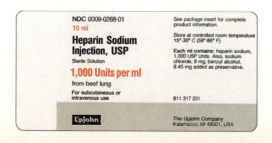

NDC 0009-0268-01
10 ml
**Heparin Sodium
Injection, USP**
Sterile Solution
1,000 Units per ml
from beef lung
For subcutaneous or
intravenous use
Upjohn

See package insert for complete
product information.
Store at controlled room temperature
15°-30°C (59°-86°F)
Each ml contains: heparin sodium,
1,000 USP Units. Also, sodium
chloride, 9 mg; benzyl alcohol,
9.45 mg added as preservative.
811 317 201
The Upjohn Company
Kalamazoo, MI 49001, USA

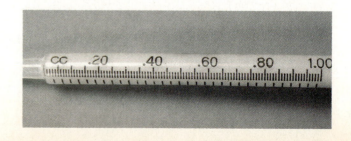

17. perphenazine 2.5 mg _____

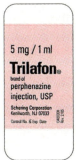

5 mg / 1 ml

Trilafon®
brand of
perphenazine
injection, USP

Schering Corporation
Kenilworth, NJ 07033

Control No. ⑥ Exp. Date

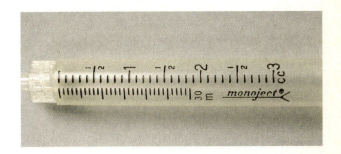

18. phenytoin Na 0.15 g _____

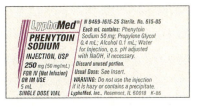

LyphoMed® | N 0469-1615-25 Sterile. No. 615-05

PHENYTOIN SODIUM
INJECTION, USP
250 mg (50 mg/mL)
FOR IV (Not Infusion)
OR IM USE
5 mL
SINGLE DOSE VIAL

Each mL contains: Phenytoin Sodium 50 mg; Propylene Glycol 0.4 mL; Alcohol 0.1 mL; Water for Injection, q.s. pH adjusted with NaOH, if necessary.
Discard unused portion.
Usual Dose: See insert.
WARNING: Do not use the injection if it is hazy or contains a precipitate.
LyphoMed, Inc., Rosemont, IL 60018 K-86

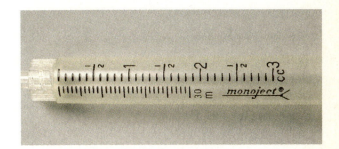

19. medroxyprogesterone 1 g _____

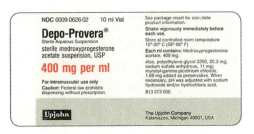

NDC 0009-0626-02   10 ml Vial

Depo-Provera®
Sterile Aqueous Suspension
sterile medroxyprogesterone acetate suspension, USP
400 mg per ml

For intramuscular use only
Caution: Federal law prohibits dispensing without prescription.

Upjohn

See package insert for complete product information.
Shake vigorously immediately before each use.
Store at controlled room temperature 15°-30° C (59°-86° F)
Each ml contains: Medroxyprogesterone acetate, 400 mg.
Also, polyethylene glycol 3350, 20.3 mg; sodium sulfate anhydrous, 11 mg; myristyl-gamma-picolinium chloride, 1.69 mg added as preservative. When necessary, pH was adjusted with sodium hydroxide and/or hydrochloric acid.
813 273 000

The Upjohn Company
Kalamazoo, Michigan 49001, USA

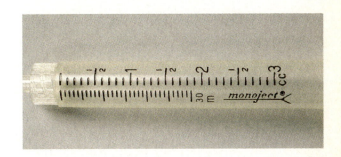

20. gentamicin 60 mg _____

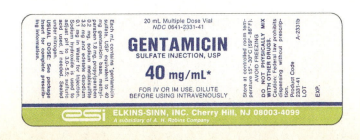

20 mL Multiple Dose Vial
NDC 0641-2331-41

GENTAMICIN
SULFATE INJECTION, USP
40 mg/mL*

FOR IV OR IM USE. DILUTE BEFORE USING INTRAVENOUSLY

Each mL contains gentamicin sulfate, USP equivalent to 40 mg gentamicin base; methylparaben 1.8 mg; propylparaben 0.2 mg; sodium metabisulfite 3.2 mg and edetate disodium 0.1 mg in Water for Injection. Sodium hydroxide is used to adjust pH to 3.0-5.5; sulfuric acid used, if needed. Sealed under nitrogen.
USUAL DOSE: See package insert for complete prescribing information.

Store at controlled room temperature 15°-30°C (59°-86°F). AVOID FREEZING. DO NOT PHYSICALLY MIX WITH OTHER DRUGS. Caution: Federal law prohibits dispensing without prescription.
Product Code 2331-41
LOT   EXP.
A-2331b

esi ELKINS-SINN, INC. Cherry Hill, NJ 08003-4099
A subsidiary of A. H. Robins Company

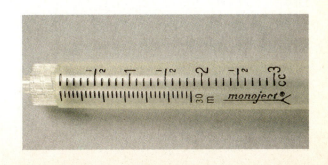

21.   lidocaine HCl 50 mg _____

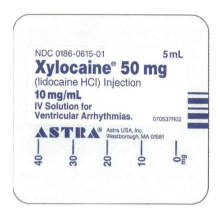

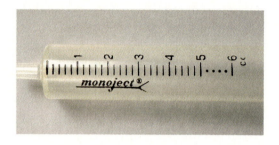

22.   sodium chloride 40 mEq _____

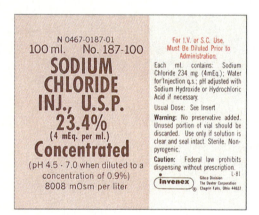

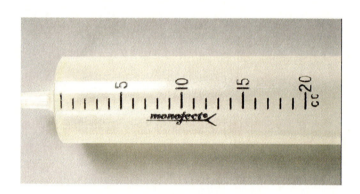

23.   atropine 0.4 mg _____

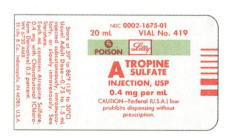

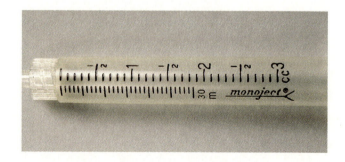

24. meperidine 50 mg _____

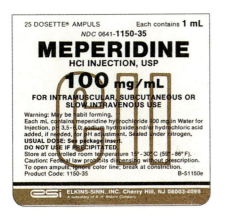

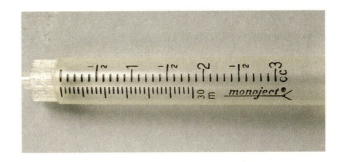

25. cimetidine 150 mg _____

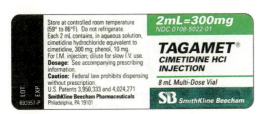

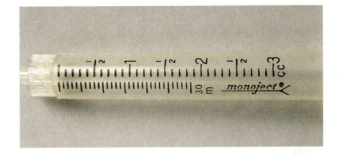

26. clindamycin 0.3 g _____

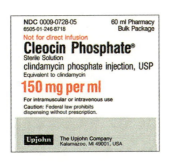

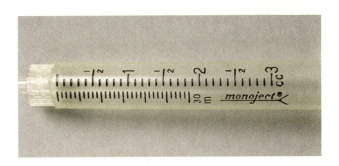

27. morphine sulfate 15 mg _____

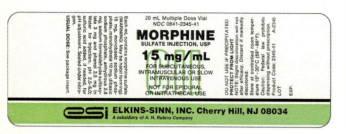

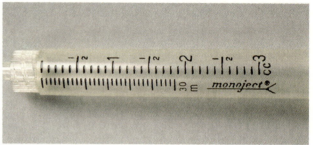

28. Compazine 10 mg _____

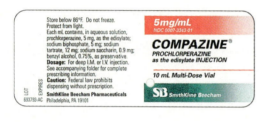

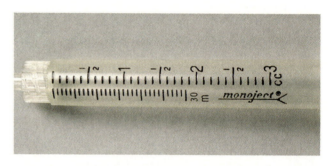

29. nitroglycerin 10 mg _____

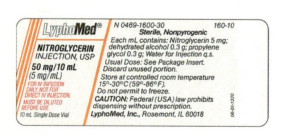

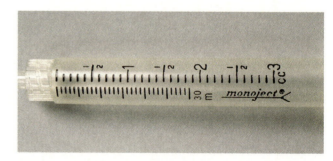

30. doxorubicin HCl 20 mg _____

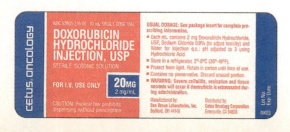

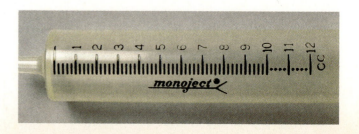

31. meperidine 50 mg _____

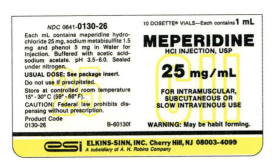
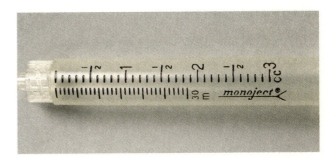

32. methadone HCl 15 mg _____

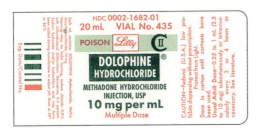
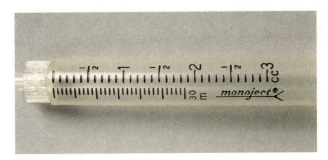

33. Celestone® 12 mg _____

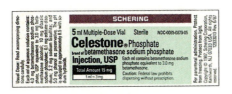
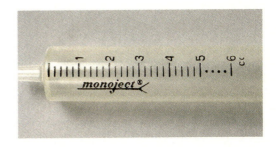

34. naloxone 0.8 mg _____

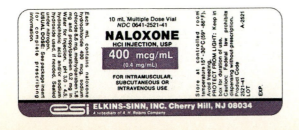
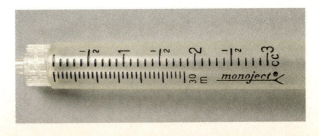

35.   dexamethasone 2 mg   _____

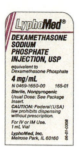

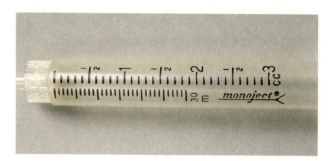

36.   chlorpromazine 50 mg   _____

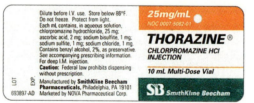

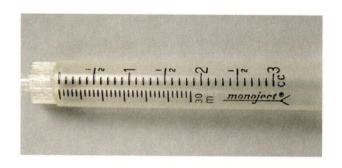

37.   Pronestyl® 0.5 g   _____

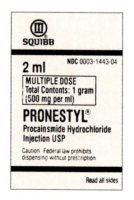

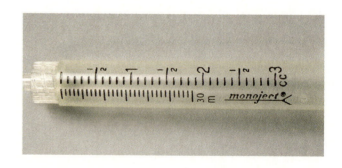

38. ergotrate maleate 0.2 mg _____

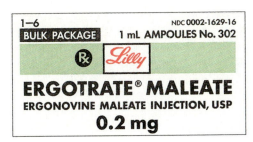

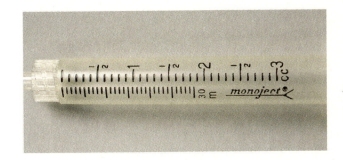

39. morphine 15 mg _____

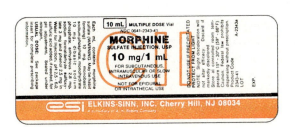

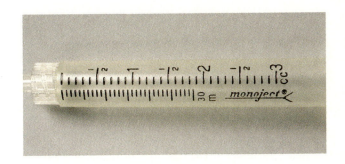

40. Betalin® 0.2 mg _____

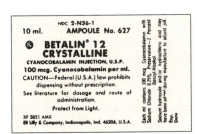

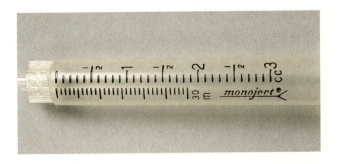

ANSWERS **1.** 2 mL **2.** 1 mL **3.** 0.5 mL **4.** 6 mL **5.** 0.5 mL **6.** 1 cc **7.** 0.5 mL **8.** 2 mL **9.** 10 mL **10.** 1 mL **11.** 10 mL **12.** 2 mL **13.** 3 mL **14.** 2 mL **15.** 1.5 mL **16.** 1 mL **17.** 0.5 mL **18.** 3 mL **19.** 2.5 mL **20.** 1.5 mL **21.** 5 mL **22.** 10 mL **23.** 1 mL **24.** 0.5 mL **25.** 1 mL **26.** 2 mL **27.** 1 mL **28.** 2 mL **29.** 2 mL **30.** 10 mL **31.** 2 mL **32.** 1.5 mL **33.** 4 mL **34.** 2 mL **35.** 0.5 mL **36.** 2 mL **37.** 1 mL **38.** 1 mL **39.** 1.5 mL **40.** 2 mL

Reconstitution of Powdered Drugs

OBJECTIVES

The student will

1. prepare solutions from powdered drugs using directions printed on vial labels
2. prepare solutions from powdered drugs using drug literature or inserts
3. determine expiration dates and times for reconstituted drugs
4. calculate simple dosages from reconstituted drugs

INTRODUCTION

Many drugs are shipped in powdered form because they retain their potency only a short time in solution. Reconstitution of these drugs is often the responsibility of hospital pharmacies, but this does not eliminate the need for nurses to know how to read and follow reconstitution directions, and how to label drugs with an expiration date and time once they have been reconstituted. The drug label, or instructional package insert, will give specific directions for reconstitution of the drug. Reading these requires care, and this chapter will take you step by step through the entire process.

Reconstitution of a Single Strength Solution

Let's start with the simplest type of reconstitution instructions, for a single strength solution. Examine the label for the oxacillin 2 g vial in figure 53.

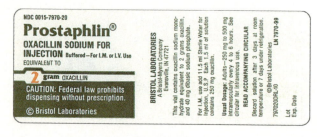

Figure 53

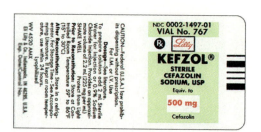

Figure 54

The first step in reconstitution is to locate the directions. They are on this label at the right side, printed sideways. Notice that the instructions read "for IM use add 11.5 mL sterile water." This would be done using a sterile syringe and aseptic technique. The vial is then rotated and upended until **all the medication is dissolved.**

Next notice the information which relates to the length of time the reconstituted solution may be stored. You are instructed to "discard solution after 3 days at room temperature, or 7 days under refrigeration."

 The person who reconstitutes a drug is responsible for labeling it with the date and time of expiration, and with her/his name or initials.

Let's assume this oxacillin solution was mixed at 2 p.m. on January 3rd. What expiration information would you print on the vial if it is stored in the refrigerator? "Exp (expires) Jan 10th 2 p.m.," which is 7 days from the time mixed. If it is stored at room temperature it must be labeled "Exp Jan 6th 2 p.m.," which is 3 days.

Once the solution is prepared and labeled with your name or initials and the expiration date, you can concentrate on the dosage strength. Notice that the label indicates that "Each 1.5 mL of solution contains 250 mg oxacillin." There is a total dosage of 2 g in this vial, or eight dosages of 250 mg at 1.5 mL each, for a total volume of 12 mL. You added only 11.5 mL to the vial to reconstitute the drug, and the reason for the increased volume is that the powder itself occupies space. **The total volume of the prepared solution will always exceed the volume of the diluent you add,** because it consists of the diluent plus the powder volume. Refer to the dosage strength again, which is 250 mg per 1.5 mL. If a 250 mg dosage is ordered you would prepare 1.5 mL; for a 0.5 g dosage prepare 3 mL.

Problem

Another medication prepared in powdered form is Kefzol® (cefazolin Na). Refer to the label in figure 54 and answer the following questions about this medication.

1. How much diluent is added to the vial for reconstitution? _____

2. What type of diluent is used? _____

3. What is the dosage strength per mL of the prepared solution? _____

4. If the order is for 450 mg what volume must you give? _____

5. What is the dosage strength of the total vial? _____

6. How many mL is the total solution after reconstitution? _____

7. How long will the drug retain its potency at room temperature? _____

8. If the drug is reconstituted at 0800 on Oct 3rd and stored at room temperature, what expiration date will you print on the label? _____

ANSWERS   1. 2 mL   **2.** sterile water, or 0.9% sodium chloride   **3.** 225 mg per mL   **4.** 2 mL   **5.** 500 mg
6. 2.2 mL   **7.** 24 hrs   **8.** 0800 Oct 4th.

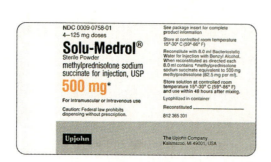

Figure 55

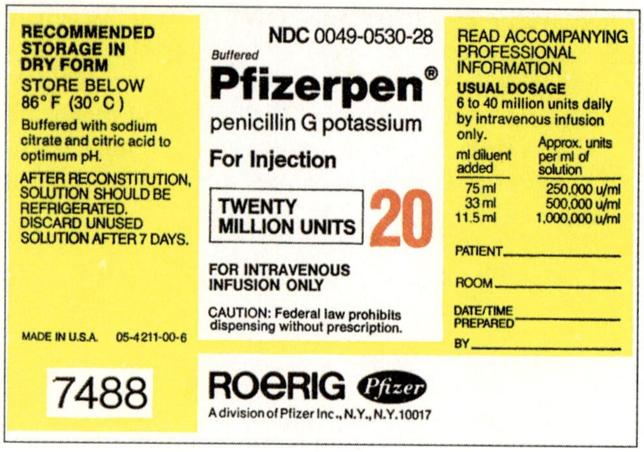

Figure 56

Problem

Read the Solu-Medrol® label in figure 55 and answer the following questions.

1. What volume of diluent must be used to reconstitute this vial? _____

2. What kind of diluent is specified? _____

3. How long will the reconstituted solution retain its potency at room temperature? _____

4. If the Solu-Medrol is reconstituted at 11 a.m. Feb 26th what expiration date and time will you print on the label? _____

5. What else will you print on the label? _____

6. What will be the dosage strength per mL of this reconstituted solution?
_____

7. If a dosage of 125 mg of methylprednisolone is ordered how much solution will you prepare? _____

ANSWERS   1. 8 mL   **2.** Bacteriostatic Water with Benzyl Alcohol   **3.** 48 hours   **4.** Exp 11 a.m. Feb 28th
5. your name or initials   **6.** 62.5 mg per mL   **7.** 2 mL

Reconstitution of a Multiple Strength Solution

Some powdered drugs offer a choice of dosage strengths. When this is the case you must choose the strength most appropriate for the dosage ordered. For example, refer to the penicillin label in figure 56. The dosage strengths which can be obtained are listed on the right.

Notice that three dosage strengths are listed: 250,000 U, 500,000 U and 1,000,000 U per mL. If the dosage ordered is 500,000 U, the most appropriate strength to mix would be 500,000 U per mL. Read across from this strength, and determine how much diluent must be added to obtain it. The answer is 33 mL. If the dosage ordered is 1,000,000 U, what would be the most appropriate strength to prepare, and how much diluent would this require? The answer is 1,000,000 U/mL, and 11.5 mL.

Notice that this label does not tell you what type of diluent to use. **When information is missing from the label look for it on the package information insert which comes with the drug.** Don't start guessing. All the information you need is in print somewhere, just take your time and locate it.

 A multiple strength solution such as this one requires that you add one additional piece of information to the label after you reconstitute it: the dosage strength you have just mixed.

Problem

Refer to the Pfizerpen® label in figure 56 to answer these additional questions.

1. If you add 75 mL of diluent to prepare a solution of penicillin, what dosage strength will you print on the label? _____

2. Does this prepared solution require refrigeration? _____

3. If you reconstitute it on June 1st at 2 p.m. what expiration date will you put on the label? _____

4. What is the total dosage strength of this vial? _____

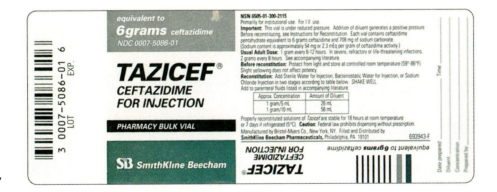

Figure 57

Refer to the Tazicef® label in figure 57 and answer the following questions.

5. What is the total strength of ceftazidime in this vial? _____

6. What kind of diluent is recommended for reconstitution? _____

7. If you wish to prepare a 1g/10 mL strength, how much diluent will you add to the vial? _____

8.   How much diluent will you add for a 1g/5 mL strength? _____

9.   What is the expiration time for this drug if it is stored at room temperature? _____

10.   If you reconstitute this drug at 0915 on April 17th and store it under refrigeration what will you print on the label? _____

ANSWERS   1. 250,000 U/mL   **2.** Yes   **3.** Exp 2 p.m. June 8th   **4.** twenty million units   **5.** 6 grams
6. Sterile Water; Bacteriostatic Water; Sodium Chloride   **7.** 56 mL   **8.** 26 mL   **9.** 18 hours
10. Exp 0915 April 24th

Reconstitution from Package Insert Directions

If the label does not contain reconstitution directions you must obtain these from the information insert which accompanies the vial. The labels for Claforan® in figures 58 and 59 fall into this category. Refer to these now, and to the portion of the package insert directions reproduced in figure 60. Notice that the insert instructions are for three vial strengths: 1 g, 2 g and 500 mg, but that only the labels for the 1 g and 2 g vials are included.

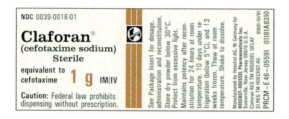

Figure 58

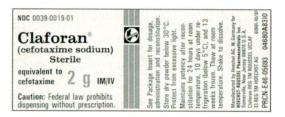

Figure 59

Preparation of Solution: Claforan for IM or IV administration should be reconstituted as follows:

Strength	Amount of Diluent To Be Added (mL)	Approximate Withdrawable Volume (mL)	Approximate Average Concentration (mg/mL)
Intramuscular			
500 mg vial	2	2.2	230
1 g vial	3	3.4	300
2 g vial	5	6.0	330
Intravenous			
500 mg vial	10	10.2	50
1 g vial	10	10.4	95
2 g vial	10	11.0	180

Shake to dissolve, inspect for particulate matter and discoloration prior to use. Solutions of Claforan range from light yellow to amber, depending on concentration, diluent used, and length and condition of storage.
For intramuscular use: Reconstitute with Sterile Water for Injection or Bacteriostatic Water for Injection as described above.

Figure 60

Problem

Read the Claforan® labels and package insert provided and answer the questions below on dosage strength and diluent quantities which pertain to them.

	Vial Strength	Amount of Diluent	Dosage Strength of Prepared Solution
1.	cefotaxime 1 g (prepare for IM injection)	a) _____	b) _____
2.	cefotaxime 2 g (prepare for IM injection)	a) _____	b) _____
3.	cefotaxime 1 g (prepare for IV administration)	a) _____	b) _____
4.	cefotaxime 2 g (prepare for IV administration)	a) _____	b) _____

5. What diluent is recommended for IM reconstitution? _____

6. How long will the solution retain its potency after reconstitution?

_____

ANSWERS 1. *a)* 3 mL *b)* 300 mg/mL 2. *a)* 5 mL *b)* 330 mg/mL 3. *a)* 10 mL *b)* 95 mg/mL 4. *a)* 10 mL *b)* 180 mg/mL 5. Sterile Water or Bacteriostatic Water 6. 24 hours at room temperature; 10 days if refrigerated below 5°C; 13 weeks frozen

Problem

Refer to the Tazicef® label and insert and answer the following questions.

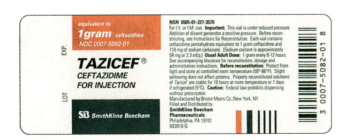

RECONSTITUTION
Single Dose Vials:
For I.M. injection, I.V. direct (bolus) injection, or I.V. infusion, reconstitute with Sterile Water for Injection according to the following table. The vacuum may assist entry of the diluent. SHAKE WELL.

Table 5

Vial Size	Diluent to Be Added	Approx. Avail. Volume	Approx. Avg. Concentration
Intramuscular or Intravenous Direct (bolus) Injection			
1 gram	3.0 ml.	3.6 ml.	280 mg./ml.
Intravenous Infusion			
1 gram	10 ml.	10.6 ml.	95 mg./ml.
2 gram	10 ml.	11.2 ml.	180 mg./ml.

Withdraw the total volume of solution into the syringe (the pressure in the vial may aid withdrawal). The withdrawn solution may contain some bubbles of carbon dioxide.

NOTE: As with the administration of all parenteral products, accumulated gases should be expressed from the syringe immediately before injection of 'Tazicef'.

These solutions of 'Tazicef' are stable for 18 hours at room temperature or seven days if refrigerated (5°C). Slight yellowing does not affect potency.

For I.V. infusion, dilute reconstituted solution in 50 to 100 ml. of one of the parenteral fluids listed under COMPATIBILITY AND STABILITY.

1. How much diluent must be added to this vial for IV reconstitution?

   _____

2. What kind of diluent must be used? _____

3. If you reconstitute the drug at 3 p.m. on May 24th and the solution is stored at room temperature, what expiration information will you print on the label? _____

4. What expiration information will you print if the solution is refrigerated?

   _____

5. What is the concentration per mL of this solution? _____

6. What is the dosage of the total vial? _____

ANSWERS   1. 10 mL   **2.** sterile water   **3.** Exp 9 a.m. May 25th   **4.** Exp 3 p.m. May 31st   **5.** 95 mg/mL   **6.** 1 gram

Summary

This concludes the chapter on reconstitution of powdered drugs. The important points to remember from this chapter are:

if the label does not contain reconstitution directions these may be found on the vial package insert

the type and amount of diluent to be used for reconstitution must be exactly as specified in the instructions

if directions are given on labels for both IM and IV reconstitution, be careful to read the correct set for the solution you are preparing

the person who reconstitutes a powdered drug must initial the vial and print the expiration date on the label, unless all the drug is used immediately

if a multiple strength solution is prepared the strength of the reconstituted drug also must be printed on the label

Summary Self Test

Refer to the nafcillin Na label, and answer the following questions about reconstitution.

1. What is the total dosage of this vial? _____

2. What volume of diluent must be used for reconstitution? _____

3. What will be the dosage strength of 1 mL of reconstituted solution?

   _____

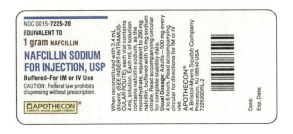

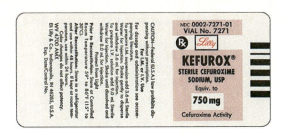

Refer to the Kefurox® label and answer the following questions.

4. What is the total dosage of this vial? _____

5. How much diluent will you add for IM preparation? _____

6. How much diluent is recommended for IV preparation? _____

7. What kind of diluent is to be used? _____

8. How long will the solution retain its potency if stored at room temperature?
   _____

9. If you reconstitute the cefuroxime at 0730 on Nov 1st and it is refrigerated for reuse, what expiration information will you print on the label?
   _____

Refer to the Velosef® label and answer the following questions.

10. What is the dosage strength of this vial? _____

11. What volume of diluent must you add to prepare the solution for IM use?
    _____ For IV use? _____

12. How long will this reconstituted cephradine retain its potency at room temperature? _____

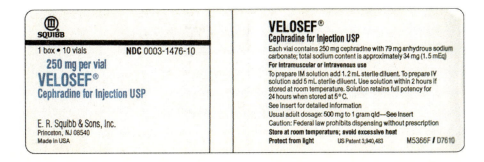

ZOSYN™ label:

NDC 0206-8620-11
ZOSYN™
40.5 GRAM
Sterile Piperacillin Sodium and Tazobactam Sodium
PHARMACY BULK VIAL

Contains no preservative.
Reconstitute with exactly 152 mL of a suitable diluent to achieve a concentration of 200 mg/mL of piperacillin and 25 mg/mL of tazobactam. Discard any unused portion after 24 hours if stored at room temperature or after 48 hours if refrigerated.
See package circular for complete directions for use.

Control No. ___   Exp. Date ___
Date Prepared _____
Diluent Used _____
Prepared by _____

Each vial provides sterile piperacillin sodium and tazobactam sodium cryodesiccated powders equivalent to 36 grams of piperacillin, 4.5 grams of tazobactam and 84.54 mEq (1,944 mg) of sodium.
CAUTION: Federal law prohibits dispensing without prescription.

Prior to Reconstitution: Store at Controlled Room Temperature 15-30°C (59-86°F). After Reconstitution: DO NOT FREEZE RECONSTITUTED SOLUTION
See package circular for stability of reconstituted solution.

For IV Use

32324-93 D1
LEDERLE PIPERACILLIN, INC.
Carolina, Puerto Rico 00987

Lederle

Refer to the Zosyn™ label and answer the following questions.

13. How much diluent is used to reconstitute this solution? _____

14. What is the total strength of the vial? _____

15. What is the strength of this Zosyn solution per mL? _____

16. How long will the solution retain its potency at room temperature? _____ If refrigerated? _____

Refer to the penicillin G Na label and answer the following questions.

17. How much diluent must be added to obtain a 250,000 U/mL concentration? _____ To obtain a 1,000,000 U/mL concentration? _____

18. The type of diluent is not specified. Where would you find this information? _____

19. If this solution is reconstituted at 8:10 p.m. Nov 30th, and stored under refrigeration, what expiration information will you print on the label?

_____

PENICILLIN G Na label:

SQUIBB® MARSAM™
1 box • 10 vials   NDC 0003-0668-05
5,000,000 units per vial
PENICILLIN G SODIUM for INJECTION USP
Caution: Federal law prohibits dispensing without prescription

PENICILLIN G SODIUM for INJECTION USP
Each vial provides 5,000,000 units penicillin G sodium with approx. 140 mg citrate buffer (composed of sodium citrate and not more than 4.6 mg citric acid). One million units penicillin contains approx. 2.0 mEq sodium.
Sterile • For intramuscular or intravenous drip use
Usual dosage: See insert
PREPARATION OF SOLUTION: Add 23 mL, 18 mL, 8 mL, or 3 mL diluent to provide 200,000 u, 250,000 u, 500,000 u, or 1,000,000 u per mL, respectively.
Sterile solution may be kept in refrigerator 1 week without significant loss of potency.
Store at room temperature prior to constitution
© 1986 Squibb-Marsam, Inc.
For information contact:
Squibb-Marsam, Inc., Cherry Hill, NJ 08034
Made by Glaxochem, Ltd., Greenford, Middlesex, England.
Filled in Italy by Squibb S.p.A. Dist. by
E. R. Squibb & Sons, Inc., Princeton, NJ 08540   C5277 / 66805

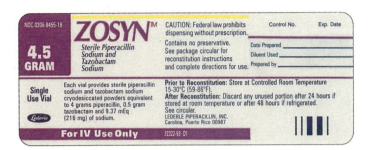

Intravenous Administration
Reconstitute ZOSYN per gram of piperacillin with 5 mL of a suitable diluent from the list provided below. Shake well until dissolved. Single dose vials should be used immediately after reconstitution. Discard any unused portion after 24 hours if stored at room temperature, or after 48 hours if stored at refrigerated temperature [2 to 8°C (36 to 46°F)]. It may be further diluted to the desired final volume with the diluent.

Compatible Intravenous Diluents
0.9% Sodium Chloride for Injection
Sterile Water for Injection
Dextran 6% in Saline
Dextrose 5%
Potassium Chloride 40 mEq
Bacteriostatic Saline/Parabens
Bacteriostatic Water/Parabens
Bacteriostatic Saline/Benzyl Alcohol
Bacteriostatic Water/Benzyl Alcohol
LACTATED RINGERS SOLUTION IS NOT COMPATIBLE WITH ZOSYN
Intermittent Intravenous Infusion - Reconstitute as previously described with 5 mL of an acceptable diluent per 1 gram of piperacillin and then further dilute in the desired volume (at least 50 mL). Administer by infusion over a period of at least 30 minutes. During the infusion it is desirable to discontinue the primary infusion solution.

Refer to the 4.5 g Zosyn™ label and insert and answer the following questions. Read all information very carefully.

20. How much diluent will be required to reconstitute this medication?

    _____

21. How many different diluents are listed as being acceptable for reconstitution? _____

22. The package insert specifically lists the name of an IV solution which may not be used as a diluent. Which solution is this? _____

23. Almost all IV medications are further diluted in IV fluids for administration. What does the package insert say about this in regards to administration of Zosyn? _____

24. The infusion time is also specified on the insert literature. What is it?

    _____

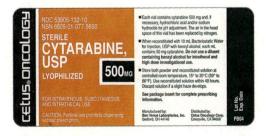

Refer to the cytarabine label and answer the following questions.

25. What is the strength of this medication? _____

26. What diluent must be used for reconstitution? _____

How much? _____

27. There is a special precaution on the label about a diluent not to be used. What is it? _____

28. How long does the reconstituted cytarabine solution retain its potency at room temperature? _____

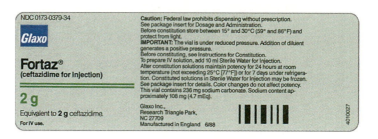

Refer to the Fortaz® label and answer the following questions.

29. What type of diluent is recommended for reconstitution? _____

How much? _____

30. If this drug is reconstituted at 0200 on March 23rd and stored at room temperature what expiration information will you print on the label?

_____

31. If it is stored under refrigeration, what date and time will you print?

_____

32. What is the dosage strength of this vial of ceftazidime? _____

PREPARATION AND STABILITY

At the time of use, reconstitute by adding either 10 mL of Sterile Water for Injection to the 500-mg vial or 20 mL of Sterile Water for Injection to the 1-g vial of dry, sterile vancomycin powder. Vials reconstituted in this manner will give a solution of 50 mg/mL. **FURTHER DILUTION IS REQUIRED.**

After reconstitution, the vials may be stored in a refrigerator for 14 days without significant loss of potency. Reconstituted solutions containing 500 mg of vancomycin must be diluted with at least 100 mL of diluent. Reconstituted solutions containing 1 g of vancomycin must be diluted with at least 200 mL of diluent. The desired dose, diluted in this manner, should be administered by intermittent intravenous infusion over a period of at least 60 minutes.

Refer to the vancomycin HCl label and insert preparation directions and answer the following questions.

33. What is the total strength of this vial? _____

34. What is the dosage strength per mL? _____

35. How much diluent must be added to reconstitute this powdered medication? _____

36. What type of diluent? _____

37. How must the reconstituted solution be stored? _____

38. If you reconstituted this medication at 1:15 p.m. on April 15th what information will you print on the label? _____

39. Prior to IV administration this solution must be further diluted. What minimum amount of additional diluent will be required? _____

40. What time factor is mentioned regarding the IV administration of this drug? _____

ANSWERS 1. 1 g **2.** 3.4 mL **3.** 250 mg **4.** 750 mg **5.** 3.6 mL **6.** 9 mL **7.** Sterile Water **8.** 24 hours **9.** Exp 0730 Nov 3rd **10.** 250 mg **11.** 1.2 mL; 5 mL **12.** 2 hours **13.** 152 mL **14.** 40.5 g **15.** 200 mg **16.** 24 hours; 48 hours **17.** 18 mL; 3 mL **18.** package insert information sheet **19.** Exp 8:10 p.m. Dec 7th **20.** 22.5 mL (5 mL/g) **21.** 9 **22.** Lactated Ringers soln **23.** dilute in at least 50 mL of additional fluid **24.** at least 30 min **25.** 500 mg **26.** Bacteriostatic Water; 10 mL **27.** No diluents containing benzyl alcohol **28.** 48 hrs **29.** sterile water; 10 mL **30.** Exp 0200 March 24th **31.** Exp 0200 March 30th **32.** 2 g **33.** 500 mg **34.** 50 mg/mL **35.** 10 mL **36.** sterile water **37.** under refrigeration **38.** Exp 1:15 p.m. April 29th **39.** 100 mL **40.** minimum of 60 min

SECTION

FOUR

Calculating Medication Dosages

13

Dosage Calculation Using Ratio and Proportion

OBJECTIVES

The student will

1. read drug labels to identify dosage strengths
2. set up proportions and determine the volume of medication required for specified dosages
3. assess answers obtained to determine if they are logical

INTRODUCTION

In an earlier chapter you were given a thorough review of the math of ratio and proportion, and an introduction to its use in dosages. In this chapter we will concentrate on the use of ratio and proportion to set up and solve dosage problems in metric/international measures, for parenteral medications. Three basic rules govern all calculations: 1. routinely double check all math; 2. assess each answer obtained to determine if it is logical; and 3. seek help if you have any question of your accuracy.

Parenteral Dosage Calculation

It is easier and safer to solve dosage problems if you are consistent in the way you set a proportion up. A good way to do this is to **write the complete or known ratio first.** This will always be the dosage strength of the drug available, which you will read from the drug label. **The incomplete or unknown ratio is the dosage ordered, and it is written second.** Let's review some examples.

EXAMPLE 1 Order: Administer 700 mg of a drug which has a dosage strength of 500 mg per 2 mL. Express your answer to the nearest tenth.

$$500 \text{ mg} : 2 \text{ mL} = 700 \text{ mg} : X \text{ mL} \quad \text{or} \quad \frac{500 \text{ mg}}{2 \text{ mL}} = \frac{700 \text{ mg}}{X \text{ mL}}$$

$$\left(\begin{array}{cc} \text{complete ratio} & \text{incomplete ratio} \\ \text{drug strength} & \text{dosage ordered} \end{array} \right) \qquad \left(\begin{array}{cc} \text{complete ratio} & \text{incomplete ratio} \\ \text{drug strength} & \text{dosage ordered} \end{array} \right)$$

Do not forget the critical step of **writing the ratios in the same sequence of measurement units.** In the examples above this was done; **mg : mL = mg : mL.** With the proportion correctly set up the math is exactly as you have practiced.

$$500 \text{ mg} : 2 \text{ mL} = 700 \text{ mg} : X \text{ mL} \quad \text{or} \quad \frac{500 \text{ mg}}{2 \text{ mL}} = \frac{700 \text{ mg}}{X \text{ mL}}$$

$$500X = 2 \times 700 \qquad\qquad\qquad 500X = 2 \times 700$$

$$X = \frac{2 \times 700}{500} = \textbf{2.8 mL} \qquad\qquad X = \frac{2 \times 700}{500} = \textbf{2.8 mL}$$

After you have double checked your math, assess the answer to determine if it is logical. If 500 mg equals 2 mL it will require more than 2 mL to obtain a dosage of 700 mg. Your answer, 2.8 mL is larger, therefore it is logical.

EXAMPLE 2 A drug label reads 100 mg per 2 mL. The medication order is for 130 mg. How many mL must you administer?

$$100 \text{ mg} : 2 \text{ mL} = 130 \text{ mg} : X \text{ mL} \quad \text{or} \quad \frac{100 \text{ mg}}{2 \text{ mL}} = \frac{130 \text{ mg}}{X \text{ mL}}$$

$$100X = 2 \times 130 \qquad\qquad\qquad 100X = 2 \times 130$$

$$X = \frac{2 \times 130}{100} = \textbf{2.6 mL} \qquad\qquad X = \frac{2 \times 130}{100} = \textbf{2.6 mL}$$

130 mg is a larger dosage than the 100 mg per 2 mL available, and must be contained in a larger volume. The answer, 2.6 mL, is a larger volume.

EXAMPLE 3 The order is to give 0.15 g of medication. The dosage strength available is 200 mg/mL.

This problem cannot be solved as it is now written because the **drug weights are in different units of measure:** g and mg. In a previous chapter you learned that it may be safer to convert down the scale, higher units to lower, to eliminate or avoid decimals. **Convert the g to mg.**

$$200 \text{ mg} : 1 \text{ mL} = \textbf{0.15 g} : X \text{ mL} \quad \text{or} \quad \frac{200 \text{ mg}}{1 \text{ mL}} = \frac{\textbf{0.15 g}}{X \text{ mL}}$$

$$200 \text{ mg} : 1 \text{ mL} = \textbf{150 mg} : X \text{ mL} \qquad \frac{200 \text{ mg}}{1 \text{ mL}} = \frac{\textbf{150 mg}}{X \text{ mL}}$$

$$200X = 1 \times 150 \qquad\qquad\qquad 200X = 1 \times 150$$

$$X = \frac{150}{200} = 0.75 = \textbf{0.8 mL} \qquad X = \frac{150}{200} = 0.75 = \textbf{0.8 mL}$$

The answer should be a smaller quantity, and it is.

EXAMPLE 4 You have a dosage strength of 200 mcg/mL. The order is to give 0.5 mg.

$$200 \text{ mcg} : 1 \text{ mL} = \textbf{0.5 mg} : X \text{ mL} \quad \text{or} \quad \frac{200 \text{ mcg}}{1 \text{ mL}} = \frac{\textbf{0.5 mg}}{X \text{ mL}}$$

$$200 \text{ mcg} : 1 \text{ mL} = \textbf{500 mcg} : X \text{ mL} \qquad \frac{200 \text{ mcg}}{1 \text{ mL}} = \frac{\textbf{500 mcg}}{X \text{ mL}}$$

$$200X = 500 \qquad\qquad 200X = 500$$

$$X = \textbf{2.5 mL} \qquad\qquad X = \textbf{2.5 mL}$$

500 mcg is a larger quantity than 200 mcg so it must be contained in a larger quantity than 1 mL. The answer, 2.5 mL, is logical.

Ratio and proportion is also used to solve dosage calculations for **international units and mEq dosages.**

EXAMPLE 5 The order is to give 1200 U. The available dosage strength is 1000 U per 1.5 mL.

$$1000 \text{ U} : 1.5 \text{ mL} = 1200 \text{ U} : X \text{ mL} \quad \text{or} \quad \frac{1000 \text{ U}}{1.5 \text{ mL}} = \frac{1200 \text{ U}}{X \text{ mL}}$$

$$1000X = 1.5 \times 1200 \qquad\qquad 1000X = 1.5 \times 1200$$

$$X = \frac{1.5 \times 1200}{1000} = \textbf{1.8 mL} \qquad X = \frac{1.5 \times 1200}{1000} = \textbf{1.8 mL}$$

1200 U is a larger dosage than 1000 U so the answer in mL should be larger, which it is.

EXAMPLE 6 A drug has a dosage strength of 2 mEq/mL. You are to give 10 mEq.

$$2 \text{ mEq} : 1 \text{ mL} = 10 \text{ mEq} : X \text{ mL} \quad \text{or} \quad \frac{2 \text{ mEq}}{1 \text{ mL}} = \frac{10 \text{ mEq}}{X \text{ mL}}$$

$$2X = 10 \qquad\qquad 2X = 10$$

$$X = \textbf{5 mL} \qquad\qquad X = \textbf{5 mL}$$

10 mEq is considerably larger than 2 mEq, so the answer should also be significantly larger, and it is.

Problem

Solve the following dosage problems. Express answers to the nearest tenth.

1. The drug label reads 1000 mcg in 2 mL. The order is 0.4 mg. _____

2. The ordered dosage is 275 mg. The available drug is labeled 0.5 g per 2 mL. _____

3. A dosage strength of 0.2 mg in 1.5 mL is available. Give 0.15 mg. _____

4. The strength available is 1 g in 3.6 mL. Prepare a 600 mg dosage. _____

5. A 10,000 U dosage has been ordered. The dosage strength available is 8,000 U in 1 mL. _____

6. The dosage available is 20 mEq per 20 mL. You are to prepare 15 mEq.

   _____

7. The order is for 200,000 U. The strength available is 150,000 U per 2 mL.

   _____

ANSWERS **1.** 0.8 mL **2.** 1.1 mL **3.** 1.1 mL **4.** 2.2 mL **5.** 1.3 mL **6.** 15 mL **7.** 2.7 mL

Summary

This chapter has reviewed key concepts in dosage calculation covered earlier, and added several others. The important points to remember from this chapter are:

the available dosage strength provides the complete or known ratio for calculations

the dosage to be given provides the incomplete or unknown ratio

the ratios in a proportion must be set up in the same sequence of measurement units, for example mg : mL = mg : mL

if the measurement units in a calculation are different, for example mg and g, one of these must be converted before the problem can be solved

the math of all calculations is routinely double checked

a logical assessment of the answer you obtain is a routine step in your calculations

if you have any doubt of your accuracy in calculations seek help

Summary Self Test

Directions: Read the medication labels provided and calculate the volume necessary to provide the dosage ordered. Express your answers as decimal fractions to the nearest tenth.

PART I

1. Prepare a dosage of 20 mg of Zantac® _____

2. Prepare a 300 mcg dosage of naloxone _____

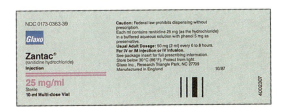

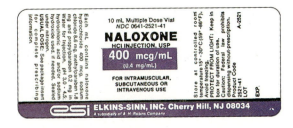

3. Prepare a 50 mg dosage of gentamicin _____

4. Furosemide 15 mg has been ordered _____

5. A dosage of perphenazine 7 mg is ordered _____

6. The order is for 70 mg of tobramycin _____

7. An order reads: dexamethasone 5 mg _____

8. Draw up 30 mEq of sodium bicarbonate _____

9. Prepare nitroglycerine 12 mg _____

10. The dosage is Depo-Provera® 140 mg _____

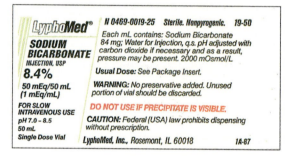

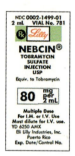

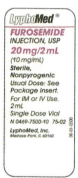

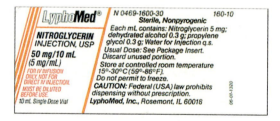

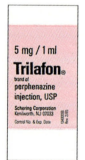

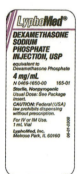

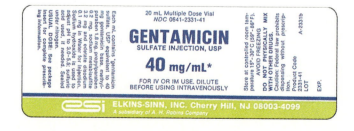

PART II

11. Draw up a 60 mg dosage of chlorpromazine _____

12. Prepare Cogentin 1.5 mg _____

13. Draw up a 400 mg dosage of aminophylline _____

14. Prepare a 35 mg dosage of amikacin _____

15. Compazine 12 mg has been ordered _____

16. Prepare 80 mg meperidine for IM injection _____

17. Atropine 0.2 mg has been ordered _____

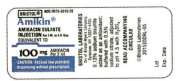

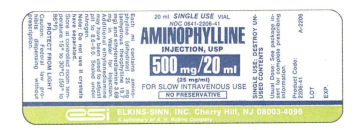

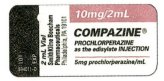

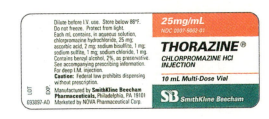

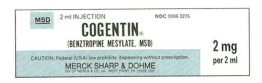

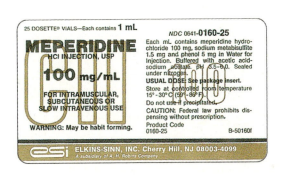

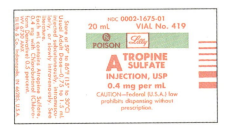

18.   Tigan® 250 mg has been ordered _____

19.   Garamycin® 100 mg has been ordered _____

20.   Prepare a 200 mg dosage of cimetidine. _____

21.   Prepare cyanocobalamin 1500 mcg _____

22.   Draw up 50 mg of tobramycin _____

23.   A dosage of Pronestyl® 600 mg is to be prepared _____

24.   Prepare a 400,000 U dosage of Duracillin® AS _____

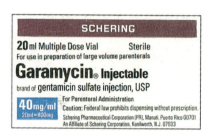

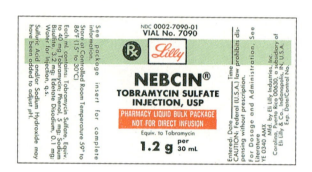

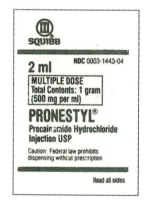

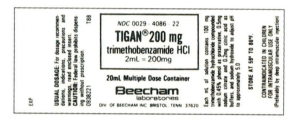

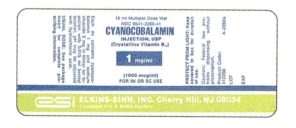

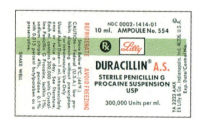

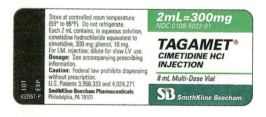

PART III

25. Draw up 75 mg of Dilantin®. _____

26. Prepare a 5 mg dosage of Celestone® _____

27. Pitocin® 25 U has been ordered. _____

28. Prepare an 8 mg dosage of morphine _____

29. Prepare 20 mEq of potassium chloride _____

30. A dosage of diazepam 7.5 mg has been ordered _____

31. Prepare an 8 mg dosage of Trandate® _____

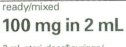
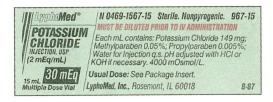
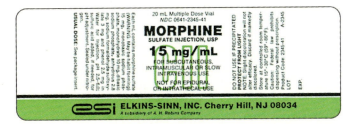
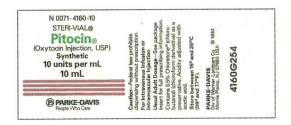
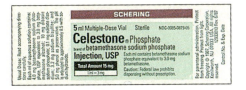
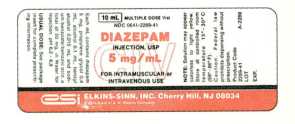
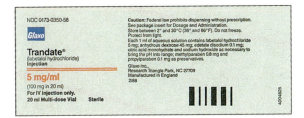
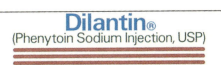
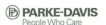

PART IV

32. Methadone 16 mg has been ordered. _____

33. Prepare a 100 mcg dosage of ergonovine _____

34. Measure a 15 mg dosage of furosemide _____

35. Atropine 600 mcg has been ordered. _____

36. Measure a 450 mg dosage of Depo-Provera® _____

37. Compazine® 8 mg has been ordered _____

38. Prepare a 90 mg dosage of phenytoin Na _____

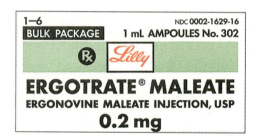

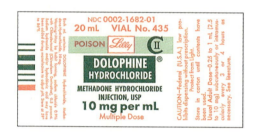

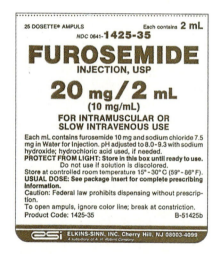

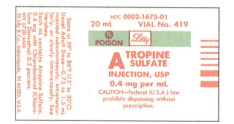

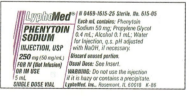

39. Give Vistaril® 70 mg IM _____

40. Measure a 275 mg dosage of clindamycin _____

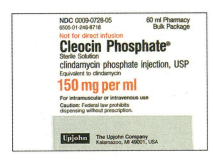

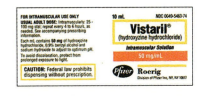

14

Dosage Calculation Using the Formula Method

OBJECTIVE

The student will

use the formula method to solve dosage problems containing metric, international unit, and mEq dosages.

INTRODUCTION

This chapter will teach you how to use a formula for ratio and proportion to set up and solve simple dosage problems. This formula is useful for uncomplicated calculations, and may save a little time in setting problems up. However it will not replace the ratio and proportion method for solving the majority of advanced clinical calculations. The formula is easy to remember and use, so let's take a look at it, and see how it works.

Formula Method of Dosage Calculation

The formula is as follows:

> **FORMULA**
>
> $$\frac{D}{H} \times Q = X$$

Here is what these initials mean.

D = desired. The dosage **ordered,** in mg, g, etc.

H = have. The dosage strength **available,** in mg, g, etc.

Q = quantity. The **volume** the dosage strength **available** is contained in, mL, cc, etc.

X = the unknown. The **volume** the **desired** dosage will be contained in.

It is necessary to memorize this formula. Stop and do so now. Print the formula several times to help yourself remember it.

The same three rules which governed calculations using ratio and proportion also apply to the use of the formula: 1. routinely double check all math; 2. assess each answer to determine if it is logical; and, 3. seek help if you have any doubt of your accuracy. Now let's look at some examples of how the formula is used, so you can begin to be comfortable with it.

EXAMPLE 1 A dosage of 80 mg is ordered. The dosage strength available is 100 mg in 2 mL. The desired dosage (D) is 80 mg. You have (H) 100 mg in (Q) 2 mL available. X will always be expressed in the same units of measure as Q, which in this problem is mL. **Always set up the formula with the units of measure included.**

$$\frac{\text{(D)}\ 80\ \text{mg}}{\text{(H)}\ 100\ \text{mg}} \times \text{(Q)}\ 2\ \text{mL} = \text{X mL}$$

$$\frac{80}{100} \times 2 = \text{X} = \textbf{1.6 mL}$$

To give a dosage of 80 mg you must administer 1.6 mL. After you have double checked your math look at your answer to see if it is logical. The dosage strength available is 100 mg in 2 mL. To prepare 80 mg, which is a smaller dosage, you will need a smaller volume. Your answer, 1.6 mL, is smaller, therefore it is logical.

EXAMPLE 2 The dosage ordered is 0.4 mg. The strength available is 0.25 mg in 1.2 mL. The desired dosage (D), is 0.4 mg. You have (H) 0.25 mg in (Q) 1.2 mL.

$$\frac{0.4\ \text{mg}}{0.25\ \text{mg}} \times 1.2\ \text{mL} = \text{X mL}$$

$$\frac{0.4}{0.25} \times 1.2 = \text{X} = \textbf{1.9 mL}$$

0.4 mg is a larger dosage than 0.25 mg and the volume which contains it must be larger, which it is, 1.9 mL.

EXAMPLE 3 A dosage of 750 mcg has been ordered. The strength available is 1000 mcg per mL.

$$\frac{750\ \text{mcg}}{1000\ \text{mcg}} \times 1\ \text{mL} = \text{X mL}$$

$$\frac{750}{1000} \times 1 = \text{X} = 0.75 = \textbf{0.8 mL}$$

The answer should be a smaller quantity than 1 mL, and it is, 0.8 mL.

Problem

Determine the volume which will contain the dosage ordered in the following problems. Express answers as decimal fractions to the nearest tenth.

1. A dosage of 0.8 g has been ordered. The strength available is 1 g in 2.5 mL.

   _____

2. You have available a dosage strength of 250 mg in 1.5 mL. The order is for 200 mg. _____

3. The strength available is 1 g in 5 mL. The order is for 0.2 g. _____

4. A dosage of 300 mcg has been ordered. The strength available is 500 mcg in 1.2 mL. _____

ANSWERS   1. 2 mL   2. 1.2 mL   3. 1 mL   4. 0.7 mL

 D and H, the drug strengths, must be expressed in the same units of measure.

EXAMPLE 4   A dosage of 200 **mcg** is ordered. The strength available is 0.3 **mg** in 1.5 mL. This problem cannot be solved as it is now written. D and H, the drug strengths, are in different units of measure. One of them must be changed before the problem can be solved. As in earlier chapters where you practiced conversions it may be somewhat less confusing to change the higher unit to a lower one, for example, the 0.3 **mg** to **mcg,** in order to eliminate a decimal point.

$$0.3 \text{ mg} = 300 \text{ mcg}$$

$$\frac{200 \text{ mcg}}{300 \text{ mcg}} \times 1.5 \text{ mL} = X \text{ mL}$$

$$\frac{200}{300} \times 1.5 = \textbf{1 mL}$$

Your answer must be a smaller quantity, and it is. To administer 200 mcg you must give 1 mL of the 0.3 mg in 1.5 mL dosage strength.

EXAMPLE 5   A dosage of 0.7 g has been ordered. Available is a strength of 1000 mg in 1.5 mL.

$$0.7 \text{ g} = 700 \text{ mg}$$

$$\frac{700 \text{ mg}}{1000 \text{ mg}} \times 1.5 \text{ mL} = X \text{ mL}$$

$$\frac{700}{1000} \times 1.5 = \textbf{1.1 mL}$$

The answer should be less than 1.5 mL, which it is, 1.1 mL.

Problem

Determine the volume which will be required to prepare the following dosages. Express answers to the nearest tenth.

1. The dosage ordered is 780 mcg. The strength available is 1 mg per mL.

   _____

2. The available dosage strength is 0.1 g per mL. The dosage ordered is 250 mg.

   _____

3. Prepare a dosage of 0.6 mg from an available strength of 1000 mcg per 2 mL.

_____

4. A dosage of 0.4 g has been ordered. The strength available is 500 mg per 1.3 mL. _____

ANSWERS **1.** 0.8 mL **2.** 2.5 mL **3.** 1.2 mL **4.** 1 mL

EXAMPLE 6 A dosage of 7500 U is ordered. The available strength is 10,000 U per mL.

$$\frac{7500 \text{ U}}{10,000 \text{ U}} \times 1 \text{ mL} = \text{X mL}$$

$$\frac{7500}{10,000} \times 1 = 0.75 = \textbf{0.8 mL}$$

The dosage ordered is less than the strength available, and must be contained in a smaller volume of solution than 1 mL, which it is, 0.8 mL.

EXAMPLE 7 A dosage strength of 40 mEq in 5 mL is available. You are to prepare 30 mEq.

$$\frac{30 \text{ mEq}}{40 \text{ mEq}} \times 5 \text{ mL} = \text{X mL}$$

$$\frac{30}{40} \times 5 = 3.75 = \textbf{3.8 mL}$$

The dosage ordered, 30 mEq, is less than the dosage of the solution available. It must be contained in a smaller volume than 5 mL, and the answer, 3.8 mL, indicates that it is.

Problem

Determine the volume which will contain the following dosages. Express answers to the nearest tenth.

1. A dosage strength of 1000 U per 1.5 mL is available. Prepare a 1250 U dosage.

_____

2. A dosage of 45 U has been ordered. The strength available is 80 U per mL.

_____

3. The IV solution available has a strength of 200 mEq per 20 mL. You are to prepare a 50 mEq dosage. _____

4. The strength available is 80 mEq per 5 mL. Prepare 30 mEq. _____

ANSWERS **1.** 1.9 mL **2.** 0.6 mL **3.** 5 mL **4.** 1.9 mL

Summary

This concludes the chapter on using the formula method to solve simple dosage calculations. The important points to remember from this chapter are:

the formula method can be used to solve problems expressed in metric, unit, and mEq dosages

when the formula method is used, D and H, the dosage strengths, must be expressed in the same units of measure

the answer obtained, X, will always be in the same unit of measure as Q, the quantity

the math of all calculations is routinely double checked

a logical assessment of the answer you obtain is a routine step in calculations

if you are unsure of your calculations seek help

Summary Self Test

Directions: Calculate the volume of medication (in mL, cc) necessary to administer the dosages ordered in the following problems. Express your answers as decimal fractions to the nearest tenth.

1. A 50 mg dosage has been ordered. The strength available is 60 mg in 1.5 mL. _____

2. Prepare a 300 mcg dosage. The dosage available is 0.4 mg/mL. _____

3. Prepare 0.45 g. The strength available is 300 mg/mL. _____

4. The medication is labeled 5 mg/mL. An 8 mg dosage has been ordered. _____

5. Prepare a 70 mg dosage from a solution labeled 250 mg in 5 mL. _____

6. The drug is labeled 25 mg per mL; 30 mg has been ordered. _____

7. The label reads 50 mg/mL. Prepare a 60 mg dosage. _____

8. The order is for 12 mg. The vial is labeled 5 mg per mL. _____

9. A dosage of 7 mg has been ordered. The vial label reads 10 mg per mL. _____

10. The dosage strength is 10 mg/1 mL; 8 mg has been ordered. _____

11.   Prepare a 0.3 g dosage from a medication labeled 900 mg per 6 mL.

_____

12.   Prepare a 300 mg IV dosage from a vial labeled 0.5 g/20 mL. _____

13.   The vial is labeled 0.5 g per 2 mL. A dosage of 750 mg has been ordered.

_____

14.   Prepare a dosage of 0.2 mg from an available dosage of 250 mcg/5 mL.

_____

15.   The order is for 130 mg and the single use ampule is labeled 0.1 g per 2 mL.

_____

16.   Draw up a 12 mg dosage from a vial labeled 15 mg in 5 mL. _____

17.   The ampule is labeled 20 mg/2 mL. Prepare 14 mg. _____

18.   The medication is labeled 1.2 g per 30 mL. Draw up an 800 mg dosage for IV

administration. _____

19.   Prepare an 80 mg dosage of a medication labeled 100 mg in 2 mL.

_____

20.   The solution strength is 0.4 mg per mL. A dosage of 300 mcg has been or-

dered. _____

21.   Prepare a 600 mg dosage from an available dosage strength of 0.4 g/mL.

_____

22.   Draw up a 60 mEq dosage for addition to an IV from a solution labeled

40 mEq per 20 mL. _____

23.   The label reads 400 mcg/mL; 0.6 mg has been ordered. _____

24.   Prepare a 60 mg dosage from a 75 mg/mL strength. _____

25.   Prepare a 0.1 g dosage from a vial labeled 40 mg/mL. _____

26.   The drug is labeled 50 mg/10 mL. The order is for 8 mg. _____

27. Measure a 0.8 mg dosage from an available strength of 1000 mcg/cc. _____

28. Prepare 40 mg from a vial labeled 25 mg per mL. _____

29. A dosage of 10 mg has been ordered. You have available a strength of 4000 mcg per mL. _____

30. Prepare 200 mg for IV use of a medication labeled 0.25 g per 25 mL. _____

31. The dosage strength available is 15 mg in 1 mL; 10 mg has been ordered. _____

32. Prepare a 4 mg dosage from a dosage available of 5 mg/mL. _____

33. A dosage of 75 U has been ordered from an available strength of 90 U in 1.5 mL. _____

34. You are to prepare 100 mEq for addition to an IV solution. The solution available is labeled 80 mEq per 20 mL. _____

35. Prepare a dosage of 180 mg from a 0.15 g in 1 mL solution. _____

36. Prepare a 750 U dosage from an available strength of 1000 U/mL. _____

37. Draw up a 60 mEq dosage for addition to IV solution from a vial labeled 40 mEq/20 mL. _____

38. 400,000 U has been ordered and you have available 300,000 U in 1 mL. _____

39. A dosage of 0.2 mg per 2 mL is available. Prepare a 250 mcg dosage. _____

40. A dosage of 35 mEq has been ordered for addition to an IV solution. The solution is labeled 50 mEq per 50 mL. _____

ANSWERS 1. 1.3 mL   2. 0.8 mL   3. 1.5 mL   4. 1.6 mL   5. 1.4 mL   6. 1.2 mL   7. 1.2 mL   8. 2.4 mL   9. 0.7 mL
10. 0.8 mL   11. 2 mL   12. 12 mL   13. 3 mL   14. 4 mL   15. 2.6 mL   16. 4 mL   17. 1.4 mL   18. 20 mL   19. 1.6 mL
20. 0.8 mL   21. 1.5 mL   22. 30 mL   23. 1.5 mL   24. 0.8 mL   25. 2.5 mL   26. 1.6 mL   27. 0.8 cc   28. 1.6 mL
29. 2.5 mL   30. 20 mL   31. 0.7 mL   32. 0.8 mL   33. 1.3 mL   34. 25 mL   35. 1.2 mL   36. 0.8 mL   37. 30 mL
38. 1.3 mL   39. 2.5 mL   40. 35 mL

Measuring Insulin Dosages

15

OBJECTIVES

The student will

1. distinguish between insulins of animal and human origin
2. discuss the difference between rapid, intermediate and long acting insulins
3. read insulin labels to identify origin and type
4. read calibrations on U-100 insulin syringes
5. measure single insulin dosages
6. measure combined insulin dosages

INTRODUCTION

Insulin dosages are measured in units (U), with the 100 U per cc (U-100) strength being used almost exclusively. Dosages are measured using special insulin syringes which are calibrated to match the dosage strength of insulin being used. For example U-100 syringes are used to prepare U-100 strength dosages. This chapter will show you a variety of U-100 syringes to illustrate how to measure dosages. However, let's begin with an introduction to the types of insulin in use.

Types of Insulin

Insulins are classified by **origin** (animal or human) and by **action** (rapid, intermediate or long acting). The origin or source of insulins is printed on every label, and it is important to know where to locate this information as physicians may specify origin when writing insulin orders. Notice the small print on the Regular insulin label in figure 61 which identifies its pork (animal) origin, and the Regular insulin label in figure 62 which identifies its human (semi-synthetic) origin. Also notice how similar these labels

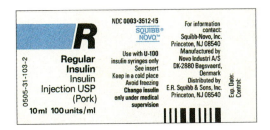

Figure 61

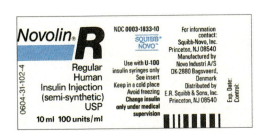

Figure 62

are. Careful reading of insulin labels is essential for correct identification. Insulins are prepared in multiple use vials and routinely labeled with each patient's name. However this does not eliminate the need to read the entire label prior to dosage preparation.

Next look at the labels in figures 63 and 64. Both of these insulins are of human origin and use the trade name Humulin®. Then notice the initials which follow the trade name: L (Lente) and U (Ultralente). These identify the type of insulin by action time. There are three basic action times of insulins. Regular and Semilente have the most rapid action, beginning in ½ hr, peaking in 2½–5 hr, and ending in 8 hr. In the intermediate range are the Lente and NPH insulins, beginning in 1½–2½ hr, peaking in 4–15 hr, and ending in 16–24 hr. Among the long acting insulins are the Ultralente whose action begins in 4 hr, peaks in 10–30 hr, and ends in 36 hr. Insulin types and dosages are prescribed to correlate with life style, diet and activity schedule.

Figure 63

Figure 64

Problem

Identify the type, and origin of the insulin from the following labels.

Type of Insulin	Origin
1. _____	_____
2. _____	_____
3. _____	_____
4. _____	_____
5. _____	_____
6. _____	_____

1

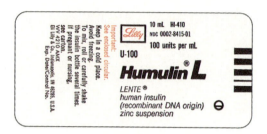

2

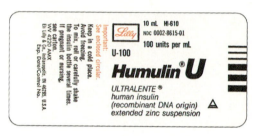

3
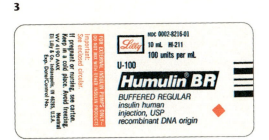

4
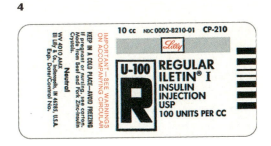

5
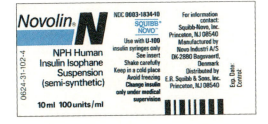

6
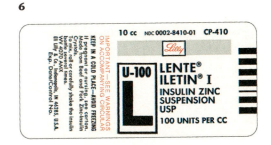

ANSWERS **1.** Ultralente; beef **2.** NPH; beef and pork **3.** Buffered Regular; human **4.** Regular; beef and pork **5.** NPH; human **6.** Lente; beef and pork

Insulin Syringes

Refer back to each of the labels you have just read and you will notice that all have a U-100 strength.

 To prepare U-100 insulin dosages you must use a U-100 calibrated syringe.

Refer to the U-100 syringe pictured in figure 65 and you will notice that it is very small. In order to read the calibrations and number of units it is necessary to rotate insulin syringes from side to side. To make it possible for you to practice measuring insulin dosages in this chapter the syringe calibrations have been flattened out. These are the identical calibrations which appear on the syringes, so your dosage practice will be authentic.

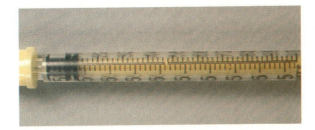

Figure 65

The designation U-100 means that the insulin dosage strength is 100 U per cc. Insulin syringes are calibrated to this 100 U/cc dosage, but they do not all have a 1 cc capacity. There are actually several sizes (capacities) of U-100 syringes in use. The easiest of these to read and use are the Lo-Dose® syringes.

Lo-Dose® Syringes

Lo-Dose syringes have a capacity of 30 or 50 U. Lo-Dose insulin syringes do exactly what their name implies: they measure low dosages, but on an enlarged and easier to read scale. This larger scale is an important safety feature for diabetic patients, who frequently have vision problems, as well as for ease of use by medical personnel.

Refer to the calibrations on the 50 U (½ cc) Lo-Dose capacity syringes in figure 66. Notice that each calibration measures 1 U, and that each 5 U increment is numbered.

Problem

Refer to the syringe calibrations for the 50 U Lo-Dose syringes below and identify the dosages indicated by the shaded areas.

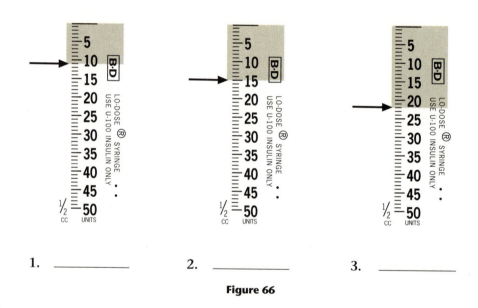

1. _____   2. _____   3. _____

Figure 66

Problem

Use the U-100 Lo-Dose calibrations in figure 67 to shade in the following dosages. Have your instructor check your accuracy.

1.   33 U   2.   38 U   3.   18 U

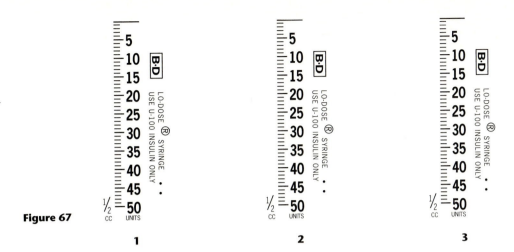

Figure 67

1 cc Capacity Syringes

There are two 100 U (1 cc) insulin syringes in common use. Refer to the first of these in figure 68. Notice the 100 U capacity, and that each 10 U increment is numbered, 10, 20, etc. Next notice the number of calibrations in each 10 U increment, which is five, indicating that **this syringe is calibrated in 2 U increments. Odd numbered units are measured between the even calibrations.** For example the shading on syringe 4 identifies 85 U.

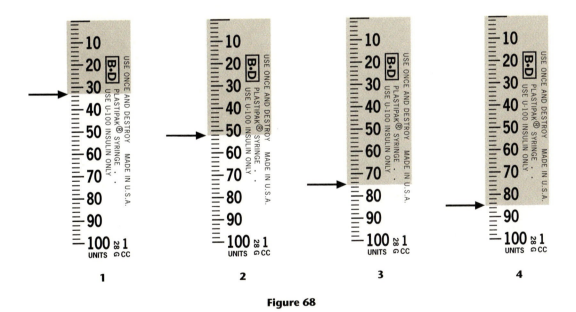

Figure 68

Problem

Identify the dosages indicated on the U-100 1 cc syringes in figure 68.

1. _____   2. _____   3. _____

Problem

Shade in the syringes in figure 69 to measure the following dosages.

1. 67 U   2. 84 U   3. 28 U   4. 45 U

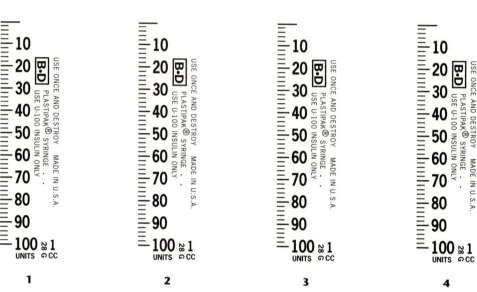

Figure 69

The second type of U-100 1 cc capacity syringe is illustrated in figure 70. Notice that this syringe has a **double scale, the odd numbers are on the left, and the even are on the right.** Each 5 U increment is numbered, but on opposite sides of the syringe. This syringe does have a calibration for each 1 U increment, but in order to count them all to measure a dosage, the syringe would have to be rotated back and forth, which could cause confusion. There is a safer way to read the calibrations. To measure uneven numbered dosages, for example 7, 13, 27, etc., use the uneven (left) scale only; for even numbered dosages such as 6, 10, 56, etc., use the even (right) scale only. **Count each calibration (on one side only) as 2 U, because that is what it is measuring.**

EXAMPLE 1   To prepare an 89 U dosage start at 85 U on the uneven left scale, count the first calibration above this as 87 U, the next as 89 U **(each calibration on the same side measures 2 U).**

EXAMPLE 2   To measure a 26 U dosage, use the even numbered right side calibrations. Start at 20 U, move up one calibration to 22 U, another to 24 U, and one more to 26 U **(each calibration is 2 U).**

Problem

Identify the dosages measured on the U-100 1 cc syringes provided.

Figure 70

1. _____   2. _____   3. _____

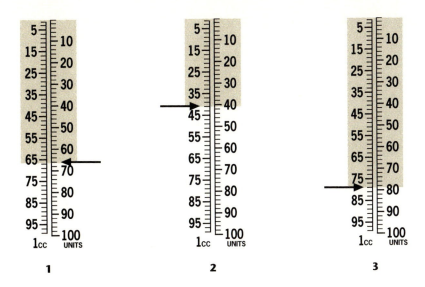

1   **2**   **3**

ANSWERS   **1.** 66 U   **2.** 41 U   **3.** 79 U

Problem

Shade in each U-100 syringe provided to identify the following dosages.

1.   55 U   2.   94 U   3.   69 U

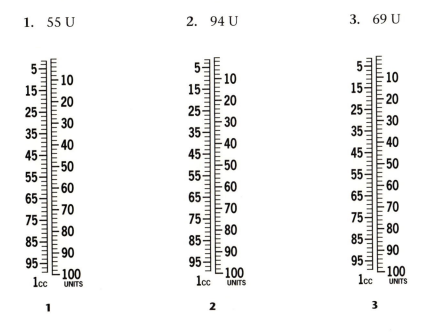

1   **2**   **3**

Combining Insulin Dosages

Insulin dependent individuals must have at least one, and sometimes several subcutaneous injections of insulin per day. In order to reduce the number of injections as much as possible it is common to combine two insulins in a single syringe, for example a short acting with either an intermediate or long acting insulin.

 When two insulins are combined in the same syringe the regular (shortest acting) insulin is drawn up first.

Both insulins will be withdrawn from sealed 10 mL vials, which requires that an amount of air equal to the insulin to be withdrawn be injected first. This keeps the pressure inside the vials equalized. An additional step concerns preparation of the insulin itself. Regular insulin does not need to be mixed prior to withdrawal, but intermediate and long acting insulins precipitate out. They need to be rotated and mixed before withdrawal from the vial. **The smallest capacity syringe possible should be selected to prepare the dosage,** as the enlarged scale is easier to read and therefore more accurate.

The actual step by step procedure for combining insulins is as follows:

EXAMPLE 1 A dosage of 10 U of Regular and 48 U of NPH insulin has been ordered.

STEP 1 Locate the correct insulins and rotate the NPH until it is thoroughly mixed.

STEP 2 Use an alcohol wipe to cleanse both vial tops.

STEP 3 The combined dosage (10 U + 48 U = 58 U) requires the use of a 1 cc U-100 syringe. Draw up 48 U of air and insert the needle into the NPH vial. Keep the needle tip above the insulin and inject the air.

STEP 4 Draw up 10 U of air and inject this into the Regular insulin vial. Draw up the 10 U of Regular insulin.

STEP 5 Insert the needle back into the NPH vial and draw up 48 U of NPH insulin. This will require that you draw the plunger back until the total insulin in the syringe is 58 U (10 U Regular + 48 U NPH). Withdraw the needle and administer the insulin promptly so that the NPH does not have time to precipitate out.

EXAMPLE 2 The order is to give 16 U of Regular insulin and 22 U of Lente insulin.

STEP 1 Locate the correct insulins and rotate the Lente to mix it.

STEP 2 Cleanse both vial tops.

STEP 3 Use a 50 U capacity syringe to draw up 22 U of air. Insert the needle into the Lente vial. Keep the needle tip above the insulin as you inject the air into the vial.

STEP 4 Draw up 16 U of air and inject it into the Regular insulin vial. Draw up the 16 U of Regular insulin.

STEP 5 Insert the needle back into the Lente vial and draw up Lente insulin until the syringe capacity is 38 U (16 U Regular + 22 U Lente). Administer the dosage promptly.

Problem

For each of the following combined insulin dosages indicate the total volume of the combined dosage, and the smallest capacity syringe you can use to prepare it (30 U, 50 U and 100 U capacity syringes are available).

		Total Volume	**Syringe Size**
1.	28 U Regular, 64 U NPH	_____	_____
2.	16 U Ultralente, 6 U Regular	_____	_____

3. 33 U Regular, 41 U Lente   _____   _____

4. 21 U Regular, 52 U NPH   _____   _____

5. 13 U Regular, 27 U Ultralente   _____   _____

Summary

This concludes the chapter on measuring insulin dosages. The important points to remember from this chapter are:

read insulin labels very carefully to be sure you have obtained the correct type

U-100 insulins are measured using U-100 calibrated syringes

the smallest capacity syringe possible is used to increase accuracy of dosage preparation

calibrations on 30 U and 50 U syringes are in 1 U increments

calibrations on 100 U syringes may be in 1 U or 2 U increments

when insulin dosages are combined the Regular insulin is drawn up first

the intermediate and long acting insulins precipitate out and must be thoroughly mixed before measurement, and administered promptly after measurement

Summary Self Test

Directions: Use the syringe calibrations provided to measure the following dosages. For combined insulin dosages use arrows to indicate the exact calibration to be used for each insulin ordered. Have your instructor check your answers.

1. 37 U Regular

2. 17 U Regular
   12 U Lente

3. 48 U NPH

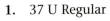
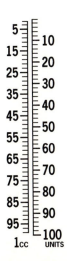

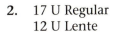
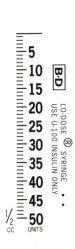

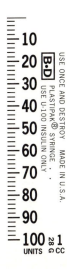

4.   14 U Regular
     58 U NPH

5.   12 U NPH

6.   18 U Regular
     8 U Lente

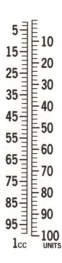

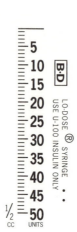

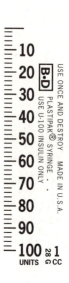

7.   23 U Regular
     14 U Humulin BR

8.   8 U Regular
     20 U Protamine Zinc

9.   23 U Lente

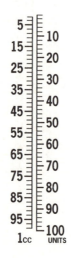

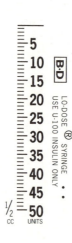

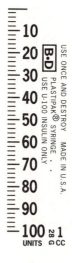

10.   57 U NPH

11.   22 U Regular
      8 U Lente

12.   15 U Regular
      43 U NPH

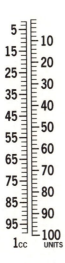

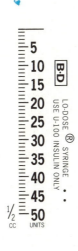

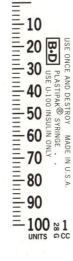

13.   24 U Regular
      27 U Lente

14.   33 U Regular
      10 U Humulin L

15.   55 U Regular

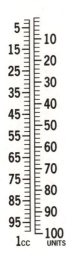

Directions: Identify the dosages measured on the following syringes.

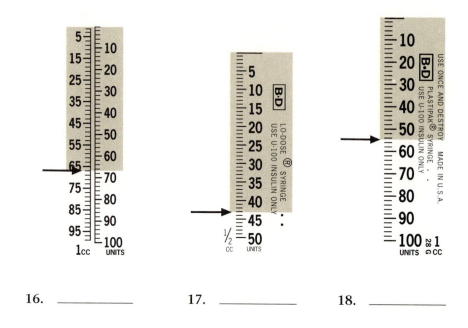

16. _____   17. _____   18. _____

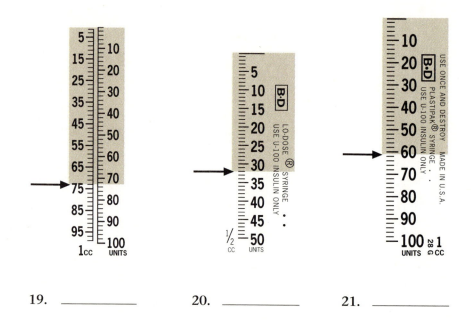

19. _____   20. _____   21. _____

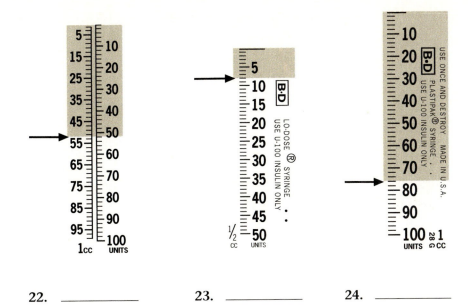

22. _____   23. _____   24. _____

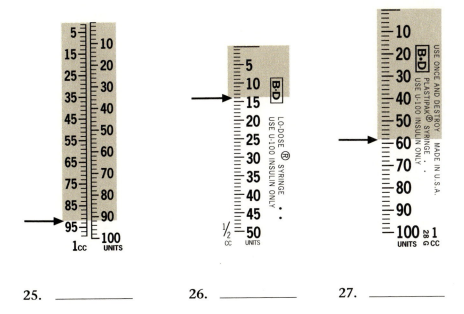

25. _____   26. _____   27. _____

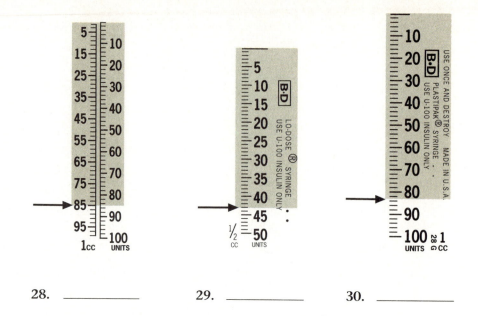

28. _____   29. _____   30. _____

SECTION

FIVE

Medication Administration Systems

CONTINUING MEDICATION RECORD

Veterans Administration

MONTH: **MAY**   YEAR: **19___**

DATE:

ORIG. ORD. DATE	START DATE	STOP DATE	MEDICATIONS DOSE/ROUTE/FREQUENCY	ADMIN. TIMES:	3	4	5	6	7	8	9	10	11	12	13	14	15	16
4-28	4-28	5-28	Digoxin 0.25 mg p.o. q.d.	0900	JD PGY													
5-1	5-1	5-15	Furosemide 40 mg p.o. b.i.d.	0900	JD													
				1700														
5-1	5-1	6-1	Ferrous sulfate 300 mg p.o. q.d.	0900	JD													
5-1	5-1	6-1	Allopurinal 300 mg p.o. b.i.d.	0900	JD													
				1700														
5-3	5-3	5-13	Amoxicillin 250 mg p.o. q.6.h.	0600														
				1200														
				1800														
				2400														

ADDRESSOGRAPH

PATIENT IDENTIFICATION

INJECTION SITES

INDICATE RIGHT (R)
OR LEFT (L)
1. DELTOID
2. ABDOMEN
3. ILIAC CREST
4. GLUTEAL
5. THIGH

SIGNATURE/TITLE   INIT.   ALLERGIES

Jennifer Bailey, R.N.   JD

VA FORM AUG 1982 **10-2970**   SUPERSEDES VA FORM 10-2970, JAN 1973, WHICH WILL NOT BE USED.

NAME: BED #   PAGE ____ OF ____

Medication Administration Records

16

OBJECTIVES

The student will read medication records to identify

1. drugs ordered on a continuing basis
2. dosage ordered
3. time of administration
4. route of administration

INTRODUCTION

The system of drug administration most commonly used in hospitals is the medication record system. In this system all the drugs a patient is receiving on a continuing basis are listed on a single record. In some hospitals p.r.n. and IV medications are also listed on this record, in others these are on a separate record, or records. A wide variety of records are in use, and the purpose of this chapter is to provide an introduction to a sufficient number so that you will not be confused by the differences, but rather will recognize and locate essential information which is common to all. The focus will be on identifying the drug, dosage, time and route of medications being administered on a continuing basis.

Medication Record 1

On the opposite page is the Continuing Medication Record currently being used at Veterans Hospitals in the U.S.A. Notice that from left to right the columns identify the original order date of the drug; the date administration was started; the date the order expires; the drug name, dosage, route and frequency of administration; the time of administration; and finally, the date columns used by the person administering to initial, indicating that the dosage was given. For example, Jennifer Daley has initialed for the 0900 dosages on May 3rd, and has identified her initials in the Signature/Title column on the lower right of the form. This hospital uses the 24 hour military time clock (0–2400).

Refer back to the drug information. The first drug, furosemide 40 mg, has been ordered p.o. b.i.d., to be given at 0900 and 1700. The administration time column is set up beginning with the earliest administration for the day, and includes all dosages to be given on a continuing basis. The patient identification would be stamped in the lower left corner.

185

PHARMACY USE ONLY		PHARMACY USE ONLY	
FILLED BY	CHECKED BY	FILLED BY	CHECKED BY
1. *as.*	*AB.*	5.	
2. *as.*	*AB.*	6.	
3.		7.	
4.			

THE TORONTO HOSPITAL

THE
TORONTO
HOSPITAL

THE TORONTO HOSPITAL
MEDICATION
ADMINISTRATION
RECORD

TWD ☐   TGD ☐

SCHEDULED MEDICATIONS

PHARM USE ONLY	DATE D/M/Y			TIME	1 7/3/94	2 8/3/94	3 9/3/94	4 10/3/94	5 11/3/94	6 12/3/94	7 13/3/94
FILL QTY. *CD*	T. R.	MEDICATION *HUMULIN LENTE*	DOSE 22								
1. 2. 3. 4. 5. 6.	✓ BY RN *mm* ✓ BY PHM *as*	FREQUENCY & DIRECTIONS *9 AM*	u	08	*mm* *mm* *mm*						
7.			ROUTE *SQ*								
		ORDERED DATE 7·3·94	STOP DATE / /								
FILL QTY. *CD*	T. R.	MEDICATION *DIGOXIN*	DOSE 0.125	09	*mm* *mm* *mm*						
1. 2. 3. 4. 5. 6.	✓ BY RN *mm* ✓ BY PHM *as*	FREQUENCY & DIRECTIONS *o.d.*	mg								
7.			ROUTE *po*								
		ORDERED DATE 7·3·94	STOP DATE / /								
FILL QTY. *CD*	T. R.	MEDICATION *ENALAPRIL*	DOSE 2.5	09	*mm* *mm* *mm*						
1. 2. 3. 4. 5. 6.	✓ BY RN *mm* ✓ BY PHM *as*	FREQUENCY & DIRECTIONS *o.d.*	mg		BP=160/10 BP=145/90 BP=138/80						
7.			ROUTE *po*								
		ORDERED DATE 7·3·94	STOP DATE / /								
FILL QTY. *CD*	T. R.	MEDICATION *COLACE*	DOSE 100	09	*mm* *mm* *mm*						
1. 2. 3. 4. 5. 6.	✓ BY RN *mm* ✓ BY PHM *as*	FREQUENCY & DIRECTIONS *BID*	mg								
7.			ROUTE *po*	21	*BJ* *BJ* *B.J.*						
		ORDERED DATE 7·3·94	STOP DATE / /								
FILL QTY. *CD*	T. R.	MEDICATION *HEPARIN*	DOSE 5000	09	*mm①* *mm⑤* *mm⑫*		/ D/C /			
1. 2. 3. 4. 5. 6.	✓ BY RN *mm* ✓ BY PHM *as*	FREQUENCY & DIRECTIONS *o.d.*	u								
7.			ROUTE *SQ*								
		ORDERED DATE 7·3·94	STOP DATE 10·3·94								
FILL QTY. *CD*	T. R.	MEDICATION *COUMADIN*	DOSE 2								
1. 2. 3. 4. 5. 6.	✓ BY RN *mm* ✓ BY PHM *as*	FREQUENCY & DIRECTIONS *o.d.*	mg	18	*BJ* *BJ* *B.J.*						
7.			ROUTE *po*								
		ORDERED DATE 7·3·94	STOP DATE / /								

Problem

Read the VA record and identify for each drug listed the name, dosage, route and time of administration.

	DRUG	DOSAGE	ROUTE	TIME
1.	_____	_____	_____	_____
2.	_____	_____	_____	_____
3.	_____	_____	_____	_____
4.	_____	_____	_____	_____
5.	_____	_____	_____	_____

6. If it was your responsibility to administer the drugs to this patient at 1700, which ones would you give? _____

ANSWERS **1.** digoxin 0.25 mg p.o. 0900 **2.** furosemide 40 mg p.o. 0900, 1700 **3.** ferrous sulfate 300 mg p.o. 0900 **4.** allopurinal 300 mg p.o. 0900, 1700 **5.** amoxicillin 250 mg p.o. 0600, 1200, 1800, 2400 **6.** At 1700 you would give furosemide 40 mg and allopurinal 300 mg

Medication Record 2

Take a close look at the record on the opposite page from the Toronto Hospital. You can see that the information it contains is very similar to the VA record, only the arrangement is different. The scheduled (continuing) medications are listed on the left, with the time and date of administration columns to the right. This medical center also uses military time, but omits the hourly zeros (for example 1900 is written as 19). The columns for initials are on this page, but the signature identification is on the reverse of the record, as are the p.r.n. medications.

Problem

Read the Toronto Hospital record and list the drug, dosage, route, and time of all medications ordered.

	DRUG	DOSAGE	ROUTE	TIME
1.	_____	_____	_____	_____
2.	_____	_____	_____	_____
3.	_____	_____	_____	_____
4.	_____	_____	_____	_____
5.	_____	_____	_____	_____
6.	_____	_____	_____	_____

7. Which drugs were given by BJ on 7-3? _____

ANSWERS **1.** Humelin Lente 22 U s.q. 08 **2.** Digoxin 0.125 mg p.o. 09 **3.** Enalapril 2.5 mg p.o. 09 **4.** Colace 100 mg p.o. 09, 21 **5.** Heparin 5000 U s.q. 09 **6.** Coumadin 2 mg p.o. 18 **7.** Colace 100 mg at 21, Coumadin 2 mg at 18

MEDICATION ADMINISTRATION RECORD - 14 DAY

Enter Here
IN PENCIL
Number of
Forms in Use

NAME
ADM. NO.   PATIENT IDENTIFICATION

IMPRINT HERE

DIAGNOSES: _____

ALLERGIC TO: _____   DIET: _____
(Record in Red)

Scheduled Medications

OR. DATE / INITIALS	EXP.DATE / TIME	MEDICATION-DOSAGE-FREQUENCY-RT. OF ADM.	HR.	5/3	5/4	5/5	5/6	5/7	5/8	5/9	5/10	5/11	5/12	5/13	5/14	5/15	5/16
5-3 AMC		Tagamet 300 mg p.o. q.6.h.	6 12 6 12														
5-2 AMC	5-16 8q2	Blocadren 10 mg p.o. b.i.d.	9 9														
5-3 AMC		Nitro-Bid ung 1" (top) apply to chest q.6.h. while awake	6 12 6 12														
5-3 AMC		Dialose cap ī p.o. t.i.d.	9 1 9														
5-3 AMC		Bactrim DS ī p.o. b.i.d.	6 6														

Single Orders + Pre-Operatives

USE RED ASTERISK *TO INDICATE DOSES
NOT GIVEN - EXPLAIN IN NURSE'S NOTES

OR. DATE / INITIALS	MEDICATION-DOSAGE-RT. OF ADM.	TO BE GIVEN DATE	TIME	NURSE INITIAL	OR. DATE / INITIALS	MEDICATION-DOSAGE-RT. OF ADM.	TO BE GIVEN DATE	TIME	NURSE INITIAL

AGE _____ RELIGION _____ DOCTOR _____   DATE/TIME ADMITTED _____

RM. _____ NAME _____

Lionville Systems, Inc.
© Parke, Davis & Company, 1978
P/N 10104 Rev. H

Medication Record 3

Medication record 3 is produced by Lionville Systems of Parke-Davis & Co. Notice that it provides space at the lower left for Single Order and Pre-Operative drugs. The previous records you examined listed these, and p.r.n. drugs, on separate records. IV drugs are also often listed on separate records. The nurse signature identification is not shown, as it is on the back of this particular form.

Problem

Read the medication record on the opposite page and list the drug, dosage, and route of each drug that will be administered at 6 p.m.

ANSWERS   Tagamet 300 mg p.o.; Nitro-Bid ung 1″ topical to chest; Bactrim DS 1 p.o.

151-265 (R7-82) 6

MEDICATION ADMINISTRATION
RECORD

UNIVERSITY HOSPITAL
UNIVERSITY OF CALIFORNIA MEDICAL CENTER
SAN DIEGO

Start / Stop	Medication and Dose	Schedule	Route / Nurse		Date 5-3	Date 5-4	Date 5-5	Date 5-6
5-1	Capoten (captopril) 25 mg t.i.d.	08 14 20	p.o. / BW	Time Site Initials				

Initials	Signature	Initials	Signature	Initials	Signature	Initials	Signature
BW	BPardin, RN						

Physician

Allergies

Room #   Name

Medication Record 4

The final record, from the University of California Medical Center, San Diego, also uses military time. Once again you can see the similarities with the previous records, however this record lists both trade and generic drug names in the "Medication and Dose" column.

Problem

Use the drug entry on Medication Record 4 as reference to enter the following drugs, dosages, frequency, and route of administration on the form. Record your initials in the "Nurse" column to indicate you have done the transcribing, and identify your initials appropriately on the record. Have your instructor check your completed record.

1. Coumadin (warfarin Na) 5 mg p.o. q.d. 1800

2. Pronestyl (procainamide) 1000 mg q.6.h. p.o. 0600 1200 1800 2400

3. Mefoxin (cefoxitan Na) 1.5 g q.8.h. IM 0600 1400 2200

4. Ansaid (flurbiprofen) 100 mg p.o. b.i.d. $\overline{c}$ meals 0800 1800

5. Hismanal (astemizole) 10 mg p.o. q.h.s. 2200

Summary

This concludes your introduction to Medication Administration Records. The important points to remember from this chapter are:

all the drugs the patient is receiving on a continuing basis are entered on a single record

the record contains columns for drug, dosage, route, frequency, and times of administration

dosages are charted and initialed for each calendar day in the appropriate time slots

initials are identified with full signature on each record

p.r.n. and IV medications are frequently recorded on a separate record, or separate section of the continuing medication record

17 Medication Card Administration

OBJECTIVES

The student will read medication cards to identify

1. drug
2. dosage
3. time of administration
4. route of administration

INTRODUCTION

In the medication card system a **separate card is made for each drug** the patient is to receive. These are usually combined with the medicine cards for all other patients on a unit, and stored in a card rack under **the time of next administration.** If your assignment was to give the 9 a.m. medications you would pull all the cards from the 9 a.m. slot, prepare, administer, and chart them, then sort and return the cards to the time slot of the **next administration;** 1 p.m., 9 p.m., and so on. P.R.N. cards are kept separate.

There are several recognized weaknesses in this system, lost or misplaced cards being one of the more serious. For this reason many hospitals have phased out this system in favor of the medication record system. However, you should still know how to read a medicine card correctly.

Reading Medication Cards

Examine the medication cards labeled A and B in figure 71. Notice that both cards contain the patient's name, surname first. The room and bed number (frequently written in pencil, so that it can be changed if the patient is moved) is next. Both contain the name of the drug, acetaminophen, the dosage, 600 mg, and the frequency and route of administration, t.i.d. p.o. The time of administration is designated by an X in the appropriate time slot. The shaded areas on these cards identify the evening/night hours. Card B has a built-in weakness in that the time of administration is X'ed in a separate column, leaving open the possibility of misreading the 2100 dosage, for example, as 0900 (this card uses military time).

This information is all you will need to read medication cards. Take the time to read them carefully. Many will be hand printed, as in the examples provided, and not always easy to read. Abbreviations also will vary. The summary self test will provide a representative sampling.

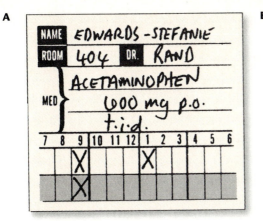

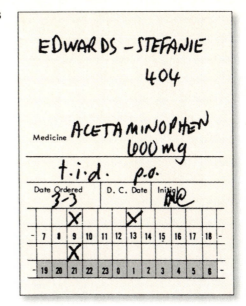

Figure 71

Summary

The important points to remember about reading medication cards are:

in the medication card system a card is made for each drug the patient is to receive

the patient's name, room number, drug, dosage, frequency and route of administration are all printed on the card

the time of administration is X'ed in the appropriate time space for each dosage to be administered

when the medications for a given time have been administered and charted, the cards are returned to the time slot of the next administration

Summary Self Test

Directions: For each of the following medication cards identify the drug, dosage, route and time of administration. Indicate a.m. or p.m. for dosages given at standard time, but omit these designations if military time is used.

	DRUG	DOSAGE	ROUTE	TIME
1.				
2.				
3.				
4.				
5.				
6.				

7. _____ _____ _____ _____

8. _____ _____ _____ _____

9. _____ _____ _____ _____

10. _____ _____ _____ _____

11. _____ _____ _____ _____

12. _____ _____ _____ _____

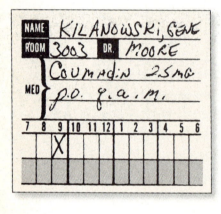

NAME: KILANOWSKI, GENE
ROOM: 3003 DR. MOORE
MED: Coumadin 2.5mg
p.o. q.a.m.

7 8 9 10 11 12 1 2 3 4 5 6

1

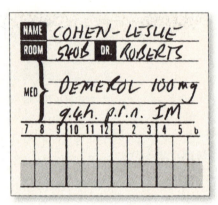

NAME: COHEN - LESLIE
ROOM: 540B DR. ROBERTS
MED: Demerol 100mg
q.4.h. p.r.n. IM

7 8 9 10 11 12 1 2 3 4 5 6

2

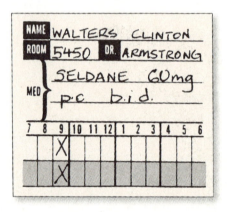

NAME: WALTERS CLINTON
ROOM: 5450 DR. ARMSTRONG
MED: SELDANE 60mg
p.c b.i.d.

7 8 9 10 11 12 1 2 3 4 5 6

3

44D

MEINZER, ROBERT

Medicine PROZAC 40mg

p.o. 9am

Date Ordered 2-10 D. C. Date Initial BTB

- 7 8 9 10 11 12 13 14 15 16 17 18 -
- 19 20 21 22 23 0 1 2 3 4 5 6 -

4

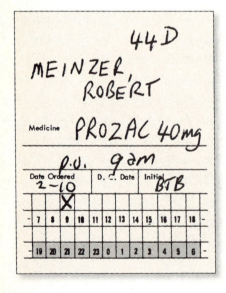

Young. Dennis
43A

Medicine COMPAZINE 10mg
q4h PRN IM

Date Ordered D. C. Date Initial ees

- 7 8 9 10 11 12 13 14 15 16 17 18 -
- 19 20 21 22 23 0 1 2 3 4 5 6 -

5

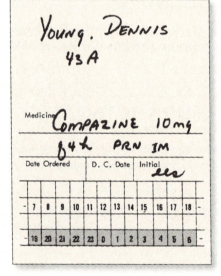

ISAACS, DALE
3033

Medicine XANAX 0.25 mg
tid po

Date Ordered D. C. Date Initial Raf

- 7 8 9 10 11 12 13 14 15 16 17 18 -
- 19 20 21 22 23 0 1 2 3 4 5 6 -

6

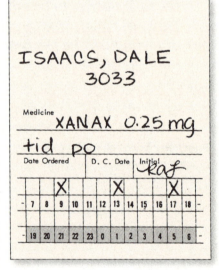

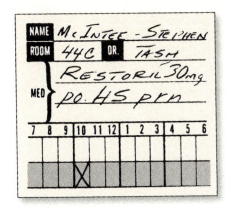

7

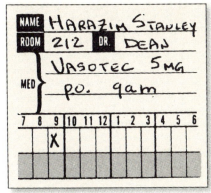

8

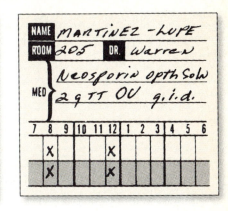

9

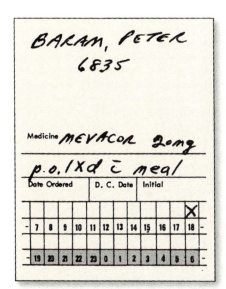

10

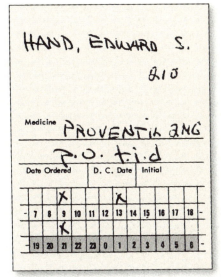

11

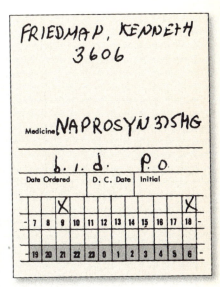

12

ANSWERS	1.	Coumadin	2.5 mg	p.o.	9 a.m.
	2.	Demerol	100 mg	IM	q.4.h. p.r.n.
	3.	Seldane	60 mg	p.o.	9 a.m.–9 p.m.
	4.	Prozac	40 mg	p.o.	0900
	5.	Compazine	10 mg	IM	q.4.h. p.r.n.
	6.	Xanax	0.25 mg	p.o.	0900–1300–1700
	7.	Restoril	30 mg	p.o.	h.s. p.r.n. 10 p.m.
	8.	Vasotec	5 mg	p.o.	9 a.m.
	9.	Neosporin opth. soln	2 gtt	OU	8 a.m.–12 p.m.–8 p.m.–12 a.m.
	10.	Mevacor	20 mg	p.o. c̄ meal	1800
	11.	Proventil	2 mg	p.o.	0900–1300–2100
	12.	Naprosyn	375 mg	p.o.	0900–1800

SIX

Dosage Determination by Body Weight and BSA

18

Pediatric & Adult Dosages Based on Body Weight

OBJECTIVES

The student will

1. convert body weight from lb to kg
2. convert body weight from kg to lb
3. calculate dosages using mg/kg, mcg/kg, mg/lb
4. determine if dosages ordered are within the normal range

INTRODUCTION

Body weight is a major factor in calculating drug dosages for both adults and children. It is the most important determiner of dosages for infants and neonates, whose ability to metabolize drugs is not fully developed. The dosage which will produce optimum therapeutic results for any particular individual, either child or adult, depends not only on dosage, but on individual variables, including drug sensitivities and tolerance, as well as age, weight, sex, and metabolic, pathologic or psychologic conditions.

The doctor will, of course, order the drug and dosage. However it is a nursing responsibility to check each dosage to be sure the order is correct. Each drug label or drug package insert provides specific dosage details, but more complete information is readily available in drug formularies, the PDR, and other nursing or medical references. The hospital pharmacist is an excellent resource person who can also supply you with additional information.

Individualized dosages may be calculated in terms of mcg per kg, mg per kg, or mg per lb, per day. The total daily dosage is usually administered in divided (more than one) doses, for example q.6.h. (4 doses), or t.i.d. (3 doses). In this chapter you will learn how to calculate dosages based on body weight so that, at any time, you can check an order that appears questionable, or incorrect.

However, a preliminary step is necessary to understand conversions between kg and lb, since dosages may be specified in one measure, while body weight is recorded in the other.

Converting lb to kg

Many hospitals still record body weight in lb, but most drug literature states dosages in terms of kg. The most common conversion is therefore from lb to kg. Weights are rounded to the nearest tenth kg.

 There are 2.2 lb in 1 kg

To convert from lb to kg **divide by 2.2.** Since you are dividing the answer, in kg, will be **smaller** than the lb you are converting. Answers are expressed to the nearest tenth.

EXAMPLE 1 A child weighs 41 lb. Convert to kg.

41 lb = 41 ÷ 2.2 = **18.6 kg**

Your answer should be a smaller number because you are dividing, and it is (41 lb = 18.6 kg).

EXAMPLE 2 Convert the weight of a 144 lb adult to kg.

144 lb = 144 ÷ 2.2 = 65.45 = **65.5 kg**

EXAMPLE 3 Convert the weight of a 27 lb child to kg.

27 lb = 27 ÷ 2.2 = 12.27 = **12.3 kg**

Problem

Convert the following body weights from lb to kg. Round weight to the nearest tenth kg.

1. 14.5 lb = _____ kg
2. 19 lb   = _____ kg
3. 163 lb = _____ kg
4. 31 lb   = _____ kg
5. 100 lb = _____ kg

ANSWERS **1.** 6.6 kg **2.** 8.6 kg **3.** 74.1 kg **4.** 14.1 kg **5.** 45.5 kg

Converting kg to lb

To convert in the opposite direction, from kg to lb, always **multiply by 2.2.** Because you are multiplying the answer, in lb, will be **larger** than the kg you started with. Express weight to the nearest tenth.

EXAMPLE 1 A child weighs 23 kg. Convert to lb.

23 kg = 23 × 2.2 = **50.6 lb**

Your answer must be larger because you are multiplying, and it is, 23 kg = 50.6 lb.

EXAMPLE 2 Convert an adult weight of 73 kg to lb.

$$73 \text{ kg} = 73 \times 2.2 = \textbf{160.6 lb}$$

EXAMPLE 3 Convert the weight of a 14 kg child to lb.

$$14 \text{ kg} = 14 \times 2.2 = \textbf{30.8 lb}$$

Problem

Convert the following body weights from kg to lb. Round weights to the nearest tenth lb.

1. 21 kg = _____ lb
2. 99 kg = _____ lb
3. 18 kg = _____ lb
4. 71 kg = _____ lb
5. 10 kg = _____ lb
6. 5 kg   = _____ lb

ANSWERS   **1.** 46.2 lb   **2.** 217.8 lb   **3.** 39.6 lb   **4.** 156.2 lb   **5.** 22 lb   **6.** 11 lb

Calculating Dosages from Drug Label Information

The sources for the information you will need to calculate dosages may be on the actual drug label, which is common for pediatric oral liquid medications.

Calculating the dosage is a two step procedure. First the total daily dosage is calculated, then it is divided by the number of doses per day to obtain the actual dose administered at one time.

Let's start by looking at some pediatric oral antibiotic labels which contain the mg/kg/day dosage guidelines.

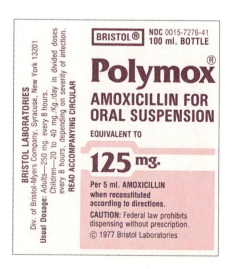

Figure 72

EXAMPLE 1 Refer to the information written sideways on the left of the Polymox® label in Figure 72 for children's dosages. Notice that the average dosage range is 20–40 mg/kg/day. This dosage is to be given in divided doses every 8 hours, or a total of 3 doses (24 hr ÷ 8 hr).

Once you have located the dosage information you can move ahead and calculate the dosage. Let's assume you are checking the dosage ordered for an 18 kg child. Start by calculating the **recommended dosage range.**

Lower dosage = 20 mg/kg   **Upper dosage** = 40 mg/kg

20 mg × 18 kg (wt of child) = 360 mg/day

40 mg × 18 kg = 720 mg/day

The recommended range for this 18 kg child is **360–720 mg/day.**

The drug is to be given in 3 divided doses.

Lower dosage 360 mg ÷ 3 = 120 mg per dose

Upper dosage 720 mg ÷ 3 = 240 mg per dose

The dosage range is **120 mg to 240 mg per dose q.8.h.**

Now that you have the dosage range for this child you are able to assess the accuracy of physician orders. Let's look at some and see how you can use the dosage range you just calculated.

1. If the order is to give 125 mg q.8.h. is this within the recommended dosage range? Yes, 125 mg q.8.h. is within the average range of 120–240 mg per dose.

2. If the order is to give 375 mg q.8.h. is this a safe dosage? No, this is an overdosage. The maximum recommended dosage is 240 mg per dose. The 375 mg dose should not be given; the doctor must be called and the order questioned.

3. If the order is for 75 mg q.8.h. is this an accurate dosage? The recommended lower limit for an 18 kg child is 120 mg. While 75 mg might be safe, it will probably be ineffective. Notify the doctor that the dosage appears to be too low.

4. If the order is for 250 mg q.8.h. is this accurate? Since 240 mg per dose is the recommended upper limit 250 mg q.8.h. is essentially within normal range. The drug strength is 125 mg per 5 mL and a 250 mg dosage is 10 mL. The doctor has probably ordered this dosage based on available dosage strength, and ease of preparation.

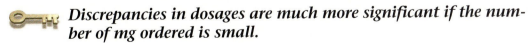 *Discrepancies in dosages are much more significant if the number of mg ordered is small.*

For example the difference between 4 mg and 6 mg is much more critical than the difference between 240 mg and 250 mg since the drug potency is obviously greater. Additional factors which must be considered are age, weight, and medical condition. While these factors cannot be dealt with at length keep in mind that **the younger, the older, or more compromised by illness the patient is, the more critical a discrepancy is likely to be.**

5. If the dosage ordered is 125 mg q.4.h. is this an accurate dosage? In this order the frequency of administration, q.4.h., does not fit the recommendations of q.8.h. The total daily dosage of 750 mg (125 mg × 6 doses = 750 mg) is higher than the 720 mg maximum. There may be a reason the doctor ordered this dosage but call to verify the order.

Problem

Refer to the cloxacillin (Tegopen®) label in figure 73 and answer the following questions.

1. What is the average children's dosage? _____

2. How is this dosage to be administered? _____

3. How many divided doses will this be in 24 hours? _____

4. What will the total daily dose be for a child weighing 10 kg? _____

5. The dosage strength of this oral cloxacillin solution is 125 mg per 5 mL, and the doctor has ordered 125 mg q.6.h. for this 10 kg child. Is there any need to question this order? _____

ANSWERS   1. 50 mg/kg/day   **2.** equal doses q.6.h.   **3.** 4 doses in 24 hrs.   **4.** 500 mg   **5.** No

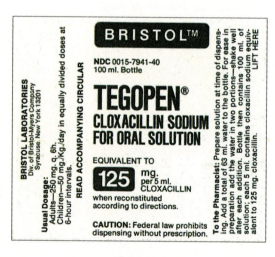

Figure 73

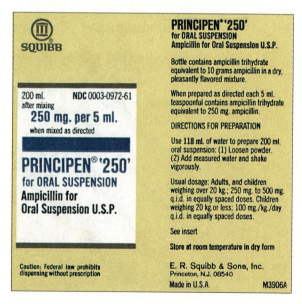

Figure 74

Problem

Refer to the ampicillin (Principen®) label in figure 74. Answer the following questions for a 12 lb infant.

1. What is the child's body weight in kg to the nearest tenth kg? _____
2. What is the recommended dosage in mg per day for this infant? _____

3. How many doses will this be divided into? _____

4. How many mg will this be per dose? _____

5. The order is to give 125 mg q.6.h. Is this dosage accurate? _____

6. How many mL would you need to administer a 125 mg dosage? _____

ANSWERS 1. 5.5 kg **2.** 550 mg **3.** 4 doses **4.** 137.5 mg **5.** Yes **6.** 2.5 mL

Calculating Dosages from Drug Literature

The labels you have just been reading were from oral syrups and suspensions, but the same calculation steps are necessary for dosages to be administered by the IV or IM route. Parenteral labels are much smaller in size and usually do not include dosage recommendations. To obtain these you will have to refer to the drug package inserts, or the PDR, or similar references. These references will contain extensive details about each drug's chemistry, actions, adverse reactions, recommended administration, etc. so it will be necessary for you to search for and select the information you need under the heading "Dosage and Administration." In the following exercises we have done the searching for you, and presented only those excerpts necessary for your calculations.

KEFZOL®, STERILE CEFAZOLIN SODIUM, USP

ADMINISTRATION AND DOSAGE

In children, a total daily dosage of 25 to 50 mg/kg (approximately 10 to 20 mg/lb) of body weight, divided into 3 or 4 equal doses, is effective for most mild to moderately severe infections (Table 5). Total daily dosage may be increased to 100 mg/kg (45 mg/lb) of body weight for severe infections.

TABLE 5. PEDIATRIC DOSAGE GUIDE

Weight		25 mg/kg/Day Divided into 3 Doses		25 mg/kg/Day Divided into 4 Doses	
lb	kg	Approximate Single Dose (mg q8h)	Vol (mL) Needed with Dilution of 125 mg/mL	Approximate Single Dose (mg q6h)	Vol (mL) Needed with Dilution of 125 mg/mL
10	4.5	40 mg	0.35 mL	30 mg	0.25 mL
20	9	75 mg	0.6 mL	55 mg	0.45 mL
30	13.6	115 mg	0.9 mL	85 mg	0.7 mL
40	18.1	150 mg	1.2 mL	115 mg	0.9 mL
50	22.7	190 mg	1.5 mL	140 mg	1.1 mL

Weight		50 mg/kg/Day Divided into 3 Doses		50 mg/kg/Day Divided into 4 Doses	
lb	kg	Approximate Single Dose (mg q8h)	Vol (mL) Needed with Dilution of 225 mg/mL	Approximate Single Dose (mg q6h)	Vol (mL) Needed with Dilution of 225 mg/mL
10	4.5	75 mg	0.35 mL	55 mg	0.25 mL
20	9	150 mg	0.7 mL	110 mg	0.5 mL
30	13.6	225 mg	1 mL	170 mg	0.75 mL
40	18.1	300 mg	1.35 mL	225 mg	1 mL
50	22.7	375 mg	1.7 mL	285 mg	1.25 mL

Figure 75

Problem

Refer to the cefazolin (Kefzol®) insert in figure 75 and locate the following information for pediatric dosages.

1. What is the dosage range in mg/kg/day for mild to moderate infections?

    _____

2. What is the dosage range for mild to moderate infections in mg/lb/day?

    _____

3. The total dosage will be divided into how many doses per day? _____

4. In severe infections what is the maximum dosage recommended in mg/kg ________ mg/lb? ________

ANSWERS **1.** 25 mg–50 mg **2.** 10 mg–20 mg **3.** 3–4 doses per day **4.** 100 mg/kg; 45 mg/lb

Notice that in this table sample dosages are provided for several kg and lb weights, for both the 25 mg and 50 mg dosage, and for both 3 and 4 doses per day. Tables of this sort may be helpful, or harmful. They are helpful if they are easy to understand and the child whose dosage you are calculating fits exactly one of the weights listed; they are harmful if they tend to confuse, which could happen.

The essential information needed to calculate recommended safe dosage ranges is the dosage range in mg/kg/day (or mg/lb/day) and the frequency of administration.

With this information you can quickly calculate what the dosages should be, and determine if the dosages ordered are correct.

Problem

Use the information you just obtained for Kefzol to calculate the following for a child who weighs 35 lb and has a moderately severe infection.

1. What is the lower daily dosage range? ________

2. What is the upper daily dosage range? ________

3. If the medication is given in 4 divided dosages what will the range be? ________

4. If a dosage of 125 mg q.6.h. is ordered will you need to question it? ________

ANSWERS **1.** 350 mg/day **2.** 700 mg/day **3.** 87.5 mg to 175 mg per dose **4.** No; within normal range

Problem

Refer to the dosage information on Mezlin® in figure 76 and answer the following questions about adult IV dosages.

DOSAGE AND ADMINISTRATION

MEZLIN® (sterile mezlocillin sodium) may be administered intravenously or intramuscularly. For serious infections, the intravenous route of administration should be used. Intramuscular doses should not exceed 2g per injection.

The recommended adult dosage for serious infections is 200-300 mg/kg per day given in 4 to 6 divided doses. The usual dose is 3g given every 4 hours (18g/day) or 4g given every 6 hours (16g/day). For life-threatening infections, up to 350 mg/kg per day may be administered, but the total daily dosage should ordinarily not exceed 24g.

[See table below.]

For patients with life-threatening infections, 4g may be administered every 4 hours (24g/day).

Dosage for any individual patient must take into consideration the site and severity of infection, the susceptibility of

Figure 76

MITHRACIN® ℞
(plicamycin)
FOR INTRAVENOUS USE

DOSAGE

The daily dose of Mithracin is based on the patient's body weight. If a patient has abnormal fluid retention such as edema, hydrothorax or ascites, the patient's ideal weight rather than actual body weight should be used to calculate the dose.

Treatment of Testicular Tumors: In the treatment of patients with testicular tumors the recommended daily dose of Mithracin (plicamycin) is 25 to 30 mcg (0.025–0.030 mg) per kilogram of body weight. Therapy should be continued for a period of 8 to 10 days unless significant side effects or toxicity occur during therapy. A course of therapy consisting of more than 10 daily doses is not recommended. Individual daily doses should not exceed 30 mcg (0.030 mg) per kilogram of body weight.

Figure 77

1. What is the recommended dosage range for serious infections? _____

2. How many divided doses and at what intervals should this dosage be given? _____   _____

3. What is the maximum daily dosage? _____

4. Calculate the dosage range in g for a 176 lb adult? _____

5. If this dosage is to be given q.6.h. what will the individual dosage range be? _____

6. If 2 g per dosage is ordered what initial assessment would you make? _____

7. If a dosage of 10 g q.6.h. is ordered what assessment would you make? _____

ANSWERS 1. 200 mg/kg to 300 mg/kg   2. 4 to 6 doses; q.6.h. or q.4.h.   3. 24 g   4. 16 g–24 g   5. 4 g–6 g
6. the dosage is too low   7. the dosage is too high

Problem

Refer to the dosage recommendations for Mithracin® in figure 77 and answer the following questions for treatment of testicular tumors in a patient weighing 240 lbs.

1. What is the recommended dosage range in mcg? _____

2. How often is this dosage to be given, and for how long? _____ _____

3. What is the exact dosage range in mg for this patient (calculate to the nearest tenth)? _____

4. If a dosage of 3 mg IV q.a.m. is ordered does this need to be questioned? _____

ANSWERS 1. 25–30 mcg/kg   2. 1× day; 8–10 days   3. 2.7–3.3 mg   4. No, within normal range

Problem

Refer to the cephradine (Velosef®) literature in figure 78 and answer the following questions.

1. What is the usual dosage range in mg/kg/day? _____

2. What is the dosage range in mg/lb/day? _____

3.   What is the recommended number of dosages per day? _____

4.   What will the daily dosage range be for a child weighing 12 kg? _____

5.   How many mg will be administered per dose? _____

6.   If the order for this child is cephradine 250 mg q.6.h. is this an accurate dosage? _____

7.   What is the dosage range for a child weighing 19 lb? _____

8.   What amount will be administered per dose? _____

9.   If 340 mg q.6.h. is ordered is this an accurate dosage? _____

VELOSEF® for INJECTION
Cephradine for Injection USP

DOSAGE AND ADMINISTRATION

Infants and Children
The usual dosage range of VELOSEF is 50 to 100 mg/kg/day (approximately 23 to 45 mg/lb/day) in equally divided doses four times a day and should be regulated by age, weight of the patient and severity of the infection being treated.

PEDIATRIC DOSAGE GUIDE				
	50 mg/kg/day		100 mg/kg/day	
Weight	Approx. single dose mg q6h	Volume needed @ 208 mg/mL dilution	Approx. single dose mg q6h	Volume needed @ 227 mg/mL dilution
lbs kg				
10 4.5	56 mg	0.27 mL	112 mg	0.5 mL
20 9.1	114 mg	0.55 mL	227 mg	1 mL
30 13.6	170 mg	0.82 mL	340 mg	1.5 mL
40 18.2	227 mg	1.1 mL	455 mg	2 mL
50 22.7	284 mg	1.4 mL	567 mg	2.5 mL

Figure 78

Summary

This concludes the chapter on calculation and assessment of dosages based on body weight. The important points to remember from this chapter are:

dosages are frequently ordered on the basis of weight, especially for children

dosages may be recommended based on mg/kg/day, mcg/kg/day or mg/lb/day, usually in divided doses body weight may need to be converted from kg to lb, or lb to kg to correlate with dosage recommendations

to convert lb to kg divide by 2.2; to convert kg to lb multiply by 2.2

calculating dosage is a two step procedure: first calculate the total daily dosage for the weight; then divide this by the number of doses to be administered

to check the accuracy of a doctor's order calculate the correct dosage and compare it with the dosage ordered

dosage discrepancies are much more critical if the dosage range is low, for example 4–6 mg, as opposed to high, for example 250 mg

factors that make discrepancies particularly serious are age, low body weight, and severity of medical condition

if the drug label does not contain all the necessary information for safe administration, additional information should be obtained from drug package inserts, the PDR, drug formularies, or the hospital pharmacist

---

Summary Self Test

Directions: Read the dosage labels and literature provided to indicate if dosages are within normal safety limits. If they are not, give the correct range. Express body weight conversions to the nearest tenth, and dosages to the nearest whole number in your calculations.

1. A 45 lb child has an order for Ilosone® (erythromycin) oral susp. 250 mg q.6.h. Read the accompanying label and decide if this is a correct dosage.

   _____

2. Zinacef® (cefuroxime) 375 mg has been ordered IV q.8.h. for a child weighing 44 lb. Determine if this is a safe dosage. _____

3. Zinacef® has also been ordered for a child weighing 84 lb. What would the dosage range be per day, and per dose if the medication is given q.6.h.?

   _____ _____

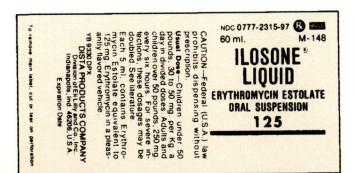

ILOSONE® LIQUID
ERYTHROMYCIN ESTOLATE
ORAL SUSPENSION
125

NDC 0777-2315-97 ℞
60 ml. M-148

CAUTION—Federal (U.S.A.) law prohibits dispensing without prescription.
Usual Dose—Children under 50 pounds, 30 to 50 mg. per Kg. a day in divided doses. Adults and children over 50 pounds, 250 mg. every six hours. For severe infections, these dosages may be doubled. See literature.
Each 5 ml. contains Erythromycin Estolate equivalent to 125 mg. Erythromycin in a pleasantly flavored vehicle.
YB 9330 DPX
DISTA PRODUCTS COMPANY
Division of Eli Lilly and Co., Inc.
Indianapolis, Ind. 46206, U.S.A.
Expiration Date
To remove main label, cut or tear on perforation

ZINACEF®
[zin 'ah-sef]
(sterile cefuroxime sodium, Glaxo)

DOSAGE AND ADMINISTRATION

Infants and Children Above 3 Months of Age: Administration of 50 to 100 mg/kg/day in equally divided doses every six to eight hours has been successful for most infections susceptible to cefuroxime. The higher dose of 100 mg/kg/day (not to exceed the maximum adult dose) should be used for the more severe or serious infections.
In bone and joint infections, 150 mg/kg/day (not to exceed the maximum adult dose) is recommended in equally divided doses every eight hours. In clinical trials a course of oral antibiotics was administered to children following the completion of parenteral administration of ZINACEF.
In cases of bacterial meningitis, larger doses of ZINACEF are recommended, 200 to 240 mg/kg/day intravenously in divided doses every six to eight hours.
In children with renal insufficiency, the frequency of dosage should be modified consistent with the recommendations for adults.

4. Oxacillin (Prostaphlin®) 250 mg q.6.h. p.o. has been ordered for a 44 lb child. Determine if this dosage is safe. _____

5. This same oral oxacillin solution has been ordered for a 16 lb infant. The dosage is 125 mg q.6.h. Is this within normal limits? _____

6. A 22 lb child has an order for IV methylprednisolone (Solu-Medrol®) 125 mg q.6.h. for 48 hours. Read the literature and decide if this dosage is within normal range. _____

7. A 7 kg infant has an order for Veetids® 125 mg q.8.h. Comment on this dosage. _____

8. A dosage of vancomycin (Vancocin®) 100 mg has been ordered q.6.h. IV for a child weighing 22 lb. Is this a safe dosage? _____

9. Another child weighing 54 lb also has an order for vancomycin IV. Determine what the dosage should be q.6.h. _____

10. Amoxil® oral amoxicillin suspension 125 mg q.8.h. has been ordered for an infant weighing 14 lb. Determine if this is a safe dosage? _____

11. Calculate the dosage range per day and per dose of the amoxicillin oral susp. for a child weighing 41 lb. Given the fact that this child has a severe infection, and that the dosage of the solution is 250 mg per 5 mL, what would you expect the order to be q.8.h? _____ _____
    _____

12. A child weighing 15 kg with a diagnosis of bacterial meningitis has an order for cefuroxome (Kefurox®) 750 mg IV q.6.h. From the available information calculate to determine if this is a correct dosage. _____

KEFUROX™
[kĕf′ōō-rŏcks]
sterile cefuroxime sodium)

DOSAGE AND ADMINISTRATION

Infants and Children Above 3 Months of Age —Administration of 50 to 100 mg/kg/day in equally divided doses every 6 to 8 hours has been successful for most infections susceptible to cefuroxime. The higher dose of 100 mg/kg/day (not to exceed the maximum adult dose) should be used for the more severe or serious infections.

In cases of bacterial meningitis, larger doses of Kefurox are recommended, initially 200 to 240 mg/kg/day intravenously in divided doses every 6 to 8 hours.

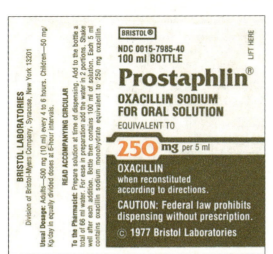

BRISTOL®

NDC 0015-7985-40
100 ml BOTTLE

Prostaphlin®

OXACILLIN SODIUM
FOR ORAL SOLUTION

EQUIVALENT TO

250 mg per 5 ml

OXACILLIN
when reconstituted
according to directions.

CAUTION: Federal law prohibits
dispensing without prescription.

© 1977 Bristol Laboratories

LIFT HERE

BRISTOL LABORATORIES
Division of Bristol-Myers Company, Syracuse, New York 13201

Usual Dosage: Adults—500 mg (10 ml) every 4 to 6 hours. Children—50 mg/Kg/day in equally divided doses at 6-hour intervals.

READ ACCOMPANYING CIRCULAR

To the Pharmacist: Prepare solution at time of dispensing. Add to the bottle a total of 66 ml water. For ease in preparation add the water in 2 portions. Shake well after each addition. Bottle then contains 100 ml of solution. Each 5 ml contains oxacillin sodium monohydrate equivalent to 250 mg oxacillin.

SOLU–MEDROL®
brand of methylprednisolone sodium succinate sterile
powder
(methylprednisolone sodium succinate for
injection, USP)
For Intravenous or Intramuscular
Administration

DOSAGE AND ADMINISTRATION
When high dose therapy is desired, the recommended dose of SOLU-MEDROL Sterile Powder (methylprednisolone sodium succinate) is 30 mg/kg administered intravenously over at least 30 minutes. This dose may be repeated every 4 to 6 hours for 48 hours.

Dosage may be reduced for infants and children but should be governed more by the severity of the condition and response of the patient than by age or size. It should not be less than 0.5 mg per kg every 24 hours.

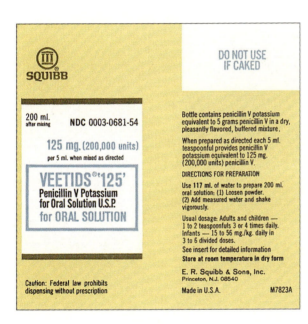

Ⅲ®
SQUIBB

DO NOT USE
IF CAKED

200 ml.
after mixing   NDC 0003-0681-54

125 mg. (200,000 units)

per 5 ml. when mixed as directed

VEETIDS®'125'
Penicillin V Potassium
for Oral Solution U.S.P.
for ORAL SOLUTION

Caution: Federal law prohibits
dispensing without prescription

Bottle contains penicillin V potassium equivalent to 5 grams penicillin V in a dry, pleasantly flavored, buffered mixture.

When prepared as directed each 5 ml. teaspoonful provides penicillin V potassium equivalent to 125 mg. (200,000 units) penicillin V.

DIRECTIONS FOR PREPARATION
Use 117 ml. of water to prepare 200 ml. oral solution: (1) Loosen powder. (2) Add measured water and shake vigorously.

Usual dosage: Adults and children — 1 to 2 teaspoonfuls 3 or 4 times daily. Infants — 15 to 56 mg./kg. daily in 3 to 6 divided doses.
See insert for detailed information
Store at room temperature in dry form

E. R. Squibb & Sons, Inc.
Princeton, N.J. 08540

Made in U.S.A.   M7823A

VANCOCIN® HCl
[văn 'kō-sĭn ăch 'sē-ĕl]
(vancomycin hydrochloride)
Sterile, USP
IntraVenous

DOSAGE AND ADMINISTRATION
Patients with Normal Renal Function
Adults—The usual daily intravenous dose is 2 g divided either as 500 mg every 6 hours or 1 g every 12 hours. Each dose should be administered over a period of at least 60 minutes. Other patient factors, such as age or obesity, may call for modification of the usual daily dose.
Children—The total daily intravenous dosage of Vancocin® HCl (vancomycin hydrochloride, Lilly), calculated on the basis of 40 mg/kg of body weight, can be divided and incorporated into the child's 24-hour fluid requirement. Each dose should be administered over a period of at least 60 minutes.
Infants and Neonates—In neonates and young infants, the total daily intravenous dosage may be lower. In both neonates and infants, an initial dose of 15 mg/kg is suggested, followed by 10 mg/kg every 12 hours for neonates in the first week of life and every 8 hours thereafter up to the age of 1 month. Close monitoring of serum concentrations of vancomycin may be warranted in these patients.

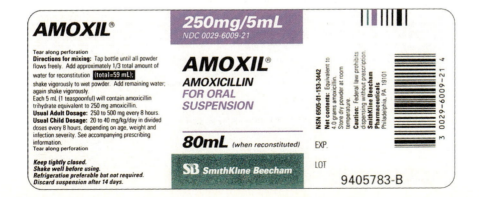

AMOXIL®

250mg/5mL
NDC 0029-6009-21

AMOXIL®
AMOXICILLIN
FOR ORAL
SUSPENSION

80mL (when reconstituted)

SB SmithKline Beecham

Tear along perforation
Directions for mixing: Tap bottle until all powder flows freely. Add approximately 1/3 total amount of water for reconstitution (total=59 mL); shake vigorously to wet powder. Add remaining water; again shake vigorously.
Each 5 mL (1 teaspoonful) will contain amoxicillin trihydrate equivalent to 250 mg amoxicillin.
Usual Adult Dosage: 250 to 500 mg every 8 hours.
Usual Child Dosage: 20 to 40 mg/kg/day in divided doses every 8 hours, depending on age, weight and infection severity. See accompanying prescribing information.
Tear along perforation

Keep tightly closed.
Shake well before using.
Refrigeration preferable but not required.
Discard suspension after 14 days.

NSN 6505-01-153-3442
Net contents: Equivalent to 4.0 grams amoxicillin
Store dry powder at room temperature
Caution: Federal law prohibits dispensing without prescription.
SmithKline Beecham
Pharmaceuticals
Philadelphia, PA 19101

EXP.

LOT

3 0029-6009-21 4

9405783-B

13.   An infant suffering from a genitourinary tract infection has an order for IV ampicillin (Omnipen-N®) 125 mg q.6.h. The infant weighs 12 lb. Is this a correct dosage? _____

14.   A 14 lb infant has ampicillin ordered for a respiratory infection. The doctor has ordered 62.5 mg IV q.6.h. Comment on this dosage. _____

15.   A dosage of Ancef® 125 mg q.6.h. has been ordered for a child weighing 16 kg. Calculate the safe dosage range and determine if this dosage is within normal limits. _____   _____

16.   Ceftazidime (Tazidime®) 1250 mg IV is ordered q.8.h. for a child weighing 55 lb. How many dosages will the child receive in 24 hr? _____

17.   What is this child's weight in kg? _____

18.   What is the normal dosage range for IV administration of this drug to this child? _____

19.   Is the dosage ordered within the normal range? _____

20.   A 198 lb adult is to be treated with IV Ticar® for a respiratory tract infection. What is the daily dosage range in g for this patient? _____

21.   If the drug is administered q.4.h. What will the range per dose be?

_____

22.   Do you need to question a 4 g per dosage order? _____

TICAR ®
brand of
sterile ticarcillin disodium
for Intramuscular or Intravenous Administration

DOSAGE AND ADMINISTRATION
Clinical experience indicates that in serious urinary tract and systemic infections, intravenous therapy in the higher doses should be used. Intramuscular injections should not exceed 2 grams per injection.
Adults:

Bacterial septicemia Respiratory tract infections Skin and soft-tissue infections Intra-abdominal infections Infections of the female pelvis and genital tract	200 to 300 mg/kg/day by I.V. infusion in divided doses every 4 or 6 hours. (The usual dose is 3 grams given every 4 hours [18 grams/day] or 4 grams given every 6 hours [16 grams/day] depending on weight and the severity of the infection.)
Urinary tract infections Complicated:	150 to 200 mg/kg/day by I.V. infusion in divided doses every 4 or 6 hours. (Usual recommended dosage for average [70 kg] adults: 3 grams q.i.d.)
Uncomplicated:	1 gram I.M. or direct I.V. every 6 hours.

PRESCRIBING INFORMATION

ANCEF®
brand of
sterile cefazolin sodium and cefazolin sodium injection

Pediatric Dosage

In children, a total daily dosage of 25 to 50 mg per kg (approximately 10 to 20 mg per pound) of body weight, divided into three or four equal doses, is effective for most mild to moderately severe infections. Total daily dosage may be increased to 100 mg per kg (45 mg per pound) of body weight for severe infections. Since safety for use in premature infants and in infants under one month has not been established, the use of Ancef (sterile cefazolin sodium) in these patients is not recommended.

Pediatric Dosage Guide

Weight		25 mg/kg/Day Divided into 3 Doses		25 mg/kg/Day Divided into 4 Doses	
Lbs	Kg	Approximate Single Dose mg/q8h	Vol. (mL) needed with dilution of 125 mg/mL	Approximate Single Dose mg/q6h	Vol. (mL) needed with dilution of 125 mg/mL
10	4.5	40 mg	0.35 mL	30 mg	0.25 mL
20	9.0	75 mg	0.60 mL	55 mg	0.45 mL
30	13.6	115 mg	0.90 mL	85 mg	0.70 mL
40	18	150 mg	1.20 mL	115 mg	0.90 mL
50	22.7	190 mg	1.50 mL	140 mg	1.10 mL

Wyeth®
Omnipen®-N
(ampicillin sodium)
For Parenteral Administration

Dosage (IM or IV)

Infection	Organisms	Adults	Children*
Respiratory tract	streptococci, pneumococci, nonpenicillinase-producing staphylococci, *H. influenzae*	250-500 mg q. 6 h.	25-50 mg/kg/day in equal doses q. 6 h.
Gastrointestinal tract	susceptible pathogens	500 mg q. 6 h.	50 mg/kg/day in equal doses q. 6 h.
Genitourinary tract	susceptible gram-negative or gram-positive pathogens	500 mg q. 6 h.	50 mg/kg/day in equal doses q. 6 h.
Urethritis (acute) in adult males	*N. gonorrhoeae*	500 mg b.i.d. for 1 day (IM)	

(In complications such as prostatitis and epididymitis, prolonged and intensive therapy is recommended. Gonorrhea cases with suspected primary lesion of syphilis should have dark-field examinations before treatment. In any case suspected of concomitant syphilis, monthly serologic tests for at least 4 months are necessary.)

Infection	Organisms	Adults	Children*
Bacterial meningitis	*N. meningitidis,* *H. influenzae*	8-14 gram/day	100-200 mg/kg/day

(Initial treatment is usually by IV drip, followed by frequent [q. 3-4 h.] IM injections.)
S. viridans

*Children's dosage recommendations are intended for those whose weight will not result in a dosage higher than for the adult.

TAZIDIME™
[tă'zĭ-dēm]
(ceftazidime)
for injection

DOSAGE AND ADMINISTRATION

The guidelines for dosage of Tazidime™ (ceftazidime, Lilly) are listed in Table 3. The following dosage schedule is recommended:

Table 3: Recommended Dosage Schedule for Ceftazidime

	Dose	Frequency
Adults		
Usual recommended dose	1 g IV or IM	q8 or 12h
Uncomplicated urinary tract infections	250 mg IV or IM	q12h
Bone and joint infections	2 g IV	q12h
Complicated urinary tract infections	500 mg IV or IM	q8 or 12h
Uncomplicated pneumonia; mild skin and skin-structure infections	500 mg–1 g IV or IM	q8h
Serious gynecologic and intra-abdominal infections	2 g IV	q8h
Meningitis	2 g IV	q8h
Very severe life-threatening infections, especially in immunocompromised patients	2 g IV	q8h
Pseudomonal lung infections in patients with cystic fibrosis with normal renal function*	30–50 mg/kg IV to a maximum of 6 g/day	q8h
Neonates (0–4 weeks)	30 mg/kg IV	q12h
Infants and Children (1 month to 12 years)	30–50 mg/kg IV to a maximum of 6 g/day†	q8h

23.   An adult weighing 77.3 kg with good cardio-renal function who tolerated a test dose of Fungizone® is to receive this drug IV. What will the dosage be to the nearest tenth mg? _____

24.   Another patient who weighs 67.4 kg is to receive Fungizone® for a severe infection. What will this dosage be to the nearest tenth mg? _____

25.   Dosages can be increased to a maximum of _____ . What would this be to the nearest tenth mg for a patient weighing 63.6 kg? _____

FUNGIZONE® INTRAVENOUS   ℞
Amphotericin B For Injection USP

WARNING
This drug should be used *primarily* for treatment of patients with progressive and potentially life-threatening fungal infections; it should not be used to treat noninvasive forms of fungal disease such as oral thrush, vaginal candidasis and esophegeal candidiasis in patients with normal neutrophil counts.

DOSAGE AND ADMINISTRATION
CAUTION: Under no circumstances should a total daily dose of 1.5 mg/kg be exceeded. Amphotericin B overdoses can result in cardio-respiratory arrest (see OVERDOSAGE).
FUNGIZONE Intravenous should be administered by *slow* intravenous infusion. Intravenous infusion should be given over a period of approximately 2 to 6 hours (depending on the dose) observing the usual precautions for intravenous therapy (see PRECAUTIONS, General). The recommended concentration for intravenous infusion is 0.1 mg/mL (1 mg/10 mL).
Since patient tolerance varies greatly, the dosage of amphotericin B must be individualized and adjusted according to the patient's clinical status (e.g., site and severity of infection, etiologic agent, cardio-renal function, etc.).
A single intravenous **test dose** (1 mg in 20 mL of 5% dextrose solution) administered over 20–30 minutes may be preferred. The patient's temperature, pulse, respiration, and blood pressure should be recorded every 30 minutes for 2 to 4 hours.
In patients with **good cardi-renal function** and a well tolerated test dose, therapy is usually initiated with a daily dose of 0.25 mg/kg of body weight. However, in those patients having **severe and rapidly progressive fungal infection**, therapy may be initiated with a daily dose of 0.3 mg/kg of body weight. In patients with **impaired cardio-renal function** or a **severe reaction to the test dose**, therapy should be initiated with smaller daily doses (i.e., 5 to 10 mg).
Depending on the patient's cardio-renal status (see PRECAUTIONS, Laboratory Tests), doses may gradually be increased by 5 to 10 mg per day to final daily dosage of 0.5 to 0.7 mg/kg.

ANSWERS 1. Yes **2.** Yes **3.** 1910–3820 mg/day; 478–955 mg/dose **4.** Yes **5.** No. Normal is 91 mg/dose **6.** No **7.** Within normal range of 35–131 mg/dose **8.** Yes **9.** 246 mg **10.** Not safe. 43–85 mg/dose is average **11.** Dosage would be 250 mg q.8.h. Range: 372–744 mg/day; 124–248 mg/dose **12.** Yes **13.** No. 69 mg/dose is normal **14.** Within normal range of 40–80 mg/dose **15.** 100–200 mg per dose; within normal limits **16.** 3 **17.** 25 kg **18.** 750–1250 mg per dose **19.** Yes **20.** 18–27 g **21.** 3–4.5 g **22.** No **23.** 19.3 mg **24.** 20.2 mg **25.** 0.7 mg/kg; 44.5 mg

Pediatric & Adult Dosages Based on Body Surface Area

19

OBJECTIVES

The student will

1. calculate BSA using formulas for weight and height
2. use BSA to calculate dosages
3. assess the accuracy of dosages prescribed on the basis of BSA
4. recognize the West nomogram as an alternative for determining BSA

INTRODUCTION

Body surface area (BSA or SA) is a major factor in calculating dosages for some drugs, because many of the body's physiologic processes are more closely related to body surface than they are to weight. One of the major drug classifications which uses body surface to calculate dosages is antineoplastic agents, for cancer chemotherapy. However, an increasing number of other drugs are also calculated using BSA. The nursing responsibility for checking dosages based on BSA varies widely among hospitals, therefore this chapter will cover all three essentials: calculation of BSA, calculation of dosages based on BSA, and assessment of physician orders based on BSA.

Body surface is calculated in **square meters (m²)** using the patient's **weight and height.** The safest way to calculate BSA is by using a calculator which has square root ($\sqrt{}$) capabilities (fortunately most do) and a simple formula. Two formulas are available, one for kg and cm measurements, and another for lb and in measurements.* We'll look at these separately.

Calculating BSA from kg and cm

The formula used to calculate BSA from kg and cm measurements is very easy to remember.

*Carol K. Taketomo, Jane Hurlburt Hodding, and Donna M. Kraus, *Pediatric Dosage Handbook.* Hudson/Cleveland/Akron: Lexi-Comp, Inc., 1993-94, p. 652

FORMULA

$$BSA = \sqrt{\frac{wt\ (kg) \times ht\ (cm)}{3600}}$$

EXAMPLE 1 Calculate the BSA of a man who weighs 104 kg and whose height is 191 cm. Express BSA to the nearest hundredth.

$$\sqrt{\frac{104\ (kg) \times 191\ (cm)}{3600}}$$

$$= \sqrt{5.517}$$

$$= 2.348 = \mathbf{2.35\ m^2}$$

Calculators may vary in the way square root must be obtained, but here's how this BSA was calculated:

104. × 191. ÷ 3600. = 5.517, then immediately enter $\sqrt{\quad}$.

Only the final m² BSA is rounded to hundredths. Your answers may vary slightly depending on how your calculator is set. Consider answers within 2–3 hundredths correct. Fractional weights and heights are also simple to calculate.

EXAMPLE 2 Calculate the BSA of an adolescent who weighs 59.1 kg and is 157.5 cm in height. Express BSA to the nearest hundredth.

$$\sqrt{\frac{59.1\ (kg) \times 157.5\ (cm)}{3600}}$$

$$= \sqrt{2.585}$$

$$= 1.607 = \mathbf{1.61\ m^2}$$

EXAMPLE 3 A child who is 96.2 cm tall weighs 15.7 kg. What is his BSA in m² to the nearest hundredth?

$$\sqrt{\frac{15.7\ (kg) \times 96.2\ (cm)}{3600}}$$

$$= \sqrt{0.4195}$$

$$= 0.647 = \mathbf{0.65\ m^2}$$

Problem

Calculate the BSA in m² for the following patients. Express to the nearest hundredth.

1. An adult weighing 59 kg whose height is 160 cm. _____

2. A child whose weight is 35.9 kg and height 63.5 cm. _____

3. A child whose weight is 7.7 kg and height 40 cm. _____

4. An adult whose weight is 92 kg and height 178 cm. _____

5. A child whose weight is 46 kg and height 102 cm. _____

ANSWERS 1. 1.62 m² 2. 0.8 m² 3. 0.29 m² 4. 2.13 m² 5. 1.14 m²

Calculating BSA from lb and in

The formula for calculating BSA from lb and in measurements is equally easy to use. **The only difference is the denominator, which is 3131.**

FORMULA

$$BSA = \sqrt{\frac{wt\ (lb) \times ht\ (in)}{3131}}$$

EXAMPLE 1 Calculate BSA to the nearest hundredth of a child who is 24 in tall weighing 34 lb.

$$\sqrt{\frac{34\ (lb) \times 24\ (in)}{3131}}$$

$$= \sqrt{0.260}$$

$$= 0.510 = \mathbf{0.51\ m^2}$$

EXAMPLE 2 Calculate BSA to the nearest hundredth of an adult who is 61.3 in tall and weighs 142.7 lb.

$$\sqrt{\frac{142.7\ (lb) \times 61.3\ (in)}{3131}}$$

$$= \sqrt{2.793}$$

$$= 1.671 = \mathbf{1.67\ m^2}$$

EXAMPLE 3 A child weighs 105 lb and is 51 in tall. Calculate BSA to the nearest hundredth.

$$\sqrt{\frac{105\ (lb) \times 51\ (in)}{3131}}$$

$$= \sqrt{1.71}$$

$$= 1.307 = \mathbf{1.31\ m^2}$$

Problem

Determine the BSA for the following patients. Express to the nearest hundredth.

1. A child weighing 92 lb who measures 35 in. _____

2. An adult of 175 lb who is 67 in tall. _____

3. An adult who is 70 in tall and weighs 194 lb. _____

4. A child who is 72.4 lb and 40.5 in tall. _____

5. A child who measures 26 in and weighs 36 lb. _____

ANSWERS **1.** 1.01 m² **2.** 1.94 m² **3.** 2.08 m² **4.** 0.97 m² **5.** 0.55 m²

Dosage Calculation Based on BSA

Once you know the BSA, dosage calculation is simple multiplication.

EXAMPLE 1 Dosage recommended is 5 mg per m². The child has a BSA of 1.1 m².

$$1.1 \times 5 \text{ mg} = \textbf{5.5 mg}$$

EXAMPLE 2 The recommended child's dosage is 25–50 mg per m². The child has a BSA of 0.76 m².

$$0.76 \times 25 = 19 \text{ mg}$$

$$0.76 \times 50 = 38 \text{ mg}$$

The dosage range is **19–38 mg**

Problem

Determine the child's dosage for the following drugs. Express answers to the nearest whole number.

1. The recommended child's dosage is 5–10 mg/m². The BSA is 0.43 m².

    _____

2. A child with a BSA of 0.81 m² is to receive a drug with a recommended dosage of 40 mg/m². _____

3. Calculate the dosage of a drug with a recommended child's dosage of 20 mg/m² for a child with a BSA of 0.50 m². _____

4. An adult is to receive a drug with a recommended dosage of 20–40 U per m². The BSA is 1.93 m². _____

5. The adult recommended dosage is 3–5 mg per m². Calculate dosage for 2.08 m². _____

ANSWERS **1.** 2–4 mg **2.** 32 mg **3.** 10 mg **4.** 39–77 U **5.** 6–10 mg

Determining Accuracy of Orders Based on BSA

In most situations where you will have to check a dosage against m² recommendations you will be referring to drug package inserts, medication protocols, or the PDR to determine what the dosage should be.

EXAMPLE 1 Refer to the vinblastine information insert in figure 79 and calculate the first dose for an adult whose BSA is 1.66 m². Calculations are to the nearest whole number.

Recommended first dose = 3.7 mg/m²

1.66 (m²) × 3.7 mg = 6.14 = **6 mg**

EXAMPLE 2 A child with a BSA of 0.96 m² is to receive her fourth dose of vinblastine.

Recommended fourth dose = 6.25 mg/m²

0.96 (m²) × 6.25 mg = **6 mg**

Cetus Oncology

STERILE VINBLASTINE SULFATE, USP

DOSAGE AND ADMINISTRATION

Caution: It is extremely important that the needle be properly positioned in the vein before this product is injected.

If leakage into surrounding tissue should occur during intravenous administration of vinblastine sulfate, it may cause considerable irritation. The injection should be discontinued immediately, and any remaining portion of the dose should then be introduced into another vein. Local injection of hyaluronidase and the application of moderate heat to the area of leakage help disperse the drug and are thought to minimize discomfort and the possibility of cellulitis.

There are variations in the depth of the leukopenic response which follows therapy with vinblastine sulfate. For this reason, it is recommended that the drug be given no more frequently than *once every 7 days*. It is wise to initiate therapy for adults by administering a single intravenous dose of 3.7 mg/M² of body surface area (bsa); the initial dose for children should be 2.5 mg/M². Thereafter, white-blood-cell counts should be made to determine the patient's sensitivity to vinblastine sulfate. A reduction of 50% in the dose of vinblastine is recommended for patients having a direct serum bilirubin value above 3 mg/100 mL. Since metabolism and excretion are primarily hepatic, no modification is recommended for patients with impaired renal function.

A simplified and conservative incremental approach to dosage *at weekly intervals* may be outlined as follows:

	Adults	Children
First dose	3.7 mg/M² bsa	2.5 mg/M² bsa
Second dose	5.5 mg/M² bsa	3.75 mg/M² bsa
Third dose	7.4 mg/M² bsa	5 mg/M² bsa
Forth dose	9.25 mg/M² bsa	6.25 mg/M² bsa
Fifth dose	11.1 mg/M² bsa	7.5 mg/M² bsa

The above-mentioned increases may be used until a maximum dose (not exceeding 18.5 mg/M² bsa for adults and 12.5 mg/M² bsa for children) is reached. The dose should not be increased after that dose which reduces the white-cell count to approximately 3000 cells/mm³. In some adults, 3.7 mg/M² bsa may produce this leukopenia; other adults may require more than 11.1mg/M² bsa; and, very rarely, as much as 18.5 mg/M² bsa may be necessary. For most adult patients, however, the weekly dosage will prove to be 5.5 to 7.4 mg/M² bsa.

Figure 79

Problem

Calculate the following dosages of vinblastine from the information available in figure 79. Calculate dosages to the nearest whole number.

1. The dosage for an adult's third dosage. The patient's BSA is 1.91 m².

   _____

2. The first child's dosage for a patient with a BSA of 1.2 m². _____

3. The fifth adult dosage. BSA is 1.53 m². _____

4. Calculate the second child's dosage for a BSA of 1.01 m². _____

5. Calculate the second adult dose for a BSA of 2.12 m². _____

ANSWERS **1.** 14 mg **2.** 3 mg **3.** 17 mg **4.** 4 mg **5.** 12 mg

---

BiCNU®
[bĭk 'nū]
(sterile carmustine [BCNU])   ℞

DOSAGE AND ADMINISTRATION
The recommended dose of BiCNU as a single agent in previously untreated patients is 150 to 200 mg/m² intravenously every 6 weeks. This may be given as a single dose or divided into daily injections such as 75 to 100 mg/m² on 2 successive days. When BiCNU is used in combination with other myelosuppressive drugs or in patients in whom bone marrow reserve is depleted, the doses should be adjusted accordingly.

Figure 80

Problem

Refer to figure 80 for BiCNU and locate the following information. Express all dosages to the nearest whole number.

1. What is the dosage per m² if the drug is to be given in a single dose?

   _____

2. If the patient has a BSA of 1.91 m² what will the dosage range be? _____

3. If the order for this patient is a single dosage of 325 mg is there any need to question it? _____

4. If the dosage ordered is 450 mg is there any need to question it? _____

ANSWERS **1.** 150–200 mg/m² **2.** 287–382 mg **3.** No **4.** Yes, too high

Calculation of BSA Using a Nomogram

A nomogram is a **chart of average or normal values.** In the case of nomograms used to calculate BSA, these averages are based on height and weight. A variety of BSA nomograms are in use, the best known perhaps, and the one we will explain, is the West nomogram. Nomograms are not easy to use. They contain columns of heights, weights, and BSA's which are transected with a straightedge to locate the BSA. **If the ruler is even slightly off either height or weight the BSA will be incorrect.**

Until the advent of calculators, which simplified square root calculations, the nomogram was the best tool available for determining BSA. Nomograms are still in use in some hospitals, and your instructor may wish you to do some practice calculations to understand them. However, check before you commit time and effort to this instruction.

Use of the West Nomogram

Refer to figure 81 of the West nomogram, which can be used to calculate BSA for individuals weighing up to 180 lb (80 kg).

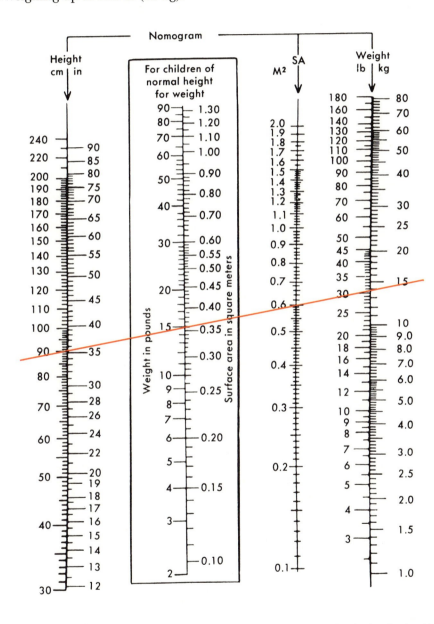

Figure 81 West Nomogram. From Behman, R. E. and Vaughan, V. C. Nelson Textbook of Pediatrics, 12th edition. Philadelphia, W. B. Saunders Co. 1987. Reprinted by permission.

If the patient is a child of roughly normal height and weight for his or her age the BSA can be determined from weight alone. If you refer to the enclosed column second from the left on the nomogram you can see, for example, that a child weighing 30 lb has a BSA of 0.60 m^2.

Before we move on to having you determine some BSA's on your own, we need to point out a peculiarity of nomograms that could cause confusion. Notice that neither the calibrations nor the numbers identifying them rise consistently from the bottom to the top of the graph. **To identify the correct values you must first read the numbers, then determine what the calibrations between them are measuring.** Refer to the column second from the left again, and notice that there is a very large space between 2 and 3 lb at the bottom, while at the top of the scale there is a very narrow space between 80 and 90 lb. Between 15 and 20 lb there are 1 lb increments in calibration representing 16, 17, 18, and 19 lb, but between 80 and 90 lb only one calibration, which represents 85 lb. Similarly, on the bottom of the m^2 scale there are four calibrations between 0.10 and 0.15, which represent 0.11, 0.12, 0.13, and 0.14 m^2. On the top of the m^2 scale there is only one calibration between 1.20 and 1.30 which represents 1.25 m^2. So once again look at the numbers and calibrations very carefully to determine what the measurements are.

Problem

Read the nomogram provided and indicate the BSA in m^2 for the following children of normal height and weight.

1. A child weighing 24 lb _____

2. A child weighing 42 lb _____

3. A child weighing 11 lb _____

4. A child weighing 52 lb _____

5. A child weighing 75 lb _____

ANSWERS   1. 0.50 m^2 **2.** 0.78 m^2 **3.** 0.29 m^2 **4.** 0.90 m^2 **5.** 1.15 m^2

The BSA can also be calculated using both weight and height. The extreme left column for height (in cm and inches), and the extreme right column for weight (in lb and kg) are used for this determination. A ruler is placed on the graph from the height column on the left to the weight column on the right, and the surface area (SA) in m^2 is indicated where this line intersects the SA column second from the right. For example the line already on the nomogram identifies a BSA of 0.59 m^2 for a child weighing 30 lb and measuring 35 inches.

Problem

Use the nomogram provided to calculate the following BSA's.

1. The child is 100 cm long and weighs 55 lb _____

2. A child whose length is 120 cm and weight 40 kg _____

3. A child whose height and weight are 65 cm and 13 kg _____

4. A child whose height is 58 in and weight 12 kg _____

5. A child whose length is 45 in and weight 18 lb _____

ANSWERS   1. 0.86 m^2 **2.** 1.2 m^2 **3.** 0.51 m^2 **4.** 0.66 m^2 **5.** 0.49 m^2

Summary

This concludes dosage calculation based on BSA. The important points to remember from this chapter are:

BSA is calculated from a patient's weight and height

BSA is more important than weight alone in calculating some drug dosages because many physiologic processes are more closely related to surface area than they are to weight

BSA is calculated in square meters (m²) using a formula

the formulas for calculation of BSA are:

$$\sqrt{\frac{wt\ (kg)\ \times\ ht\ (cm)}{3600}} \quad and \quad \sqrt{\frac{wt\ (lb)\ \times\ ht\ (in)}{3131}}$$

once the BSA has been obtained it can be used to calculate specific drug dosages, and assess accuracy of physician orders

nomograms can be used to determine BSA but they are not as accurate as the formula method

Summary Self Test

Use the formula method to calculate the following BSA's. Express BSA to the nearest hundredth.

1. The weight is 58 lb, height is 36 in. _____

2. An adult weighing 74 kg and measuring 160 cm. _____

3. A child who is 14.2 kg and measures 64 cm. _____

4. An adult weighing 69 kg whose height is 170 cm. _____

5. An adolescent who is 55 in and 103 lb. _____

6. A child who is 112 cm and weighs 25.3 kg. _____

7. An adult who weighs 55 kg and measures 157.5 cm. _____

8. An adult who weighs 65.4 kg and is 132 cm in height. _____

9. A child whose height is 58 in and weight 26.5 lb. _____

10. A child whose height and weight are 60 cm and 13.6 kg. _____

Directions: Read the drug insert information provided and answer the following questions pertaining to it. Calculate dosages to the nearest whole number.

11. Read the information on children's dosage for Periactin® syrup and calculate the dosage for a child whose BSA is 0.78 m². _____

12. If a dosage of 4 mg is ordered for this patient would you question it?

_____

13.   What would the daily dosage be for a child whose BSA is 0.29 m²?

_____

14.   What would the daily dosage be for a child with a BSA of 0.51 m²?

_____

PERIACTIN® Syrup   ℞
(Cyproheptadine HCl, MSD), U.S.P.

DOSAGE AND ADMINISTRATION

DOSAGE SHOULD BE INDIVIDUALIZED ACCORDING
TO THE NEEDS AND THE RESPONSE OF THE PATIENT.
Each PERIACTIN tablet contains 4 mg of cyproheptadine
hydrochloride. Each 5 mL of PERIACTIN syrup contains 2
mg of cyproheptadine hydrochloride.
Although intended primarily for administration to children,
the syrup is also useful for administration to adults who cannot swallow tablets.
Children
The total daily dosage for children may be calculated on the
basis of body weight or body area using approximately 0.25
mg/kg/day (0.11 mg/lb/day) or 8 mg per square meter of
body surface (8 mg/M²). In small children for whom the calculation of dosage based upon body size is most important, it
may be necessary to use PERIACTIN syrup to permit accurate dosage.

MUTAMYCIN®   ℞
[mū″-tĕ-mī′-sĭn]
(mitomycin for injection) USP

DOSAGE AND ADMINISTRATION
Mutamycin should be given intravenously only, using care to
avoid extravasation of the compound. If extravasation occurs, cellulitis, ulceration, and slough may result.
Each vial contains either mitomycin 5 mg and mannitol 10
mg, mitomycin 20 mg and mannitol 40 mg, or mitomycin 40
mg and mannitol 80 mg. To administer, add Sterile Water for
Injection, 10 mL, 40 mL or 80 mL, respectively. Shake to
dissolve. If product does not dissolve immediately, allow to
stand at room temperature until solution is obtained.
After full hematological recovery (see guide to dosage adjustment) from any previous chemotherapy, the following dosage schedule may be used at 6- to 8-week intervals:
    20 mg/m² intravenously as a single dose via a functioning
    intravenous catheter.
Because of cumulative myelosuppression, patients should be
fully reevaluated after each course of Mutamycin, and the
dose reduced if the patient has experienced any toxicities.
Doses greater than 20 mg/m² have not been shown to be
more effective, and are more toxic than lower doses.
The following schedule is suggested as a guide to dosage adjustment:

15.   A patient is to receive the antineoplastic drug Mutamycin® IV. The patient's
BSA is 1.46 m². _____

16.   Another patient with a BSA of 2.12 m² is also to receive Mutamycin. What
will the dosage be? _____

17.   A patient is to be treated with the drug Paraplatin® for ovarian carcinoma.
Her BSA is 1.61 m². What will the dosage be? _____

18.   Another patient who weighs 130 lb and measures 62 in is to receive
Paraplatin®. What will her dosage be? _____

19.   A third patient receiving Paraplatin® has a dosage of 637 mg IV ordered. She
is 161 cm tall and weighs 70 kg. Assess this dosage. _____

20.   A patient with Hodgkins disease who weighs 60 kg and is 142 cm tall is
to receive Blenoxane® IV. What is her BSA? _____ What will her
dosage range be? _____ If a dosage of 20 U is ordered must you
question it? _____

PARAPLATIN® ℞
[păr-a-plătin]
(carboplatin for injection)

DOSAGE AND ADMINISTRATION
NOTE: Aluminum reacts with carboplatin causing precipitate formation and loss of potency, therefore, needles or intravenous sets containing aluminum parts that may come in contact with the drug must not be used for the preparation or administration of PARAPLATIN.
PARAPLATIN, as a single agent, has been shown to be effective in patients with recurrent ovarian carcinoma at a dosage of 360 mg/m² IV on day 1 every 4 weeks. In general, however, single intermittent courses of PARAPLATIN should not be repeated until the neutrophil count is at least 2,000 and the platelet count is at least 100,000.
The dose adjustments shown in the table below are modified from a controlled trial in previously treated patients with ovarian carcinoma. Blood counts were done weekly, and the recommendations are based on the lowest posttreatment platelet or neutrophil value.

BLENOXANE® ℞
[blĕ-nŏk'sān]
(sterile bleomycin sulfate, USP)
vial, 15 units NSN 6505-01-060-4278(m)

DOSAGE
Because of the possibility of an anaphylactoid reaction, lymphoma patients should be treated with two units or less for the first two doses. If no acute reaction occurs, then the regular dosage schedule may be followed.
The following dose schedule is recommended: Squamous cell carcinoma, lymphosarcoma, reticulum cell sarcoma, testicular carcinoma—0.25 to 0.50 units/kg (10 to 20 units/m²) given intravenously, intramuscularly, or subcutaneously weekly or twice weekly.
Hodgkin's Disease—0.25 to 0.50 units/kg (10 to 20 units/m²) given intravenously, intramuscularly, or subcutaneously weekly or twice weekly. After a 50% response, a maintenance dose of one unit daily or five units weekly intravenously or intramuscularly should be given.
Pulmonary toxicity of Blenoxane appears to be dose related with a striking increase when the total dose is over 400 units. Total doses over 400 units should be given with great caution.

21. Another patient receiving Blenoxane® weighs 91 kg and measures 190 cm. What will his dosage range be? _____

NOVANTRONE® ℞
[nŏ-văn-trōne]
Mitoxantrone for Injection Concentrate
DOSAGE AND ADMINISTRATION
(See WARNINGS.)
NOVANTRONE SOLUTION MUST BE DILUTED PRIOR TO USE.
Combination Initial Therapy for ANLL in Adults: For induction, the recommended dosage is 12 mg/m² of NOVANTRONE daily on days 1 to 3 given as an intravenous infusion, and 100 mg/m² cytosine arabinoside for 7 days given as a continuous 24-hour infusion on days 1 to 7.
Most complete remissions will occur following the initial course of induction therapy. In the event of an incomplete antileukemic response, a second induction course may be given. NOVANTRONE mitoxantrone for Injection Concentrate should be given for 2 days and cytosine arabinoside for 5 days using the same daily dosage levels.
If severe or life-threatening nonhematologic toxicity is observed during the first induction course, the second induction course should be withheld until toxicity clears.
Consolidation therapy which was used in two large, randomized, multicenter trials consisted of NOVANTRONE 12 mg/m² given by intravenous infusion daily for days 1 and 2 and cytosine arabinoside 100 mg/m² for 5 days given as a continuous 24-hour infusion on days 1 to 5. The first course was given approximately 6 weeks after the final induction course; the second was generally administered 4 weeks after the first. Severe myelosuppression occurred. (See CLINICAL PHARMACOLOGY.)

PLATINOL® ℞
[plă'tĭ-nŏl"]
(cisplatin for injection, USP)

DOSAGE AND ADMINISTRATION
Note: Needles or intravenous sets containing aluminum parts that may come in contact with PLATINOL® (cisplatin for injection, USP) should not be used for preparation or administration. Aluminum reacts with PLATINOL, causing precipitate formation and a loss of potency.
Metastatic Testicular Tumors—The usual PLATINOL dose for the treatment of testicular cancer in combination with other approved chemotherapeutic agents is 20 mg/m² IV daily for 5 days.
Metastatic Ovarian Tumors—The usual PLATINOL dose for the treatment of metastatic ovarian tumors in combination with Cytoxan or other approved chemotherapeutic agents is 75–100 mg/m² IV once every 4 weeks, (Day 1).[1,2]
The dose of Cytoxan when used in combination with PLATINOL is 600 mg/m² IV once every 4 weeks, (Day 1).[1,2]
For directions for the administration of Cytoxan refer to the Cytoxan package insert.
In combination therapy, PLATINOL and Cytoxan are administered sequentially.
As a single agent, PLATINOL should be administered at a dose of 100 mg/m² IV once every 4 weeks.

22. A patient receiving Novantrone® is to have an induction dosage. The BSA is 1.97 m². _____

23. Cytosine arabinoside is to be given at the same time as the Novantrone®. What dosage does the Novantrone® literature specify for cytosine, and what will the dosage be for this patient? _____ _____

24. A second patient receiving these drugs has a BSA of 1.84 m². What will the dosage of Novantrone be? _____ What will the dosage of cytosine be? _____

25. Platinol® is being given for metastatic ovarian carcinoma. What is the dosage range of this drug for a patient with a BSA of 1.29 m²? _____

26. Another patient with metastatic testicular carcinoma is to receive Platinol®. He weighs 173 lb and is 65 in tall. What is his BSA? _____ What will his dosage be? _____

ZOVIRAX® Sterile Powder   ℞
[zō"vī'răx]
(Acyclovir Sodium)
FOR INTRAVENOUS INFUSION ONLY

DOSAGE AND ADMINISTRATION

CAUTION— RAPID OR BOLUS INTRAVENOUS AND INTRAMUSCULAR OR SUBCUTANEOUS INJECTION MUST BE AVOIDED. Therapy should be initiated as early as possible following onset of signs and symptoms. For diagnosis—see INDICATIONS.
Dosage:
HERPES SIMPLEX INFECTIONS
MUCOSAL AND CUTANEOUS HERPES SIMPLEX (HSV-1 and HSV-2) INFECTIONS IN IMMUNOCOMPROMISED PATIENTS —5 mg/kg infused at a constant rate over 1 hour, every 8 hours (15 mg/kg/day) for 7 days in adult patients with normal renal function. In children under 12 years of age, more accurate dosing can be attained by infusing 250 mg/m² at a constant rate over 1 hour, every 8 hours (750 mg/m²/day) for 7 days.

SEVERE INITIAL CLINICAL EPISODES OF HERPES GENITALIS —The same dose given above—administered for 5 days.
HERPES SIMPLEX ENCEPHALITIS —10 mg/kg infused at a constant rate over at least 1 hour, every 8 hours for 10 days. In children between 6 months and 12 years of age, more accurate dosing is achieved by infusing 500 mg/m², at a constant rate over at least one hour, every 8 hours for 10 days.
VARICELLA ZOSTER INFECTIONS
ZOSTER IN IMMUNOCOMPROMISED PATIENTS —10 mg/kg infused at a constant rate over 1 hour, every 8 hours for 7 days in adult patients with normal renal function. In children under 12 years of age, equivalent plasma concentrations are attained by infusing 500 mg/m² at a constant rate over at least 1 hour, every 8 hours for 7 days. Obese patients should be dosed at 10 mg/kg (Ideal Body Weight). A maximum dose equivalent to 500 mg/m² every 8 hours should not be exceeded for any patient.

27. Zovirax® is to be given IV to a child with herpes simplex encephalitis. This patient weighs 34 lb and is 24 in tall. What is the BSA? _____ What will the dosage be? _____

28. An immunocompromised 10 year old child with a herpes simplex infection is to be medicated with Zovirax®. Her weight is 72 lb and height 40 in. What is her BSA? _____ What will the hourly dosage be? _____

29. Another immunosuppressed child is to receive Zovirax® for a varicella zoster infection. His weight is 43 lb and height 28 in. What is his BSA? _____

30. What will the dosage be for this patient? _____

SECTION

SEVEN

Basic IV Therapy and Calculations

20

Introduction to IV Therapy

OBJECTIVES

The student will

1. differentiate between primary and secondary administration sets and peripheral and central IV lines
2. explain the function of drip chambers, roller and slide clamps, and on-line and indwelling injection ports
3. differentiate between volumetric pumps, controllers, syringe pumps and PCA's
4. identify the abbreviations used for IV fluid orders and charting
5. use an IV Guideline/Protocol to locate details of IV medication administration

INTRODUCTION

The calculations associated with IV therapy will be easier to understand if you have some general understanding of IV therapy. IV fluid and medication administration is one of the most challenging of all nursing responsibilities. There are currently estimated to be over 200 different IV fluids being manufactured, and at least as many additives used with IV fluids, including medications, electrolytes and nutrients. In addition there are hundreds of different types of IV administration sets and components, and dozens of different models of electronic devices used to infuse and monitor IV fluids. This would appear to make the entire subject of IV therapy overwhelming, but it is not. This chapter will present the essentials in understandable segments, and give you an excellent base of instruction on which to build. We will begin by looking at a basic sterile IV setup, which is referred to as a primary line.

Primary Line

Refer to figure 82, which shows a typical primary line connecting the IV fluid bag or bottle to the needle or cannula in a vein.

As the photo illustrates, the IV tubing is connected to the IV solution bag (using sterile technique), and the bag is hung on an IV stand. The **drip chamber,** A, is then squeezed to **half fill** it with fluid. This level is very important because IV flow rates are set and monitored by counting the drops falling in this chamber. If the chamber is too full the drops cannot be counted. On the other hand if the outlet at the bottom of the

226

chamber is not completely covered air can enter the tubing during infusions, and subsequently the vein and circulatory system. So the half full fluid level is very important.

Next notice B, the **roller clamp.** This is adjusted while the drops falling in the drip chamber are counted to set the flow rate. It provides an extremely accurate control of rate. A second type of clamp, C, called a **slide clamp,** is present on tubings. The slide clamp can be used to temporarily stop an IV without disturbing the rate set on the roller clamp.

Next notice D, the **injection ports.** Latex ports are located in several locations on the tubing, typically near the cannula end, drip chamber and middle of the line, and on most IV solution bags. Ports allow injection of medication directly into the line or bag, or the attachment of secondary IV lines containing compatible IV fluids or medications to the primary line.

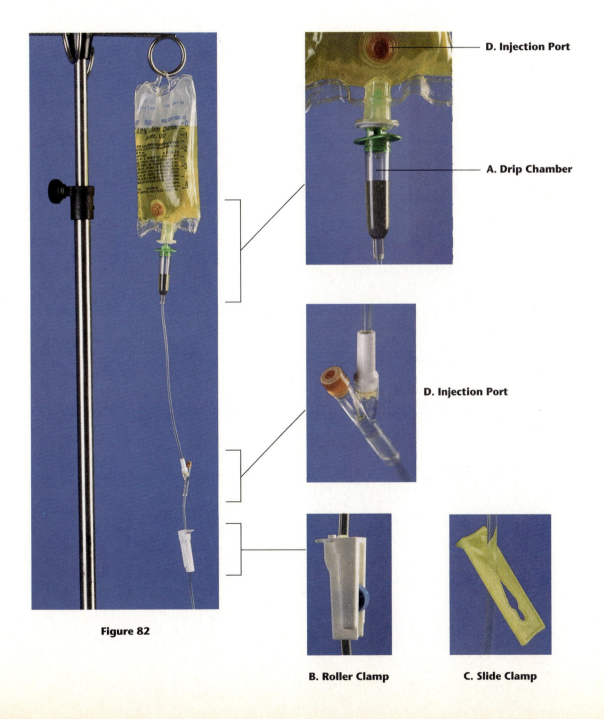

Figure 82

D. Injection Port

A. Drip Chamber

D. Injection Port

B. Roller Clamp

C. Slide Clamp

Intravenous fluids run by gravity flow. This necessitates that the IV solution bag be hung **above the patient's heart level** to exert sufficient pressure to infuse. Three feet is the average height.

 The higher an IV bag is hung, the greater the pressure, and the faster the IV will infuse.

This pressure differential also means that if the flow rate is adjusted while the patient is lying in bed it will slow down if she/he sits or stands, and in fact changes slightly with each turn from side to side. For this reason **monitoring IV flow rate is on going,** officially done every hour, but routinely checked after each major position change.

There are two additional terms relating to primary lines that you must know. If an arm (or less commonly leg) vein is used for an infusion it is referred to as a **peripheral line.** This is to distinguish it from a **central line,** in which a special catheter is used to access a large vein in the chest, either directly through the chest wall, or via a neck vein or peripheral vein in the arm.

Secondary Line

Secondary lines attach to the primary line at an injection port. They are used primarily to infuse medications, frequently on an intermittent basis, for example every 6-8 hours. They may also be used to infuse other compatible IV fluids. Secondary lines are commonly referred to as **IV piggybacks.** They are abbreviated **IVPB.** Refer to figure 83, which illustrates a primary and secondary line setup.

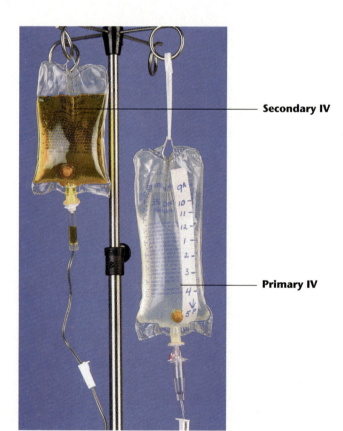

Secondary IV

Primary IV

Figure 83

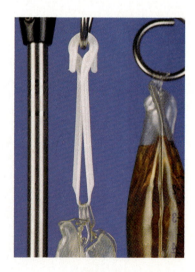

A. Extender

The IVPB is connected to a latex port located below the drip chamber on the primary line. Notice that **the IVPB bag is hanging higher than the primary.** This gives it greater pressure, and causes it to **infuse first.** Each IVPB set includes a metal or plastic **extender,** A, which is used to lower the primary solution bag to obtain this pressure differential. The flow rate for the IVPB is set by a separate roller clamp located on the secondary line. When the IVPB bag has emptied the primary line will automatically resume its flow. Secondary medication bags are usually much smaller than primary bags. Fifty, 100 and 150 cc bags are frequently used. An example is the Cefotan medication bag in figure 84, which as you can see is completely labeled with the drug name and dosage.

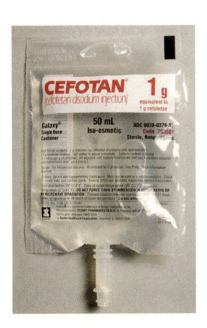

Figure 84

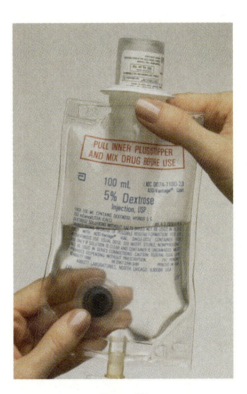

Figure 85

Another type of secondary medication setup is provided by Abbott Laboratories **ADD-Vantage® system** (figure 85).

In this system a specially designed IV fluid bag which contains a **medication vial port** is used. The medication vial containing the ordered drug and dosage is inserted into the port, and the drug (frequently in powdered form) is mixed using IV fluid as the diluent, as illustrated in figure 86. The vial contents are then displaced back into the solution bag and thoroughly mixed in the total solution prior to infusion. The vial remains in the solution bag port throughout the infusion, making it possible to cross check the vial label for drug and dosage at any time.

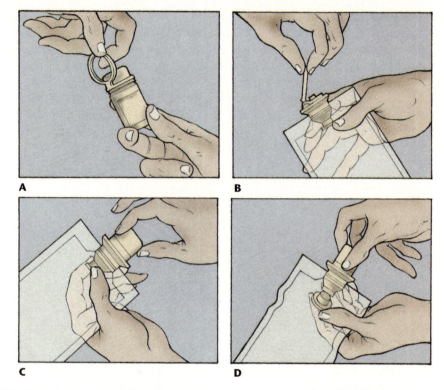

Figure 86 Abbott Laboratories ADD-Vantage® IV medication system **A.** The ADD-Vantage® Medication vial is opened first. **B.** The medication vial port on the IV bag is opened **C.** The vial top is inserted into the IV bag port and twisted to lock tightly in place **D.** The vial stopper is removed *inside* the IV bag and the medication and solution thoroughly mixed prior to infusion

If a drug is not available in either of these pre-packaged or ADD-Vantage® formats it is often totally prepared and labeled by the hospital pharmacy. And finally, an IV medication may be prepared, added to the appropriate IV fluid, thoroughly mixed, labeled and initialed, and administered by the nurse who initiates the infusion.

Volume Controlled Burettes

For greater accuracy in the measurement of **small volume** IV medications and fluids, a **calibrated burette chamber** such as the one in figure 87 may be used.

The total capacity of burettes varies from 100 to 150 mL, calibrated in 1 mL increments. Many burettes are calibrated to deliver very small drops (microdrops), which also contributes to their accuracy. Burettes are most often referred to by their trade names, for example Buretrols®, Solusets®, or Volutrols®. Burette chambers are often connected to a secondary solution bag and used as a secondary line, but they can also be primary lines. When medication is ordered it is injected into the burette through its injection port. The exact amount of IV fluid is then added as diluent. After thorough mixing the flow rate is set using a separate clamp on the burette line. Burettes are extensively used in pediatric and intensive care units, where both medication dosages and fluid volumes are critical.

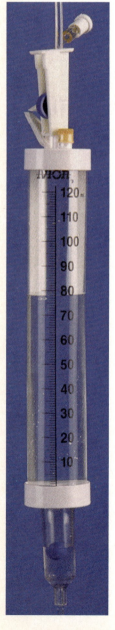

Figure 87

Indwelling Infusion Ports

When a continuous IV is not necessary, but intermittent IV medication administration is, an **infusion port adapter** (figure 88) can be attached to an indwelling cannula in a vein. To infuse the medication the latex port is cleansed and the medication line is attached. When the infusion is complete the line is disconnected until the next dosage is due. Ports are also used for **direct injection of medication using a syringe,** which is called an **IV push, or bolus.** Infusion ports are frequently referred to as **saline locks (or ports), or heplocks.** This terminology evolved because the ports must be irrigated with 1-2 cc of sterile saline every 6-8 hours to prevent clotting and blockage, and because heparin, an anticoagulant, may be used in addition to or instead of the saline flush to keep the line open.

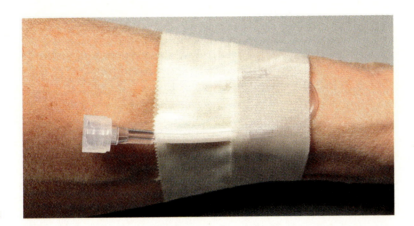

Figure 88

Problem

Answer the following questions about IV administration sets as briefly as possible.

1. What is the correct fluid level for an IV drip chamber? _____

2. Which clamp is used to regulate IV flow rate? _____

3. When might a slide clamp be used? _____

4. What is a peripheral line? _____

5. What is a central line? _____

6. What is the common abbreviation for an intravenous piggyback? _____

7. Is this a primary or secondary line? _____

8. What must the height of a primary solution bag be when a secondary bag is infusing? _____

9. When is a saline or heparin lock used? _____

Electronic Infusion Devices (EID's)

Because the flow rate of IV's can easily be altered or obstructed by a patient's positional changes, electronic infusion devices are widely used for fluid and medication infusions. There are four major categories of devices: Rate Controllers, Volumetric Pumps, Syringe Pumps, and PCA's (Patient Controlled Analgesia devices). Many different models of these devices are available, and it is only possible to talk about them in terms of their general function, rather than specific operation. How to use them must await hands on experience. The function of these devices will be discussed separately.

Electronic Rate Controllers

Controllers work on the same principle of gravity as a regular IV, with the rate of flow being maintained by rapid compression/decompression of the IV tubing by a pincher mechanism inside the controller. Refer to the controller in figure 89.

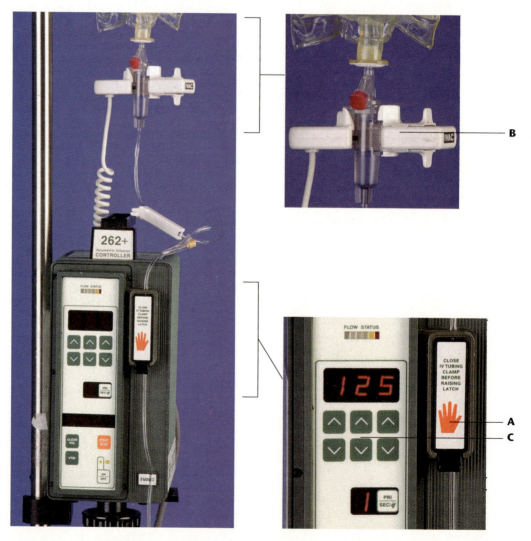

Figure 89

Notice first that the IV tubing is inserted in the controller at A, where the pincher mechanism is located. A **drop sensor,** B, is clipped to the tubing's drip chamber. This sensor monitors the flow rate, and causes the controller to adjust and compensate for flow rate changes. The desired flow rate in mL/hr is set on the controller at the flow rate panel, C (some models may be set in gtt/min).

Here is an example of how the controller would function. An IV is started, and the controller is set to deliver a rate of 125 mL/hr. Inadvertently the patient rolls on to and partially obstructs the IV tubing. The drip sensor immediately senses the slowed rate and causes the controller to adjust its compression/decompression cycle to re-establish the pre-set flow rate. **If the controller cannot maintain this rate it will alarm.**

Remember that a controller works on the principle of gravity; its control is not unlike a roller clamp, in that it adjusts the flow rate by changing the pressure on the IV tubing. The advantage of the controller is that the adjustment is instant, and continuous.

 Because controllers work by gravity the height of the solution bag is critical, and must be maintained at a minimum of 36 inches (3 feet) above the controller.

Electronic Volumetric Pumps

Volumetric pumps look very much like controllers (see figure 90), but their function is quite different.

 A volumetric pump forces fluids into the vein under pressure, and against resistance.

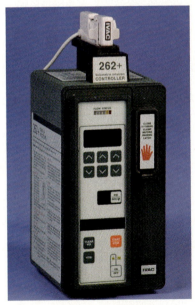 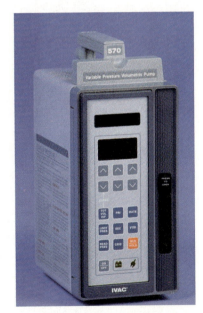

IVAC 262 Controller   IVAC 570 Volumetric Pump

Figure 90

Pumps are **always used for infusions into central veins,** where the pressure is much higher than in the peripheral veins. However, they may also be used with peripheral lines. The flow rate is set in mL/hr to be infused, or on more sophisticated models, by the drug dosage to be administered. A sensor may be used on the drip chamber with a pump, however its function is not to monitor and adjust the flow rate, but to alarm when the drip chamber (and solution bag) is empty. Gravity is not a factor in the use of a pump, and the height of the IV solution bag is not a critical factor. As with controllers, when the pre-set rate cannot be maintained the pump will alarm.

A pump will continue to force IV fluids even if the cannula becomes dislodged and is no longer in the vein.

This can not only be very painful but, depending on the type of solution infusing, can be very damaging to the tissues. For this reason when pumps are used on peripheral lines the IV site must be checked frequently for swelling, coolness or discomfort which could indicate infiltration.

Syringe Pumps

Syringe pumps, as their name implies, are devices which use a syringe to administer medications or fluids (figure 91).

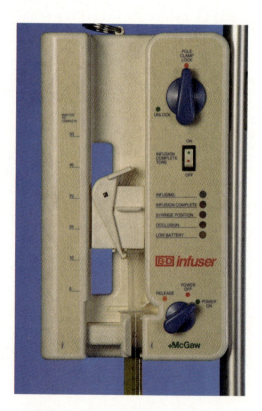

Figure 91 McGaw BD 360 Syringe Pump

Syringe pumps are particularly valuable when **drugs which cannot be mixed with other IV solutions or medications** must be administered at a controlled rate over a short period of time, for example 5, 10, or 20 minutes. The drug is measured in the syringe, which is inserted into the device, and the medication is infused at the rate set.

Patient Controlled Analgesia (PCA) Devices

PCA's allow a patient to **self administer medication to control pain.** A pre-filled syringe of pain medication is inserted into the device (figure 92) and the **dosage and frequency of administration ordered by the doctor is set.** The patient presses the control button, A, as medication is needed, and it is administered and recorded by the PCA.

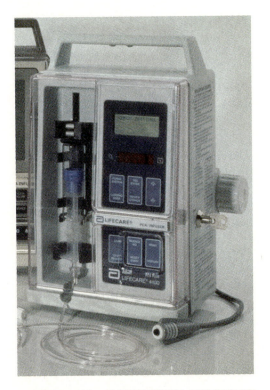

A

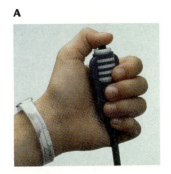

Figure 92   Abbott LIFECARE® PCA 4100 INFUSER

The device also keeps a record of the number of times a patient **attempts** to use it, and thus provides a record of the effectiveness of the dosage prescribed. If a patient's pain is not being relieved new orders must be obtained, and the PCA reset to administer the new dosage.

 All electronic devices must be monitored to be sure they are functioning properly.

Is the IV infusing at the rate which was set? Is the patient who activates a PCA getting relief of pain? If not, is it possible the PCA itself is malfunctioning? Electronic devices have been in use for many years and are relatively trouble free, but if the desired goal is not being obtained, in the absence of other obvious reasons, the possibility of malfunction must always be considered.

Problem

Answer the following questions about EID's as briefly as possible.

1.   What do electronic controllers control? _____

2.   What is the optimum height of the solution bag in relation to a controller?

_____

3.   Why? _____

4.   What is the function of a volumetric pump? _____

5.   When might a syringe pump be used? _____

6.   What is a PCA? _____

ANSWERS   1. IV flow rate   **2.** 36 inches   **3.** IV runs by gravity flow and needs pressure to infuse
4. forces fluids against resistance at a controlled rate   **5.** to infuse drugs which are not compatible with other
drugs and fluids   **6.** patient controlled analgesia device

Introduction to IV Fluids

IV fluids are prepared in plastic solution bags or glass bottles in volumes ranging from
50 cc (bags only) to 1000 cc. The 500 and 1000 cc sizes are the most commonly used. IV
bags and bottles are labeled with the **complete name** of the fluid they contain, and
fine print under the solution name identifies the exact amount of each component of
the fluid. IV **orders and charting,** however, are most often done **using abbreviations.** Some examples of frequently used fluids are: 5% Dextrose in Water, which may
be abbreviated D5W; and 5% Dextrose in Normal Saline, which may be abbreviated
D5NS.

 *In IV fluid abbreviations D always identifies dextrose;
W always identifies water; S identifies saline, NS normal
saline; and numbers identify percentage (%) strengths.*

Solutions may be abbreviated in different ways; for example in addition to D5W
you may see 5%D/W, D5%W, or other combinations. But the initials and percentage
have the identical meaning regardless of the way they are abbreviated. Normal saline solutions are frequently written with the .9 or % sign included, for example D5 .9NS, or
D5 0.9%S. IV fluids with different percentages of saline are also available: 0.45%, often
written as ½ (0.45% is half of 0.9%), and 0.33%, sometimes written as ⅓ (⅓ of 0.9) are
examples. Some typical orders might be abbreviated D5 ½S, or D5 ⅓NS.

Another commonly used solution is **Ringers Lactate,** a balanced electrolyte solution, which is also called Lactated Ringers Solution. As you would now expect, this solution is abbreviated **RL** or **LR,** and possibly RLS. Electrolytes may also be added to the
basic fluids (DW and DS) just discussed. One electrolyte so commonly added that it
must be mentioned is potassium chloride, which is abbreviated KCl. It is measured in
milliequivalents (mEq).

Problem

List as briefly as possible the components and percentage strengths of the following IV solutions.

1.   D10 NS _____

2.   D5 0.2S _____

3.   D2.5 ½S _____

4. D5 ⅓S _____

5. D20W _____

6. D5 0.9%NS _____

7. D5NS 20 mEq KCl _____

8. D5RL _____

ANSWERS 1. 10% Dextrose in 0.9% Saline **2.** 5% Dextrose in 0.2% Saline **3.** 2.5% Dextrose in 0.45% Saline **4.** 5% Dextrose in 0.33% Saline **5.** 20% Dextrose in Water **6.** 5% Dextrose in 0.9% Saline **7.** 5% Dextrose in 0.9% Saline with 20 mEq potassium chloride **8.** 5% Dextrose in Ringer's Lactate solution

Calculating Percentages in IV Fluids

The actual amount of each ingredient in an IV fluid can be calculated. You'll recall that **percent means grams of solute per 100 mL of fluid** (solvent/diluent).

EXAMPLE 1 Calculate the amount of dextrose in 1000 mL 10% DW.

This can be calculated using ratio and proportion.

% = g per 100 mL therefore 10% = 10 g per 100 mL

10 g : 100 mL = X g : 1000 mL
          X = 100 g

1000 mL 10% DW contains 100 g of dextrose

EXAMPLE 2 Determine the amount of dextrose and NaCl in 500 mL 5% DNS.

Dextrose   5 g : 100 mL = X g : 500 mL
                    X = **25 g dextrose**

NaCl   0.9 g : 100 mL = X g : 500 mL
                    X = **4.5 g NaCl**

EXAMPLE 3 Determine the amount of dextrose and NaCl in 250 mL D5 ⅓S.

Dextrose   5 g : 100 mL = X g : 250 mL
                    X = **12.5 g dextrose**

NaCl   0.33 g : 100 mL = X g : 250 mL
                    X = **0.83 g NaCl**

Problem

Calculate the amount of dextrose and NaCl in the following IV solutions.

1. 500 mL D5 ½S   dextrose = _____   NaCl = _____

2. 750 mL D5NS   dextrose = _____   NaCl = _____

ANSWERS 1. 25 g dextrose; 2.25 g NaCl **2.** 37.5 g dextrose; 6.75 g NaCl

This is not a calculation you will have to do very often because **the exact amount of each ingredient is in the fine print on all labels,** directly under the solution name. The point to keep in mind is that IV fluids may contain significant quantities of dextrose, salts and electrolytes. This highlights the importance of IV flow rates, and the considerations necessary when IV's are discovered to have infused ahead of or behind schedule.

IV Medication Guidelines or Protocols

IV drugs far outnumber those given by any other parenteral route. The number of IV drugs has become so large, and the specifics of their administration so varied, that hospitals are increasingly compiling IV **Medication Guidelines or Protocols** to cover all the pertinent details of their administration. This information is compiled from pharmaceutical manufacturers specifications, which in turn are based on clinical testing of a drug. The information contained in protocols may include usual dosage, dilution for IV administration, infusion rates and time, compatibility with other drugs and IV fluids, and patient observations specific for drug action, for example pulse or blood pressure.

Refer to the sample guidelines for adult medications in figure 93, and notice that this particular protocol has columns for Name (with trade name in parenthesis); Administration (IVPB or Push); Dosage, Rate, and Recommended Dilution; and Comments (precautions in use and administration).

GUIDELINES FOR THE ADMINISTRATION OF IV DRUGS

DRUG	ADMINISTRATION	DOSAGE, RATE, RECOMMENDED DILUTION	COMMENTS
Theophylline (Aminophyllin)	IV Drip **IVAC	500 mg/1000 cc 35–50 mg/hr (75–100 cc/hr)	1. Do not mix with any other drug
	IVPB	250 mg/50 cc (30 min) 500 mg/100 cc (50 min)	2. Do not exceed 25 mg/min 3. Assess: P for tachycardia, arrhythmias; BP for hypotension
Vancomycin (Vanocin)	IVPB	0–500 mg/100 cc (30 min) 0.5–1 g/250 cc (30 min)	
Penicillin G	IVPB	0–2 M units/50 cc (45 min) 2–6 M units/100 cc (60 min) 10–20 M units/250–1000 cc (6-8 hrs)	1. Note: Allergies
Pipracillin (Pipracil)	IVPB	< 3 g/50 mL (30 min) > 3 g/100 mL (30 min)	
	IV Push	5 cc diluent/g (3–5 min)	
Oxacillin (Prostaphlin)	IVPB	< 1 g/50 mL NS (30 min) > 1 g/100 mL NS (30 min) > 2 g/250 mL NS (60 min)	
	IV Push	1 g/10 cc in sterile water (20 min)	

Figure 93 Courtesy Scripps Memorial Hospital, La Jolla, CA.

This sample protocol provides a very simplified introduction to IV medications, but it will give you an idea of the kinds of information they contain, and what information you will be expected to locate and understand.

Problem

Examine the information contained on the IV Drug Guidelines in figure 93, and answer the following questions.

1. If Vanocin 400 mg is to be given IVPB how much solution must it be diluted in? _____ What time is specified for its administration? _____

2. When aminophyllin is administered IVPB what observations are required to monitor the patient's reaction to the drug? _____

3. If Pipracil 2.5 g is to be administered IVPB what amount of diluent is specified for its dilution? _____

4. What time is specified for the administration of a 4 g dosage of pipracillin IVPB? _____

5. What type of diluent must be used to dilute oxacillin for IVPB administration? _____ For IV Push administration? _____

6. How much diluent must be used for a 6 M (million) U penicillin dosage IVPB? _____ What time is specified for the infusion? _____

ANSWERS 1. 100 cc; 30 min **2.** P, BP **3.** 50 mL **4.** 30 min **5.** NS; Sterile Water **6.** 100 cc; 60 min

Summary

This concludes your introduction to IV therapy. The important points to remember from this chapter are:

sterile technique is used to set up all IV solutions, tubings and devices

the correct fluid level for an IV drip chamber is half full

injection ports on an IV line are used to connect secondary lines, and infuse medications

a peripheral line refers to an IV infusing in a hand, arm or leg vein

a central line refers to an IV infusing into a chest vein

IV's flow by gravity pressure, and the higher the solution bag the faster the IV will infuse

the average height for an IV solution bag above the patient's heart level is 3 feet

secondary solution bags must hang higher than the primary bag to infuse first

volume controlled burettes are used for very exact measurement of IV medications and fluids

indwelling infusion ports are used to infuse IV medications or fluids on an intermittent basis when a continuous IV is not necessary

controllers are electronic devices which regulate gravity flow IV rates

volumetric pumps are electronic devices which force fluids into a vein under pressure

syringe pumps are used to infuse medications which cannot be mixed with other fluids or medications

patient controlled analgesia (PCA) devices allow a patient to self administer pain medication

in IV fluid abbreviations D identifies Dextrose, W identifies Water, S identifies Saline, NS identifies Normal Saline, RL and LR identify Lactated Ringer's solution, and numbers identify percentage (%) strengths

IV Medication Guidelines/Protocols have been developed to clarify hospital policy on the specific details of IV medication administration

---

Summary Self Test

Directions: You are to assist with some IV procedures. Answer the following situational questions concerning these.

1. A patient is admitted and an IV of 1000 cc D5RL is started. These initials identify what type of solution? _____ This is referred to as a _____ line.

2. The IV is started in the back of the patient's left hand. This makes it a _____ line.

3. You are asked to check the fluid level in the drip chamber, and you observe that it is correct, which is _____ .

4. You are then asked to adjust the flow rate. You will use the _____ clamp to do this.

5. It is decided to use an electronic infusion control device to monitor this gravity flow IV. The device used is a _____ .

6. An IV antibiotic is ordered for the patient. This is sent from the pharmacy already prepared in a small volume IV solution bag. The setup used to infuse this medication is referred to as an IV _____, which is abbreviated _____ .

7. In order for the antibiotic to infuse first, it must be hung _____ than the original solution bag.

8. When you assisted with the IV antibiotic infusion you noticed that the staff nurse referred to a printed sheet of instructions pertaining to IV medication administration. You know that these policies are frequently called Medication _____ or _____ .

9. Some days later the patient's IV is to be discontinued, but he is to continue to receive IV antibiotics. The device used for this intermittent administration is an _____ .

10. If a central vein had been used for the infusion, what type of electronic device would it have been necessary to use? _____

11. The patient had a PCA in use for one day. You know that these initials mean _____ , and that the function of this device is to control _____ .

Directions: Answer the following questions as briefly as possible.

12. A small volume IV medication is to be diluted in 20 mL and infused. This can be most accurately measured using a _____ _____ .

13. These devices are calibrated in _____ mL increments.

14. When an IV medication is injected directly into the vein via a port it is called an IV _____ or _____ .

15. Ports may be irrigated with _____ cc of _____ to prevent blockage every _____ hr.

16. The anticoagulant which may also be used to keep the line open is _____ .

17. A volumetric pump differs from a controller in that it _____ fluids into a vein.

18. What happens if an IV infiltrates while a pump is being used? _____

19.   What is the function of the sensor on the drip chamber when a controller is being used? _____

20.   In IV fluid abbreviations D5 RL identifies what IV fluid? _____

21.   How many grams of NaCl are in 500 mL of D5 0.9NS? _____

22.   How many grams of dextrose does 1000 mL D10W contain? _____

ANSWERS   1. 5% Dextrose in Ringer's Lactate; primary   **2.** peripheral   **3.** half full   **4.** roller   **5.** controller **6.** piggyback; IVPB   **7.** higher   **8.** Guidelines or Protocols   **9.** indwelling infusion port/saline lock/heplock **10.** volumetric pump   **11.** patient controlled analgesia; pain   **12.** calibrated burette   **13.** 1 mL   **14.** Push or bolus   **15.** 1–2; Normal Saline; 6–8   **16.** heparin   **17.** forces   **18.** fluid continues to be forced into the tissues **19.** counts the drops to regulate the flow   **20.** 5% Dextrose in Ringers Lactate   **21.** 4.5 g   **22.** 100 g

IV Flow Rate Calculation

21

OBJECTIVES

The student will

1. identify calibrations in gtt/mL on IV administration sets
2. calculate flow rates by the formula method
3. calculate flow rates by the division factor method

INTRODUCTION

Intravenous fluids are most frequently ordered on the basis of **mL/hr** to be administered, for example 3000 mL/24 hr, 1000 mL/6 hr, or 125 mL/hr. Smaller volumes, usually containing IV medications, may be ordered in **mL/min,** for example 50 mL/20 min, or 10 mL/5 min. The volume ordered is administered by adjusting the rate at which the IV runs, or infuses, which is counted in drops per minute **(gtt/min).** Most flow rate calculations involve changing mL/hr or mL/min ordered into gtt/min.

The size of the drops is regulated by the size of the IV tubing, but unfortunately all tubings (and drops) are not the same size. **IV tubings are calibrated in gtt/mL,** and this calibration is needed to calculate flow rates. The first step in calculating flow rates is therefore to identify the calibration of the tubing to be used.

IV Tubing Calibration

Each hospital uses at least two sizes of IV administration tubings. The first is a **standard or macrodrip set,** for use in routine adult IV administrations. The second is called a **mini or microdrip set** and is used when more exact measurements are needed, for example to infuse medications, or in intensive care and pediatric units, where they are routinely used.

 IV tubings are calibrated in gtt/mL.

Depending on the manufacturer and type of tubing used **it will require 10, 15, or 20 gtt to equal 1 mL in standard macrodrip sets, and 60 gtt to equal 1 mL in mini or microdrip sets.** The calibration, in gtt/mL, is clearly printed on each IV package.

Problem

Refer to the IV tubing packages provided and identify the calibration in gtt/mL of each.

1. _____
2. _____
3. _____
4. _____
5. _____

1

No. 8083

PRIMARY I.V. SET
Nonvented, 100 Inch
BACKCHECK VALVE AND 3 Y-INJECTION SITES.
Piggyback MICRODRIP® with OPTION-LOK™

60 DROPS/mL

2

2C5419 s

Baxter
Vented Basic Set
10 drops/mL

10

3

Twin-Site® Venoset®
with CAIR™ Clamp

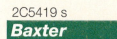
ABBOTT

No. 8957
15 drops/ml.

100 inch I.V. Set (254 cm.), with CAIR* (constant accurate infusion rate) clamp,
drip chamber providing approximately 15 drops per ml., bacterial retentive air filter,
and two Y injection sites 6 and 39 inches (15 and 99 cm.) from male adapter.
Dimensions are nominal.

*Precision roller clamp mfd. for Abbott by Adelberg R&D Laboratories. U.S. Pat. No. 3,685,787; Canadian Pat. No. 926,371.

4

code 880-02
60" (152 cm)
I.V. Set
20 ga x 11/2" (3.8 cm) needle
screw clamp
20 Drops=1ml (approx.)

Cutter

5

Catalog Number: *IV3DO6*
*Non-Vented Burette Set With Microbore Tubing
And Luer-Lock*   *Macrodrop Set: Approx. 20 drops/ml*

IVION CORPORATION
A wholly-owned subsidiary of Medex, Inc.

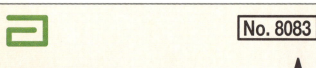

ANSWERS   1. 60 gtt/mL   **2.** 10 gtt/mL   **3.** 15 gtt/mL   **4.** 20 gtt/mL   **5.** 20 gtt/mL

Formula Method of Flow Rate Calculation

When the doctor orders an IV to be infused at a specific mL/hr volume, you will need three pieces of information in order to calculate the flow rate in gtt/min. These are the **total volume to be infused in mL, the calibration of the tubing being used** (which you just learned to locate), **and the time (in minutes) ordered for the infusion.** This information is used in the following formula.

FORMULA

$$\text{Flow Rate} = \frac{\text{Volume} \times \text{Calibration}}{\text{Time (min)}}$$

EXAMPLE 1 The doctor orders an IV to infuse at 125 mL/hr. Calculate the flow rate using a set calibrated at 10 gtt/mL.

Start by converting 1 hour to 60 minutes

$$\frac{125 \text{ (mL)} \times 10 \text{ (gtt/mL)}}{60 \text{ (min)}}$$

$$\frac{125 \times 10}{60} = 20.8 = \textbf{21 gtt/min}$$

 Flow rates are routinely rounded off, and answers within 1–2 gtt/min are considered correct.

EXAMPLE 2 Administer an IV medication of 100 mL in 40 min using a set calibrated at 15 gtt/mL.

$$\frac{100 \times 15}{40} = 37.5 = \textbf{38 gtt/min}$$

EXAMPLE 3 15 mL of an IV medication is ordered to infuse in 30 min. The set calibration is 60 gtt/mL.

$$\frac{15 \times 60}{30} = \textbf{30 gtt/min}$$

Problem

Calculate the flow rate in gtt/min for the following IV administrations.

1. Administer an IV at 110 mL/hr using a set calibrated at 20 gtt/mL.

   _____

2. An IV is ordered to run at 20 mL/hr using a microdrip set calibrated at 60 gtt/mL. _____

3. An IV medication with a volume of 20 mL is to be administered in 20 min using a microdrip set. _____

4. You are to administer 50 mL of an IV antibiotic in 15 min. The set calibration is 10 gtt/mL. _____

5. An IV is ordered to run at 90 mL/hr. The set is calibrated at 15 gtt/mL.

_____

ANSWERS   1. 37 gtt/min   2. 20 gtt/min   3. 60 gtt/min   4. 33 gtt/min   5. 23 gtt/min

The formula method is especially useful for calculating the flow rate of small volumes to be administered in less than an hour. Many medications are given IV in small volume dilutions and this formula works very well for determining the flow rate of these.

When an IV order is written specifying volume to be administered in **more** than one hour the formula can still be used. However, in order to keep the numbers you are working with as small and simple as possible it is best to add a preliminary step, and determine how many **mL/hr** the ordered volume will represent.

EXAMPLE 1 Calculate the flow rate for an IV of 1000 mL to run in over 8 hrs with a set calibrated at 20 gtt/mL.

1000 mL/8 hr = 1000 ÷ 8 = **125 mL/hr**

$$\frac{125 \ (mL) \times 20 \ (gtt/mL)}{60 \ (min)} = 41.6 = \textbf{42 gtt/min}$$

EXAMPLE 2 2500 mL are to infuse in 24 hr with a set calibrated at 10 gtt/mL

2500 ÷ 24 = **104 mL/hr**

$$\frac{104 \times 10}{60} = 17.3 = \textbf{17 gtt/min}$$

EXAMPLE 3 An IV of 1200 mL is ordered to run for 16 hours. Calculate the flow rate if the set is calibrated at 15 gtt/mL.

1200 ÷ 16 = **75 mL/hr**

$$\frac{75 \times 15}{60} = 18.7 = \textbf{19 gtt/min}$$

Problem

Calculate the flow rate in gtt/min for the following infusions.

1. A set with a calibration of 15 gtt/mL is used to infuse 2000 mL in 24 hr.

_____

2. Administer 300 mL in 6 hr. Set is calibrated at 60 gtt/mL. _____

3. Infuse 500 mL in 4 hr. The set calibration is 15 gtt/mL. _____

4. 1200 mL are to be infused in 10 hours. Set calibration is 20 gtt/mL.

   _____

5. 500 mL has been ordered to infuse in 5 hours. The set calibration is 10 gtt/mL. _____

ANSWERS **1.** 21 gtt/min **2.** 50 gtt/min **3.** 31 gtt/min **4.** 40 gtt/min **5.** 17 gtt/min

Division Factor Method of Flow Rate Calculation

A second method called **the division factor method** can be used to determine flow rates. It derives from the same formula you just learned, but **it can only be used if the volume to be administered is expressed in mL/hr (mL/60 min).** Let's start by looking at how the division factor is obtained.

Order: Administer an IV at 125 mL/hr. Calibration of the set is 10 gtt/mL (remember that the volume must be expressed as **mL/60 min**).

$$\frac{125 \text{ (mL)} \times \cancel{10}^{1} \text{ (gtt/mL)}}{\cancel{60}_{6} \text{ (min)}} = 20.8 = \textbf{21 gtt/min}$$

Notice that because you are restricting the time to 60 minutes, the set calibration (10) can be divided into 60 to obtain a constant number (6). **This (6) is the division factor.**

 The division factor can be obtained for any IV administration set by dividing 60 by the calibration of the set.

Problem

Determine the division factor of the following IV sets.

1. 20 gtt/mL   2. 15 gtt/mL   3. 60 gtt/mL   4. 10 gtt/mL

ANSWERS **1.** 3 **2.** 4 **3.** 1 **4.** 6

 Once you know the division factor, the flow rate can be calculated in one step, by dividing the mL/hr to be administered by the division factor.

DIVISION FACTOR METHOD:

Flow Rate = mL/hr ÷ Division Factor

EXAMPLE 1　Administer an IV at 100 mL/hr using a set calibrated at 10 gtt/mL

- Determine the division factor

    $60 \div 10 = \mathbf{6}$

- Calculate the flow rate

    $100 \div 6 = 16.6 = \mathbf{17\ gtt/min}$

EXAMPLE 2　Administer an IV at 125 mL/hr using a set calibrated at 15 gtt/mL.

$60 \div 15 = 4$　　$125 \div 4 = 31.2 = \mathbf{31\ gtt/min}$

EXAMPLE 3　Administer an IV of 50 mL/hr. Set is calibrated at 60 gtt/mL.

$60 \div 60 = 1$　　$50 \div 1 = \mathbf{50\ gtt/min}$

Notice that when a microdrip set calibrated at 60 gtt/mL is used, the division factor is 1. Therefore **the flow rate in gtt/min is the same as the volume in mL/hr for microdrip sets.**

EXAMPLE 4　Administer an IV of 80 mL/hr. Set is calibrated at 60 gtt/mL.

$80 \div 1 = \mathbf{80\ gtt/min}$

Problem

Calculate the flow rates for the following IV infusions using the division factor method.

1.　Administer 110 mL/hr via a set calibrated at 20 gtt/mL. _____

2.　Set is calibrated at 15 gtt/mL. Administer 130 mL/hr. _____

3.　Infuse 150 mL in 1 hour. Set calibration is 10 gtt/mL. _____

4.　A set calibrated at 60 gtt/mL is used to administer 45 mL/hr. _____

5.　Infusion is ordered at the rate of 75 mL/hr with a set calibrated at 15 gtt/mL. _____

ANSWERS　**1.** 37 gtt/min　**2.** 33 gtt/min　**3.** 25 gtt/min　**4.** 45 gtt/min　**5.** 19 gtt/min

The division factor method can be used to calculate the flow rate of **any volume that can be expressed in mL/hr.** Larger volumes can be divided and expressed in mL/hr, and smaller volumes can be multiplied and expressed in mL/hr.

EXAMPLE 1　2400 mL/24 hr = $2400 \div 24 = 100$ mL/hr

EXAMPLE 2　1800 mL/8 hr = $1800 \div 8 = 225$ mL/hr

EXAMPLE 3　10 mL/30 min = $10 \times 2\ (2 \times 30\ \text{min}) = 20$ mL/hr

EXAMPLE 4　15 mL/20 min = $15 \times 3\ (3 \times 20\ \text{min}) = 45$ mL/hr

Once converted to mL/hr equivalents, these administrations can be calculated using the division factor method.

Problem

Calculate the following IV flow rates using the division factor method.

1. An IV of 2000 mL is to infuse in 10 hours using a set calibrated at 20 gtt/mL. _____

2. An IV antibiotic in 20 mL of solution is to run over 20 minutes with a micro-drip. _____

3. 3000 mL is to infuse IV in the next 24 hours using a 15 gtt/mL set. _____

4. An IV medication diluted in 30 mL is to infuse in 40 min using a microdrip set. _____

5. An IV of 100 mL is to run in 30 minutes with a set calibrated at 20 gtt/mL. _____

ANSWERS 1. 67 gtt/min   **2.** 60 gtt/min   **3.** 31 gtt/min   **4.** 45 gtt/min   **5.** 67 gtt/min

Regulating Flow Rate

The flow rate is regulated by counting the number of drops falling in the drip chamber. The standard procedure for doing this is to hold a watch next to the drip chamber and actually count the drops for 15 seconds, while using the roller clamp to adjust the flow rate to the desired gtt/min. For example, if the required rate is 40 gtt/min you would adjust the flow rate to 10 gtt in 15 seconds (40 ÷ 4).

Problem

1. The 15 second count of an IV flow rate is 7 gtt. A 29 gtt/min rate is required. Is this rate correct? _____

2. You are to regulate a newly started IV to deliver 67 gtt/min. Using the 15 second count, how would you set the flow rate? _____

3. An IV is to run at 48 gtt/min. What must the drop rate be for 15 seconds? _____

4. How many gtt will you count in 15 sec if the rate is 55 gtt/min? _____

5. An IV is to run at 84 gtt/min. The 15 sec count will be _____

Because a patient's positional changes alter the rate slightly IV's occasionally infuse ahead of, or behind schedule. When this occurs the usual procedure is to recalculate the flow rate using the volume and time remaining, and adjust the rate accordingly. However each situation must be individually evaluated, especially if the discrepancy is large. If too much fluid has infused, immediately assess the patient's response to the increased intake, and take appropriate action. If too little fluid has infused it will first be necessary to assess the patient's ability to tolerate an increased rate, and secondly to consider the type of fluid/medication involved. Some medications in particular have restrictions on rate of administration. Both of these factors must be considered before rates can be increased to "catch up." In addition some hospitals will have specific policies to cover over or under infusion due to altered flow rates, and you are responsible for knowing these.

The following examples show how the rate would be recalculated.

EXAMPLE 1   An IV of 1000 mL was ordered to infuse over 10 hours at a rate of 25 gtt/min. The set calibration is 15 gtt/mL. After 5 hours you notice that 650 mL have infused instead of the 500 mL ordered. Recalculate the flow rate for the remaining solution.

Time remaining = 5 hours

Volume remaining = 350 mL

350 mL ÷ 5 = 70 mL/hr

Set calibration is 15 gtt/mL

70 ÷ 4 (division factor) = 17.5 = **18 gtt/min**

Slow the rate from 25 gtt/min to 18 gtt/min

EXAMPLE 2   An IV of 800 mL was to infuse over 8 hours at 20 gtt/min. After 5 hours you discover that only 300 mL have infused. Recalculate the flow rate using a set calibrated at 15 gtt/mL.

Time remaining = 3 hours

Volume remaining = 500 mL

500 ÷ 3 = 166.6 = 167 mL/hr

167 ÷ 4 = 41.8 = **42 gtt/min**

Increase the rate to 42 gtt/min

EXAMPLE 3   An IV of 500 mL is infusing at 28 gtt/min. It was to be completed in 3 hr, but after 1½ hr (1.5 hr) only 175 mL have infused. The set calibration is 10 gtt/mL.

Time remaining = 1.5 hr

Volume remaining = 325 mL

$325 \div 1.5 = 216.6 = 217$ mL/hr

$217 \div 6 = 36.1 = $ **36 gtt/min**

Increase the rate to 36 gtt/min

EXAMPLE 4 250 mL were to infuse at 56 gtt/min in 1½ hr using a set calibrated at 20 gtt/mL. After 30 min 175 mL have infused. Recalculate the flow rate.

Time remaining = 1 hr

Volume remaining = 75 mL

$75 \div 3 = $ **25 gtt/min**

Decrease the rate to 25 gtt/min

Problem

1. An IV of 500 mL was ordered to infuse in 3 hours using a 15 gtt/mL set. With 1½ hours remaining you discover only 150 mL is left in the bag. At what rate will you need to reset the flow? _____

2. An IV of 1000 mL was scheduled to run in 12 hours. After 4 hours only 220 mL have infused. The set calibration is 20 gtt/mL. Recalculate the rate for the remaining solution. _____

3. An IV of 1000 mL was ordered to infuse in 8 hours. With 3 hours of infusion time left you discover that 600 mL have infused. The set delivers 20 gtt/mL. Recalculate the drip rate and indicate how many drops you will count in 15 seconds to set the new rate. _____ _____

4. An IV of 750 mL was ordered to run over 6 hours with a set calibrated at 10 gtt/mL. After 2 hours you notice that 300 mL have infused. Recalculate the flow rate, and indicate how many drops you will count in 15 seconds to reset the rate. _____ _____

5. An IV of 800 mL was started at 9 a.m. to infuse in 4 hours. At 10 a.m. 150 mL have infused. The set is calibrated at 15 gtt/mL. Recalculate the flow rate in gtt/min. _____

ANSWERS 1. 25 gtt/min **2.** 33 gtt/min **3.** 44 gtt/min; 11 gtt/15 sec **4.** 19 gtt/min; 4–5 gtt/15 sec **5.** 54 gtt/min

Summary

This concludes the chapter on IV flow rate calculation and monitoring. The important points to remember from this chapter are:

IV's are ordered as mL/hr or mL/min to be administered

the flow rate is counted in gtt/min

IV tubings are calibrated in gtt/mL

macrodrip IV sets will have a calibration of 10, 15, or 20 gtt/mL

mini or microdrip sets have a calibration of 60 gtt/mL

the formula for calculating flow rates is:

$$\frac{Volume \times set\ calibration}{time\ (min)}$$

the division factor method can only be used to calculate flow rates if the volume to be administered is specified in mL/hr (60 min)

the division factor is obtained by dividing 60 by the set calibration

flow rate by the division factor method is determined by dividing the mL to be administered by the division factor

because micro and minidrips have a calibration of 60 gtt/mL, their division factor is 1, and the flow rate in gtt/min is the same as the mL/hr ordered

if an IV gets ahead of or behind schedule a standard procedure is to use the time and mL remaining and calculate a new flow rate

if a rate must be increased to compensate for running behind schedule, the type of fluid being infused and the patient's ability to tolerate an increased rate must be assessed

Summary Self Test

Directions: Answer the following questions as briefly as possible.

1. Write the formula used for IV flow rate calculations _____

2. Determine the division factor for the following IV sets.

    a) 60 gtt/mL _____

    b) 15 gtt/mL _____

    c) 20 gtt/mL _____

    d) 10 gtt/mL _____

3. How is the flow rate determined in the division factor method?

    _____

4. The division factor method can only be used if the volume to be administered is expressed in _____

5. An IV is to infuse at 50 gtt/min. How will you set it using a 15 second count? _____

6. You are to adjust an IV at a rate of 60 gtt/min. What will the 15 second count be? _____

Directions: Calculate the flow rate for each of the following IV solutions and medications. Do not let the types of solutions confuse you. Concentrate on locating the information you need for your calculations.

7. D5W 2000 mL has been ordered to run 16 hrs. Set calibration is 10 gtt/mL. _____

8. The order is for 500 mL 0.9% Normal Saline in 8 hrs. The set is calibrated at 15 gtt/mL. _____

9. Administer 150 mL of 5% Sodium Chloride over 3 hrs. A microdrip is used. _____

10. 1500 mL D5W with 40 mEq KCl/L has been ordered to run over 12 hrs. Set calibration is 20 gtt/mL. _____

11. An IV medication of 30 mL is to be administered over 30 min using a 15 gtt/mL set. _____

12. Administer 100 mL 0.9% NaCl in 1 hour using a 15 gtt/mL set. _____

13. Infuse 500 mL intralipids IV in 6 hours. Set calibration is 10 gtt/mL. _____

14. The doctor orders a liter of D5W to infuse over 10 hours. At the end of 8 hours you notice that there is 500 mL left in the bag. What would the new flow rate be if the set calibration is 10 gtt/mL. _____

15. An IV was started at 9 a.m. with orders to infuse 500 mL over 6 hrs. At 12 noon the IV infiltrated with 350 mL left in the bag. At 1 p.m. the IV was restarted. The set calibration is 20 gtt/mL. Calculate the new flow rate to deliver the fluid on time. _____

16. A 50 mL piggyback IV is to infuse over 15 min. The set calibration is 15 gtt/mL. After 5 minutes the IV contains 40 mL. Calculate the flow rate to deliver the volume on time. _____

17. An IV of 1000 cc D5 ¼NS with 20 mEq KCl is ordered to run at 25 mL/hr using a microdrip set. _____

18. Ringers Lactate 800 mL has been ordered to run in over 5 hours. Set calibration is 10 gtt/mL. _____

19. Administer 1500 mL D5 Lactated Ringers solution over 8 hours using a set calibrated at 20 gtt/mL. _____

20. The order is for D5 ½NS 750 mL over 6 hours. Set calibration is 15 gtt/mL. _____

21. An IV of 1000 mL was ordered to run over 8 hours. After 4 hours only 250 mL have infused. The set calibration is 20 gtt/mL. Recalculate the rate for the remaining solution. _____

22. The order is to infuse 50 mL of a piggyback antibiotic over 1 hour. The set calibration is a microdrip. _____

23. An IV of 500 mL D5W is to infuse over 6 hours. You will be using a set calibration of 10 gtt/mL. _____

24. Infuse 120 mL gentamicin via IVPB over 1 hour. Set calibration is 10 gtt/mL. _____

25. Administer 12 mL of an IV medication in 22 min using a microdrip set. _____

26. A patient is to receive 3000 mL of D5W over 20 hours. Set is calibrated at 20 gtt/mL. _____

27. Infuse 1 liter of D5W over 5 hours using a set calibration of 15 gtt/mL. _____

28. A hyperalimentation solution of 1180 mL is to infuse over 12 hours using a set calibration of 20 gtt/mL. _____

29. 150 mL of an antibiotic solution is to infuse over 30 minutes. At the end of 20 minutes you discover that 100 mL has infused. The set calibration is 10 gtt/mL. Should the flow rate be adjusted? If so, what is the new rate? _____

30. Two 500 mL units of whole blood are ordered. Both units are to be completed in 5 hours. The set calibration is 20 gtt/mL. _____

31. Infuse 15 mL of IV medication over the next 14 minutes using a 20 gtt/mL set. _____

32. The patient is to receive 1000 mL 0.9% NaCl in 10 hours using a 20 gtt/mL calibration. _____

33. A minidrip is used to administer 12 mL in 17 minutes. _____

34. Infuse 2750 mL over 20 hours using a 10 gtt/mL set. _____

35. D5W 1800 mL is to infuse in the next 15 hours with a 15 gtt/mL set. _____

36. Infuse 600 mL intralipids IV in 6 hours with a 10 gtt/mL set. _____

37. Administer 22 mL of an IV antibiotic solution in 18 minutes using a minidrip set. _____

38. 1800 mL of D5W with 30 mEq of KCl per liter has been ordered to infuse in 10 hours. Set calibration is 20 gtt/mL. _____

39. Infuse 8 mL in 9 minutes using a minidrip. _____

40. A patient is to receive 4000 mL D5W IV in the next 20 hours. A 20 gtt/mL set is used. _____

41. An IV of 500 mL D5W which was to infuse in 2 hr is discovered to have only 150 mL left after 30 min. Recalculate the flow rate. Set calibration is 15 gtt/mL. _____

42. 750 mL are to infuse in 5 hr at a rate of 150 mL/hr using a set calibrated at 20 gtt/mL. Calculate the drip rate, and indicate how many gtt you will count in 15 sec to set it. _____ _____

ANSWERS 1. volume × set calibration ÷ time (min) **2.** *a)* 1 *b)* 4 *c)* 3 *d)* 6 **3.** mL/hr ÷ division factor **4.** mL/hr (mL/60 min) **5.** 13 gtt/15 sec **6.** 15 gtt/15 sec **7.** 21 gtt/min **8.** 16 gtt/min **9.** 50 gtt/min **10.** 42 gtt/min **11.** 15 gtt/min **12.** 25 gtt/min **13.** 14 gtt/min **14.** 42 gtt/min **15.** 58 gtt/min **16.** 60 gtt/min **17.** 25 gtt/min **18.** 27 gtt/min **19.** 63 gtt/min **20.** 31 gtt/min **21.** 63 gtt/min **22.** 50 gtt/min **23.** 14 gtt/min **24.** 20 gtt/min **25.** 33 gtt/min **26.** 50 gtt/min **27.** 50 gtt/min **28.** 33 gtt/min **29.** No, rate is correct at 50 gtt/min **30.** 67 gtt/min **31.** 21 gtt/min **32.** 33 gtt/min **33.** 42 gtt/min **34.** 23 gtt/min **35.** 30 gtt/min **36.** 17 gtt/min **37.** 73 gtt/min **38.** 60 gtt/min **39.** 53 gtt/min **40.** 67 gtt/min **41.** 25 gtt/min **42.** 50 gtt/min; 13 gtt/15 sec

22 Calculating Total Infusion Times

OBJECTIVES

The student will calculate total infusion times using
1. the basic infusion time formula
2. gtt/min and set calibration using ratio and proportion
3. gtt/min and set calibration using a formula
4. an IV solution bag tape to label start, progress and finish times

INTRODUCTION

The infusion time is the **total time necessary for a given volume of solution to infuse intravenously.** The time may be in minutes, hours or days depending on the type of solution and the individual patient needs. The total time required for the infusion to be completed is determined by three factors: volume to be infused, drip rate, and set calibration. Once these factors are known the total infusion time can be quickly calculated. It is good planning to have the next solution prepared and ready to hang before the present one is completed. Determining infusion times is also important because laboratory studies are often made before, during, or after specified amounts of IV solutions have infused.

Basic Infusion Time Formula

An easy one step formula is used to determine basic infusion time.

> *FORMULA*
>
> $$\text{Infusion Time} = \frac{\text{total volume to infuse}}{\text{mL/hr being infused}}$$

To use this formula you must determine the total volume to be infused, and how many mL/hr the patient is receiving.

EXAMPLE 1 Calculate the infusion time for an IV of 500 mL D5W that is infusing at 50 mL/hr.

$$\frac{500 \text{ mL (total volume)}}{50 \text{ mL/hr (mL/hr to infuse)}} = 500 \div 50 = \textbf{10 hours}$$

Infusion time = 10 hours

EXAMPLE 2 A doctor orders 1000 mL of D5NS to infuse at 75 mL/hr. Calculate the infusion time to the nearest hundredth.

$$\frac{1000 \text{ mL}}{75 \text{ mL/hr}} = 13.33$$

In this example the 13 represents 13 hours, while **.33 represents a fraction of an additional hour.** To convert .33 to minutes multiply by 60 (min).

60 × .33 = 19.8 = **20 min**   Round off the minutes to the nearest whole number

Infusion time = 13 hr 20 min

EXAMPLE 3 A patient has an IV of 1000 mL 5% D5W infusing at 90 mL/hr. How many hours will it take this IV to complete?

$$\frac{1000 \text{ mL}}{90 \text{ mL/hr}} = 11.11$$

Remember that the 11 represents hours, but the .11 is a fraction of an additional hour. Convert to minutes by multiplying by 60.

.11 × 60 min = 6.6 or **7 min**

Infusion time = 11 hr 7 min

The second step in calculating the infusion time is to use it to determine when the IV will be completed. If the IV in example 3 was started at 7:30 a.m., at what time will it be completed? Add the 11 hr 7 min infusion time to 7:30 a.m. **The answer is 6:37 p.m.**

EXAMPLE 4 An IV of 750 mL RL is to infuse at a rate of 80 mL/hr. What is the infusion time?

$$\frac{750 \text{ mL}}{80 \text{ mL/hr}} = 9.38$$

Convert .38 to minutes by multiplying by 60

.38 × 60 = 22.8 = **23 min**

Infusion time is 9 hr 23 min

If this IV was started at 0910 when will it be completed?

0910 + 9 hr 23 min = **1833**

EXAMPLE 5 An IV of 500 mL D5W is to infuse at a rate of 75 mL/hr. What is the infusion time?

$$\frac{500 \text{ mL}}{75 \text{ mL/hr}} = 6.67$$

.67 × 60 = 40.2 = **40 min**

The infusion time is 6 hr 40 min

If this IV was started at 8:30 p.m. when will it be completed?

8:30 + 6 hr 40 min = **2:40 a.m.**

Problem

1.   What is the infusion time for an IV of 900 mL RL ordered to infuse at a rate of 80 mL/hr. _____ If this IV was started at 0810 when would it be totally infused? _____

2.   The doctor orders a volume of 250 mL to be infused at 30 mL per hour. You start the infusion at 12 noon. Calculate the infusion time. _____ When will the IV be completed? _____

3.   A volume of 180 mL of NS is ordered to infuse at 25 mL/hr. Calculate the infusion time. _____ If the infusion is started at 0240 when will it be completed? _____

4.   An IV of 1000 mL 5% DW is ordered to infuse at 60 mL/hr. What is the infusion time? _____ If this IV is started at 6:14 a.m. when will it be complete? _____

5.   An IV medication of 150 cc is to infuse at a rate of 80 cc/hr. What is the infusion time? _____ If the infusion is started at 1100 when will it be completed? _____

ANSWERS   **1.** 11 hr 15 min; 1925   **2.** 8 hr 20 min; 8:20 p.m.   **3.** 7 hr 12 min; 0952   **4.** 16 hr 40 min; 10:54 p.m.
5. 1 hr 53 min; 1253

Calculating from gtt/min and Set Calibration Using Ratio and Proportion

In some instances the only information you may have is the total volume to infuse, the gtt/min the IV is infusing at, and the set calibration of the tubing. You can still use the same infusion time formula but first must convert gtt/min to mL/hr. This is done in a 2 step procedure using ratio and proportion. Here's how.

EXAMPLE 1   Calculate the infusion time for an IV of 1000 mL of D5W running at 25 gtt/min using a set calibrated at 10 gtt/mL.

■ To determine the number of mL/hr the IV is infusing at, first **convert gtt/min to mL/min infusing**

$$10 \text{ gtt} : 1 \text{ mL} = 25 \text{ gtt} : \text{X mL}$$
$$10X = 25$$
$$X = 25 \div 10 = \textbf{2.5 mL/min}$$

- **Next, convert mL/min to mL/hr**

$$2.5 \text{ mL/min} \times 60 \text{ (min)} = \textbf{150 mL/hr}$$

- **Now determine the infusion time using the same basic formula**

$$\frac{1000 \text{ mL}}{150 \text{ (mL/hr)}} = 6.67$$

$$60 \text{ min} \times .67 = 40.2 = \textbf{40 min}$$

Infusion time = 6 hr 40 min

EXAMPLE 2 A patient is to receive 750 mL D5RL at a flow rate of 12 gtt/min using a set calibration of 10 gtt/mL. Calculate the infusion time.

- **Convert gtt/min to mL/min**

$$10 \text{ gtt} : 1 \text{ mL} = 12 \text{ gtt} : \text{X mL}$$
$$10X = 12$$
$$X = 12 \div 10 = \textbf{1.2 mL/min}$$

- **Convert mL/min to mL/hr**

$$1.2 \text{ mL/min} \times 60 \text{ min} = \textbf{72 mL/hr}$$

- **Calculate infusion time**

$$\frac{750 \text{ mL}}{72 \text{ mL/hr}} = 10.42$$

$$60 \text{ min} \times .42 = 25.2 = \textbf{25 min}$$

Infusion time = 10 hr 25 min

EXAMPLE 3 Determine the infusion time of 100 mL of D5NS infusing at a rate of 40 gtt/min using a microdrip set.

- **Convert gtt/min to mL/min**

$$60 \text{ gtt} : 1 \text{ mL} = 40 \text{ gtt} : \text{X mL}$$
$$60X = 40$$
$$X = 40 \div 60 = \textbf{0.67 mL/min}$$

- **Convert mL/min to mL/hr**

$$0.67 \text{ mL/min} \times 60 \text{ min} = 40.2 = \textbf{40 mL/hr}$$

- **Calculate infusion time**

$$\frac{100 \text{ mL}}{40 \text{ mL/hr}} = 2.5$$

60 min $\times$ .5 = **30 min**

Infusion time = 2 hr 30 min

EXAMPLE 4 Calculate the infusion time of an IV that has a volume of 150 mL and is infusing at 20 gtt/min using a set calibration of 15 gtt/mL.

- 15 gtt : 1 mL = 20 gtt : X mL
     15X = 20
         X = 20 ÷ 15 = 1.33 = **1.3 mL/min**

- 1.3 mL/min $\times$ 60 min = **78 mL/hr**

- $\dfrac{150 \text{ mL}}{78 \text{ mL/hr}} = 1.92$

- .92 $\times$ 60 min = 55.2 = **55 min**

Infusion time = 1 hr 55 min

EXAMPLE 5 The order is to infuse 1100 mL of hyperalimentation solution. The set calibration is 10 gtt/mL and the flow rate is 10 gtt/min. Calculate the infusion time.

- 10 gtt : 1 mL = 10 gtt : X mL
     10X = 10
         X = 10 ÷ 10 = **1 mL/min**

- 1 mL/min $\times$ 60 min = **60 mL/hr**

- $\dfrac{1100 \text{ mL}}{60 \text{ mL/hr}} = 18.33$

- .33 $\times$ 60 min = 19.8 = **20 min**

Infusion time = 18 hr 20 min

Problem

1. Determine the infusion time of 1 liter 5% DW at a flow rate of 33 gtt/min and a set calibration of 15 gtt/mL. _____

2. The doctor asks at what time a patient's infusion will be completed. There is 250 mL left in the IV with a flow rate of 25 gtt/min and set calibration of 10 gtt/mL. The time is now 1 p.m. _____

3. A volume of 100 mL is ordered to infuse at 10 gtt/min. The set calibration of the tubing is 10 gtt/mL. Calculate the infusion time. _____

4. Calculate the infusion time for an IV of 900 mL D5W to infuse at 30 gtt/min using a set calibrated at 20 gtt/mL. _____

5. What is the infusion time for an IV of 200 mL running at 18 gtt/min using a set calibration of 15 gtt/mL. _____

ANSWERS **1.** 7 hr 35 min **2.** 2:40 p.m. **3.** 1 hr 40 min **4.** 10 hr **5.** 2 hr 47 min

The infusion time may vary by several minutes depending on whether you round off to the nearest hundredth, or tenth. Variations of a few minutes are not significant. If you are having any difficulty with these calculations review all the examples and problems carefully once again.

Calculating from gtt/min and Set Calibration Using a Formula

For those who prefer working with formulas rather than ratio and proportion here is a second way of calculating infusion times from gtt/min and set calibration. The mL/hr rate is calculated first, then used with the total volume to be infused to obtain the infusion time.

FORMULA

$$\text{Infusion Time} = \begin{array}{c}\text{Total volume}\\\text{to infuse}\end{array} \div \left(\frac{\text{gtt/min}}{\text{set calibration}} \times 60 \text{ min}\right)$$

Let's begin with a few examples that will illustrate this method.

EXAMPLE 1 There are 250 mL of dextrose in an IV piggyback that is infusing at 33 gtt/min and the set calibration is 10 gtt/mL. Calculate the infusion time.

- $250 \text{ mL} \div \left(\dfrac{33 \text{ gtt/min}}{10 \text{ gtt/mL}} \times 60\right)$

- $250 \text{ mL} \div 198 \text{ mL/hr} = 1.26$

- $.26 \times 60 \text{ min} = 16$

   Infusion time = 1 hr 16 min

 The mL/hr must be determined first. The total volume to infuse is then divided by the mL/hr rate.

EXAMPLE 2 There are 500 mL of whole blood infusing at 40 gtt/min with a set calibration of 20 gtt/mL. Determine the infusion time.

- $500 \text{ mL} \div \left(\dfrac{40 \text{ gtt/min}}{20 \text{ gtt/mL}} \times 60 \text{ min}\right)$

- $500 \text{ mL} \div 120 \text{ mL/hr} = 4.17$

- $.17 \times 60 \text{ min} = 10.2 = 10 \text{ min}$

Infusion time = 4 hr 10 min

EXAMPLE 3 Infuse 1150 mL of hyperalimentation at 25 gtt/min using a set calibration of 10 gtt/mL. Calculate the infusion time.

- $1150 \text{ mL} \div \left(\dfrac{25 \text{ gtt/min}}{10 \text{ gtt/mL}} \times 60 \text{ min} \right)$

- $1150 \text{ mL} \div 150 \text{ mL/hr} = 7.67$

- $.67 \times 60 \text{ min} = 40.2 = 40 \text{ min}$

Infusion time = 7 hr 40 min

EXAMPLE 4 500 mL D5W are to infuse at a rate of 30 gtt/min using a 15 gtt/mL set.

- $500 \text{ mL} \div \left(\dfrac{30 \text{ gtt/min}}{15 \text{ gtt/mL}} \times 60 \text{ min} \right)$

- $500 \div 128 \text{ mL/hr} = 3.91$

- $.91 \times 60 \text{ min} = 54.6 = 55 \text{ min}$

Infusion time = 3 hr 55 min

Problem

Determine the following infusion times using the gtt/min and set calibration formula method.

1. 450 mL D5NS—set calibration 20 gtt/mL—flow rate 25 gtt/min _____

2. 1000 mL D5W—set calibration 10 gtt/mL—flow rate 33 gtt/min _____

3. 150 mL—flow rate 15 gtt/min—set calibration 15 gtt/mL _____

4. 50 mL—flow rate 10 gtt/min—set calibration 15 gtt/mL _____

5. 250 mL—flow rate 22 gtt/min—set calibration 10 gtt/mL _____

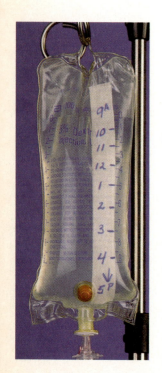

ANSWERS   1. 6 hr   2. 5 hr 3 min   3. 2 hr 30 min   4. 1 hr 15 min   5. 1 hr 53 min

Remember that this formula method will only work when you know the gtt/min and the set calibration of the tubing. After you have worked and practiced with these methods you may select the one which works the best and most consistently for you and then stick with that method.

Labeling Solution Bags with Infusion Time

IV bags are calibrated so that the amount of fluid remaining can be checked at any time. In the majority of hospitals it is also routine to **label IV solution bags when they are hung with start, finish and progress times,** to provide a visual reference of the status of the infusion. Commercially prepared labels are available for this purpose, however you can prepare one using any opaque tape available. In figure 94 you can see the calibrations on a 1000 mL solution bag, which identify each 50 mL. Only the 100 mL calibrations are numbered. This IV was started at 9 a.m. to run 8 hours (till 5 p.m.).

Figure 94

This means 125 mL are to infuse per hour. Notice that the start time of 9 a.m. and completion time of 5 p.m. are labeled, as well as each hourly 125 mL volume. This provides all staff with an ongoing and immediate reference of the IV's progress.

Problem

1. Label the IV bag in figure 95 for an infusion to run at 75 mL per hr. The IV was started at 0710.

2. Label the IV bag in figure 96 for an infusion to run at 125 mL/hr. The infusion was started at 6:30 p.m.

3. The IV in figure 97 is to run at a rate of 80 mL per hr. It was started at 0540. Have your instructor check your labeling.

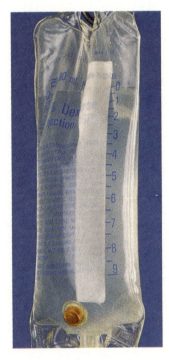
Figure 95

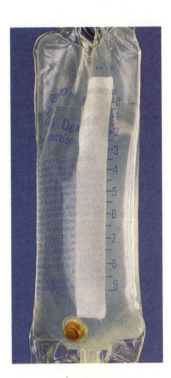
Figure 96

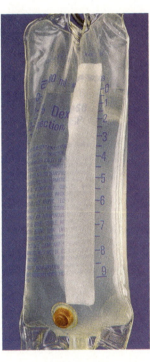
Figure 97

Summary

This concludes the chapter on calculating total infusion times. The important points to remember from this chapter are:

the infusion time is the total time necessary for a given volume of solution to infuse

the two formulas used to determine infusion times are

$$\text{Formula 1: Infusion Time} = \frac{\text{total volume to infuse}}{\text{mL/hr being infused}}$$

Formula 2: Infusion Time = Total volume $\div \left(\dfrac{\text{gtt/min}}{\text{set calibration}} \times 60 \text{ min} \right)$
to infuse

the infusion time can also be calculated from set calibration and gtt/min rate using ratio and proportion

calculating infusion times allows you to plan ahead and have the next solution ordered ready to hang

it is routine in many hospitals to label IV solution bags with start, finish and progress times to provide an instant visual record of infusion status

---

Summary Self Test

Directions: Calculate the following infusion times using whichever method you prefer.

1. Order: 50 mL D5W with 1 g Kefzol. The flow rate is 50 gtt/min, set calibration is a microdrip.

    Infusion time: _____

2. Infuse 1150 mL hyperalimentation at 80 mL per hour.

    Infusion time: _____

3. There is 280 mL left in the IV bag. The flow rate is 40 gtt/min and the set calibration is 10 gtt/mL. If it is 11:03 a.m. when you reset the flow rate when will the IV be completed?

    Infusion time: _____   Time completed: _____

4. Order: Infuse 500 mL of whole blood at 30 gtt/min using a set calibration of 20 gtt/mL.

    Infusion time: _____

5. You find 850 mL left in your patient's IV. The time is 10 a.m. The IV is infusing at 25 gtt/min with a set calibration of 10 gtt/mL. At what time will the infusion be completed?

    Infusion time: _____   Time completed: _____

6. Infuse 500 mL of Intralipids at 25 mL/hr.

    Infusion time: _____

7. A piggyback has 50 mL of solution infusing at 30 gtt/min. The set calibration is 15 gtt/mL.

    Infusion time: _____

8. There are 520 mL in the IV bag. Set calibration is 15 gtt/mL and the flow rate is 22 gtt/min. If it is now 0420 when will the infusion be complete?

    Infusion time: _____   Time completed: _____

9. The time is 12 p.m. and there is 900 mL left in the present IV. The flow rate is 50 gtt/min, and the set calibration is 10 gtt/mL. When will the IV be completed?

   Infusion time: _____   Time completed: _____

10. Infuse 150 mL of an antibiotic at 33 gtt/min. Set calibration is 10 gtt/mL.

    Infusion time: _____

11. Order: Infuse 250 mL of packed red blood cells at 20 mL/hr.

    Infusion time: _____

12. The flow rate for 1 liter of D5W is 42 gtt/min. Set calibration is 15 gtt/mL. If the IV is started at 11:05 p.m. when will it be completed?

    Infusion time: _____   Time completed: _____

13. Infuse 1 unit (250 mL) of packed cells at a flow rate of 30 gtt/min. The set calibration is 20 gtt/mL. Calculate total infusion time.

    Infusion time: _____

14. Volume to infuse is 100 mL. Flow rate is 42 gtt/min using a microdrip.

    Infusion time: _____

15. At 11 p.m. you notice that 200 mL remains in the IV. The flow rate is 20 gtt/min and the set calibration is 10 gtt/mL. What time can you expect the IV to complete?

    Infusion time: _____   Time completed: _____

16. A fluid challenge of 350 mL IV is ordered to infuse at 50 gtt/min. Set calibration is 10 gtt/mL.

    Infusion time: _____

17. An infant is to receive 25 mL of solution at 25 gtt/min. The set calibration is 60 gtt/mL.

    Infusion time: _____

18. 425 mL of D5 ½NS is infusing at 15 gtt/min. The set calibration is 10 gtt/mL. It is now 0814. When will the infusion be completed?

    Infusion time: _____   Time completed: _____

19. There are 180 mL left in an IV that is infusing at 25 mL/hr. It is 10:30 p.m. What time will it be completed?

    Infusion time: _____   Time completed: _____

20. At 2 p.m. a nurse starts 500 mL of solution, and regulates the flow rate at 20 gtt/min. The set calibration is 20 gtt/mL. At what time will the infusion be completed?

   Infusion time: _____   Time completed: _____

21. Order: Infuse 250 mL of NS at 50 gtt/min. Set calibration is 15 gtt/mL.

   Infusion time: _____

22. A physician orders an IV rate to be reduced from 50 gtt/min to 35 gtt/min. There are 525 mL left to infuse. Set calibration is 10 gtt/mL.

   Infusion time: _____

23. A liter of D5 ¼NS with 10 U regular insulin has just been started and is infusing at 22 gtt/min. Set calibration is 20 gtt/mL. It is 8:42 a.m. When will it complete?

   Infusion time: _____   Time completed: _____

24. A physician orders 2 liters of 0.9% NS to infuse at 200 mL/hr.

   Infusion time: _____

25. An antibiotic solution of 100 mL is running at 33 gtt/min with a set calibration of 10 gtt/mL.

   Infusion time: _____

26. 500 mL are infusing at a flow rate of 50 gtt/min using a microdrip set.

   Infusion time: _____

27. An IV of 1100 mL is infusing at a rate of 25 gtt/min. The calibration of the set is 15 gtt/mL.

   Infusion time: _____

28. An IV medication of 30 mL is infusing at 10 gtt/min using a set calibrated at 10 gtt/mL.

   Infusion time: _____

29. 90 mL are to be infused at a rate of 30 gtt/min using a 20 gtt/mL set.

   Infusion time: _____

30. 100 mL are to infuse on a 15 gtt/mL set at 45 gtt/min.

   Infusion time: _____

31. A total of 750 mL are to be infused using a set calibrated at 20 gtt/mL at a rate of 32 gtt/min. When will the IV complete if it is started at 3:03 p.m.?

   Infusion time: _____   Time completed: _____

Directions: Label the following IV solution bags for the times and rates indicated. Have your instructor check your labeling.

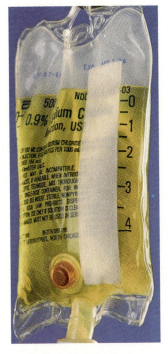

32
Started: 10:47 a.m.
Rate: 80 mL/hr

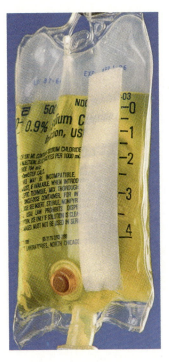

33
Started: 1315
Rate: 100 mL/hr

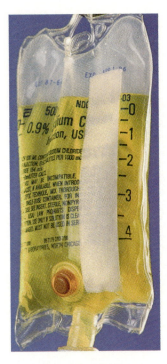

34
Started: 2:10 p.m.
Rate: 90 mL/hr

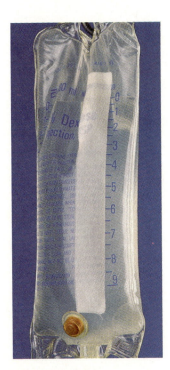

35
Started: 0440
Rate: 75 mL/hr

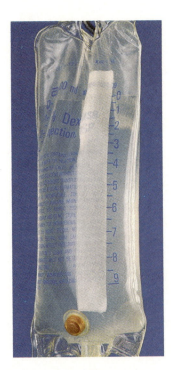

36
Started: 0730
Rate: 50 mL/hr

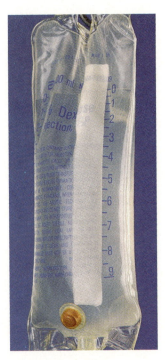

37
Started: 6:20 p.m.
Rate: 25 mL/hr

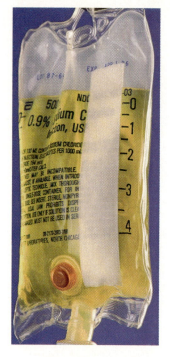

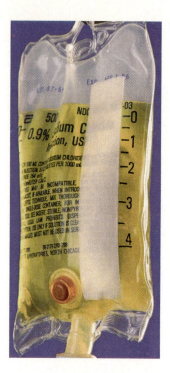

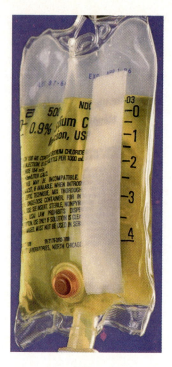

38
Started: 3:03 a.m.
Rate: 50 mL/hr

39
Started: 0744
Rate: 125 mL/hr

40
Started: 2140
Rate: 100 mL/hr

ANSWERS **1.** hr   **2.** 14 hr 23 min   **3.** 1 hr 10 min; 12:13 p.m.   **4.** 5 hr 34 min   **5.** 5 hr 40 min; 3:40 p.m.
6. 20 hr   **7.** 25 min   **8.** 5 hr 55 min; 1015   **9.** 3 hr; 3 p.m.   **10.** 46 min   **11.** 12 hr 30 min   **12.** 5 hr 57 min; 5:02 a.m.
13. 2 hr 47 min   **14.** 2 hr 23 min   **15.** 1 hr 40 min; 12:40 a.m.   **16.** 1 hr 10 min   **17.** 1 hr   **18.** 4 hr 43 min; 1257
19. 7 hr 12 min; 5:42 a.m.   **20.** 8 hr 20 min; 10:20 p.m.   **21.** 1 hr 15 min   **22.** 2 hr 30 min   **23.** 15 hr 9 min;
11:51 p.m.   **24.** 10 hr   **25.** 31 min   **26.** 10 hr   **27.** 11 hr   **28.** 30 min   **29.** 1 hr   **30.** 33 min   **31.** 7 hr 49 min;
10:52 p.m.

SECTION

EIGHT

Pediatric Medication Administration

23

Pediatric Oral and Parenteral Medications

OBJECTIVES

The student will

1. explain how suspensions are measured and administered
2. list the precautions of IM and s.c. injection in infants and children
3. calculate pediatric oral dosages
4. calculate pediatric IM and s.c. dosages

INTRODUCTION

Two differences between adult and pediatric dosages will be immediately apparent: **most oral drugs are prepared as liquids** because infants and small children cannot be expected to swallow tablets easily, if at all, and **dosages are dramatically smaller.** The oral route is used whenever possible, but when a child cannot swallow, or the drug is ineffective given orally, drugs will be administered by a parenteral route.

Both the subcutaneous and intramuscular routes may be used depending on the type of drug to be administered. However, the small muscle size of infants and children limits the use of the intramuscular route, as does the nature of the drug being used. For example, most antibiotics are administered intravenously rather than intramuscularly.

Oral Medications

Most oral pediatric drugs are prepared as liquids to facilitate ease in swallowing. If the child is old enough to cooperate these dosages may be measured in a medication cup. Solutions may also be measured using oral syringes, such as the ones shown in figure 98. Oral syringes have the same metric calibrations as hypodermic syringes, but also include household measures, for example tsp. Oral syringes have different sized tips to prevent use with hypodermic needles. On some oral syringes the tip is positioned off center (termed eccentric), to further distinguish them from hypodermic syringes, or they may be amber colored, as in the illustration.

If oral syringes are not available, hypodermic syringes **(without the needle)** can also be used for dosage measurement. In addition to accuracy syringes provide an excellent method of administering oral liquid drugs to infants and small children. Some oral liquids are prepared using a calibrated medication dropper which is an integral part of the medication bottle. These may be calibrated in mL like the dropper shown in figure 99, or in actual dosage, for example 25 mg, or 50 mg. Animal shaped measures such as those shown in figure 100 are also helpful in enticing reluctant toddlers to take necessary medications. In each instance the goal is to be sure the infant or child actually swallows the total dosage.

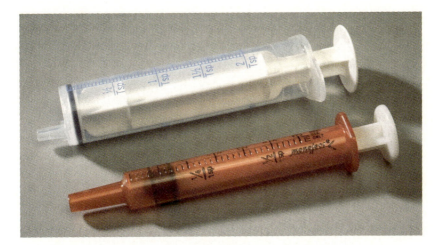

Figure 98

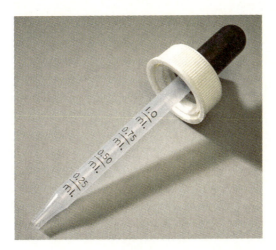

Figure 99

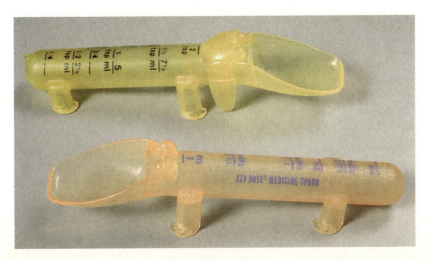

Figure 100

Care must be taken with liquid oral drugs to identify those prepared as **suspensions.** A suspension consists of an insoluble drug in a liquid base, as for example in the Augmentin® suspension in figure 101. The drug in a suspension settles to the bottom of the bottle between uses, and **thorough mixing immediately prior to pouring is mandatory.** Suspensions must also be administered to the child promptly after measurement to prevent the drug settling out again, and an incomplete dosage being administered.

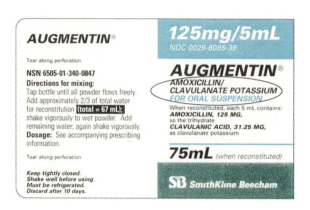

Figure 101

When a tablet or capsule is administered the child's mouth must be checked to be certain it has actually been swallowed. If swallowing is a problem some tablets can be crushed and given in a small amount of applesauce, ice cream or juice if the child has no dietary restrictions which would contraindicate this. Keep in mind however, that **enteric coated and timed release tablets or capsules cannot be crushed** since this would destroy the coating which allows them to function on a delayed action basis.

IM and s.c. Medications

The drugs most often given subcutaneously are insulin, and immunizations which specifically require the subcutaneous route. Any site with sufficient subcutaneous tissue may be used, with the upper arm being the site of choice for immunizations. The intramuscular route is used most frequently for preoperative and postoperative medications for sedation and pain, and for immunizations such as DPT (diphtheria, pertussis, tetanus) which must be administered deep IM. The intramuscular site of choice for infants and small children is the vastus lateralis or rectus femoris of the thigh, because the gluteal muscles do not develop until a child has learned to walk. Usually not more than 1 mL is injected per site, and sites are rotated regularly.

Dosage calculation is the same as for adults, except **dosages are often calculated to the nearest hundredth, and measured using a tuberculin syringe.** (Refer to Chapter 10 if you need to review the calibrations and use of a TB syringe). There is less margin for error in pediatric dosages, and calculations and measurements are routinely double checked.

Summary

This concludes the chapter on pediatric oral and IM, s.c. medication administration. The important points to remember are:

care must be taken when administering oral drugs to be positive the child has actually swallowed the dosage if liquid medications are prepared as suspensions, mix thoroughly prior to measurement, and administer promptly

care must be taken not to confuse oral syringes which are unsterile, with hypodermic syringes which are sterile

the IM site of choice for infants and children is the vastus lateralis or rectus femoris of the thigh

usually not more than 1 mL is injected per IM or s.c. site and sites are rotated regularly

pediatric dosages are frequently calculated to the nearest hundredth and measured using a TB syringe

Summary Self Test

Directions: Use the pediatric medication labels provided to measure the following oral dosages.

PART I

1. Prepare a 125 mg dosage of Augmentin®. _____

2. Prepare a 125 mg dosage of amoxicillin. _____

3. Prepare a 0.1 mg dosage of digoxin. _____

4. Prepare 3 mg of Proventil®. _____

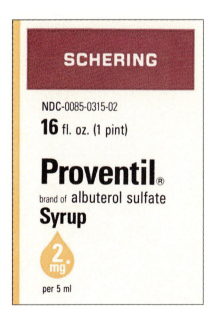

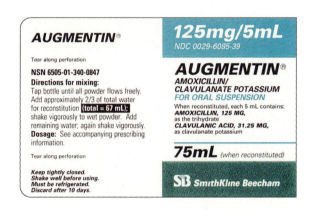

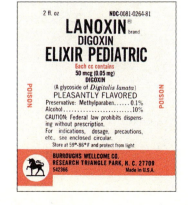

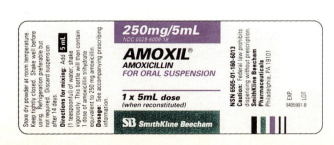

5. Prepare 400,000 U of oral penicillin V. _____

6. Prepare 40 mg of theophylline. _____

7. Prepare 62.5 mg of Dilantin®. _____

8. Prepare 250 mg of tetracycline oral suspension. _____

9. Peri-Colace® 3 tsp is ordered. How many mL will this be? _____

10. Prepare 300 mg of erythromycin. _____

11. Prepare 120 mg of acetaminophen. _____

12. Prepare 12.5 mg elixir Benadryl®. _____

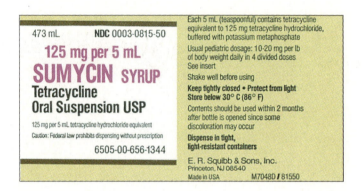

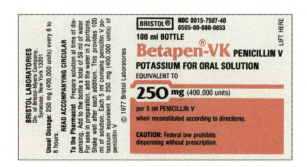

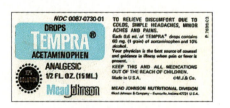

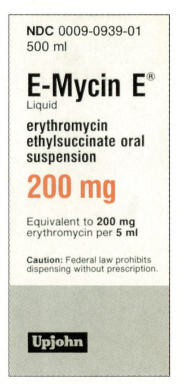

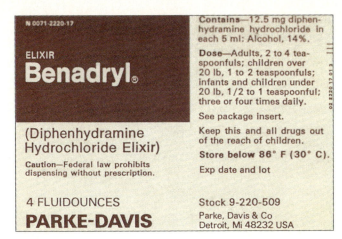

N 0071-2220-17

ELIXIR

Benadryl®

(Diphenhydramine
Hydrochloride Elixir)

Caution—Federal law prohibits
dispensing without prescription.

4 FLUIDOUNCES
PARKE-DAVIS

Contains—12.5 mg diphen-
hydramine hydrochloride in
each 5 ml: Alcohol, 14%.

Dose—Adults, 2 to 4 tea-
spoonfuls; children over
20 lb, 1 to 2 teaspoonfuls;
infants and children under
20 lb, 1/2 to 1 teaspoonful;
three or four times daily.

See package insert.

Keep this and all drugs out
of the reach of children.

Store below 86° F (30° C).

Exp date and lot

Stock 9-220-509
Parke, Davis & Co
Detroit, Mi 48232 USA

Gentle laxative and stool softener for
treating temporary constipation.
Usual dose: (preferably at bedtime).
Children over 3: 1 to 3 teaspoons.
Adults: 1 to 2 tablespoons.
Warning: Not to be used when ab-
dominal pain, nausea, or vomiting are
present.
Frequent or prolonged use of this preparation may result in dependence on
laxatives.

**Keep this and all medication out
of reach of children.**

NDC 0087-0721-01

SYRUP

PERI-COLACE®

CASANTHRANOL AND DIOCTYL SODIUM SULFOSUCCINATE

LAXATIVE PLUS STOOL SOFTENER

8 FL. OZ. (½ PT.)

Mead Johnson

Each tablespoon (15 ml., 3 teaspoons)
contains 30 mg. Peristim® (casanthranol, Mead Johnson) and 60 mg.
COLACE® (dioctyl sodium sulfosuccinate, Mead Johnson).

Contains alcohol 10%.

**PERI-COLACE is also available in 1-
pint bottles of syrup and in bottles
of 30 and 60 capsules.**

Made in U.S.A.   ©M. J. & Co.

Mead Johnson
PHARMACEUTICAL DIVISION
Mead Johnson & Company
Evansville, Indiana 47721 U.S.A.

℗ **PARKE-DAVIS**
People Who Care

N 0071-2214-20

Dilantin-125®
(Phenytoin Oral
Suspension, USP)

125 mg per 5 mL potency

Important—Another strength available;
verify unspecified prescriptions.

Caution—Federal law prohibits
dispensing without prescription.

**IMPORTANT—SHAKE WELL
BEFORE EACH USE**

8 fl oz (237 mL)

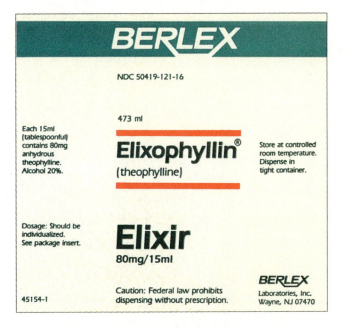

BERLEX

NDC 50419-121-16

Each 15ml
(tablespoonful)
contains 80mg
anhydrous
theophylline.
Alcohol 20%.

473 ml

Elixophyllin®
(theophylline)

Store at controlled
room temperature.
Dispense in
tight container.

Dosage: Should be
individualized.
See package insert.

Elixir
80mg/15ml

BERLEX
Laboratories, Inc.
Wayne, NJ 07470

45154-1

Caution: Federal law prohibits
dispensing without prescription.

PART II

Directions: Use the labels provided to calculate the following IM/s.c. dosages. Calculate to hundredths.

13.   Prepare a 20 mg dosage of meperidine. _____

14.   A dosage of morphine 10 mg has been ordered. _____

15.   Prepare a 0.1 mg dosage of atropine. _____

16.   Draw up a 100 mg dosage of clindamycin. _____

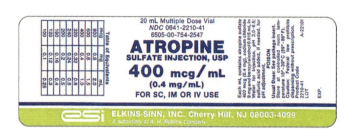

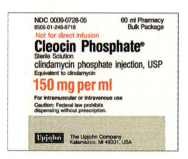

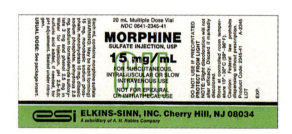

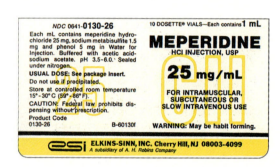

PART III

17.   Prepare a 40 mg dosage of meperidine. _____

18.   Draw up a 75 mg dosage of kanamycin. _____

19.   A dosage of Garamycin® 15 mg has been ordered. _____

20.   Prepare a 6 mg dosage of morphine. _____

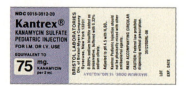

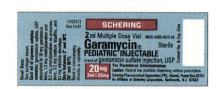

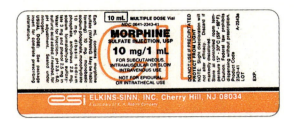

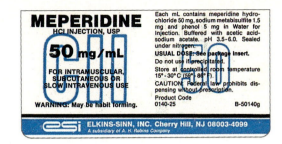

ANSWERS **1.** 5 mL **2.** 2.5 mL **3.** 2 cc **4.** 7.5 mL **5.** 5 mL **6.** 7.5 mL **7.** 2.5 mL **8.** 10 mL **9.** 15 mL **10.** 7.5 mL **11.** 1.2 mL **12.** 5 mL **13.** 0.8 mL **14.** 0.67 mL **15.** 0.25 mL **16.** 0.67 mL **17.** 0.8 mL **18.** 1 mL **19.** 1.5 mL **20.** 0.6 mL

24

Pediatric Intravenous Medications

OBJECTIVES

The student will

1. list the steps in preparing and administering IV medications using a solution bag
2. list the steps in preparing and administering IV medications using a calibrated burette
3. explain why a flush is included in IV medication administration
4. calculate flow rates for administration of IV medications using the formula or division factor method
5. use normal daily and hourly dosage ranges to calculate and assess dosages ordered

PREREQUISITES

Chapters 18 and 20

INTRODUCTION

Pediatric IV medication administration involves a challenge and a responsibility that is multi-faceted. Infants and children, particularly under the age of four, are incompletely developed physiologically and drug tolerance, absorption and excretion are ongoing concerns. In addition infants and acutely ill children can tolerate only a narrow range of hydration, making administration of IV drugs, which are diluted for administration, a critical and exact skill. Drug dilution protocols may specify a range for dilution, and on many occasions the smallest possible volume may have to be used in order not to overhydrate a child. Dosage and dilution decisions may have to be made on a day to day or even dose to dose basis, and will involve the team effort of nurse, physician and pharmacist. In addition the suitability of any flow rate calculated for administration must be made on an individual basis. For example a calculated flow rate of 100 gtt/min for a 2 year old child is too high a rate to administer.

The fragility of infants' and children's veins and the irritating nature of many medications mandates careful site inspection for signs of inflammation and infiltration. This should be done immediately before, during and after each infusion. Signs of inflammation would include redness, heat, swelling and tenderness. Signs of infiltration include swelling, coldness, pain, and lack of blood return. Either complication necessitates discontinuance of the IV and a restart at a new site.

IV Medication Guidelines or Protocols are always used to determine drug dosages, dilutions, and administration rates. In this chapter all examples and problems are representative of actual protocols.

Let's start by looking at the different methods of IV medication administration.

Methods of IV Medication Administration

Intravenous medications may be administered over a period of several hours, for example aminophylline; or on an **intermittent** basis involving several dosages in a 24 hour period, for example antibiotics. When ordered to infuse over several hours medications are usually added to an IV solution bag. Adding the drug to the IV bag may be a hospital pharmacy or staff nurse responsibility, but in any event it is not a complicated procedure. The steps for adding the drug to the solution are as follows:

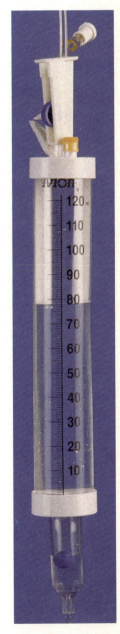

STEP 1   Locate the type and volume of IV solution ordered.

STEP 2   Measure the dosage of drug to be added.

STEP 3   Use strict aseptic technique to add the drug to the solution bag through the medication port.

STEP 4   Mix the drug thoroughly in the solution.

STEP 5   Label the IV solution bag with the name and dosage of the drug added.

STEP 6   Add your initials with the time and date you added the drug.

STEP 7   Hang the IV and set the flow rate for the infusion. Chart the administration when it has completed.

For intermittent administrations the medication may also be prepared in small volume solution bags, or using a **calibrated burette,** such as the one illustrated in figure 102. Because the total capacity of burettes is between 100 to 150 mL, calibrated in 1 mL increments, exact measurement of small volumes is possible.

Regardless of the method of intermittent administration, the medication infusion is **routinely followed by a flush,** to make sure the medication has cleared the tubing, and that the total dosage has been administered. A **15 mL flush** is standard for **peripheral lines,** and a **20 mL flush** for **central lines.** The volume of the flush is included in the flow rate calculation for the medication administration. For example, a drug may be diluted in 15 mL of solution and followed by a 15 mL flush. The total volume of medication plus flush is 30 mL, and it is this volume which will be used to calculate the flow rate for administration. If a primary line exists, the medication may be administered IVPB (IV piggyback) via a secondary line. If no IV is infusing a saline or heparin lock (heplock) is frequently in place and used for administration.

When IV medications are diluted for administration it is necessary to determine hospital policy on **inclusion of the medication volume as part of the volume specified for dilution.** For example if 20 mg has a volume of 2 mL, and it is to be diluted in 30 mL, does this mean you must add 28 mL of diluent to the burette, or 30 mL?

Figure 102

Hospital policies may vary, but in all examples and problems in this chapter the drug volume will be treated as part of the total diluent volume. The sequencing of medication and flush administration covered next for burette use is also representative of the procedure which might be followed for IVPB administrations.

Medication Administration via Burette

When a burette is used for medication administration the entire preparation is done by staff nurses. Electronic controllers and pumps are used extensively to administer intermittent IV medications. When these are used the alarm will sound each time the burette empties to signal when each successive step is necessary. For example it will alarm when the medication has infused and the flush must be started, and again when the flush is completed.

Let's look at some sample orders and go step-by-step through one procedure which may be used.

EXAMPLE 1   A dosage of 250 mg in 15 mL D5 ½NS is to be infused over 30 minutes. It is to be followed with a 15 mL D5 ½NS flush. An infusion controller will be used, and the tubing is a microdrip.

STEP 1   Read the drug label and determine what volume the 250 mg dosage is contained in. This is 1 mL.

STEP 2   The dilution is to be 15 mL. Run a total of 14 mL D5 ½NS into the burette, then add the 1 mL containing the dosage of 250 mg. This gives the ordered volume of 15 mL. Roll the burette between your hands to mix the drug thoroughly with the solution.

STEP 3   Determine the mL/hr so that you can set the controller rate.

Total volume = 30 mL (15 mL medication + 15 mL flush)

Infusion time = 30 min

30 mL : 30 min = X mL : 60 min

= 60 mL/hr

STEP 4   Label the burette to identify the drug and dosage added. Attach a label which states "medication infusing." This makes it possible for others to know the status of the administration if you are not present when the controller alarms.

STEP 5   When the medication has infused add the 15 mL D5 ½NS flush. Remove the "medication infusing" label and attach a "flush infusing" label. Continue to infuse at 60 mL/hr rate until the burette empties for the second time.

STEP 6   When the flush has been completed restart the primary IV, or disconnect from the saline lock. Remove the "flush infusing" label. Chart the dosage and time.

EXAMPLE 2   An antibiotic dosage of 125 mg in 1 mL is to be diluted in 20 mL D5 ¼NS and infused over 30 min. A flush of 15 mL D5 ¼NS is to follow. A volumetric pump will be used.

STEP 1   125 mg has a volume of 1 mL. Add 19 mL of D5 ¼NS to the burette, add the 1 mL of medication and mix thoroughly.

STEP 2   Determine the mL/hr volume.

Total volume = 35 mL (20 mL medication + 15 mL flush)

Infusion time = 30 min

35 mL in 30 min = 70 mL in 60 min

or use ratio and proportion

35 mL : 30 min = X mL : 60 min

= 70 mL/hr

STEP 3   Set the flow rate at 70 mL/hr. Label the burette with the drug and dosage, and attach a "medication infusing" label.

STEP 4   When the medication has infused start the 15 mL flush. Remove the "medication infusing" label, and add the "flush infusing" label.

STEP 5   When the flush has completed restart the primary IV or disconnect from the saline lock. Remove the "flush infusing" label. Chart the dosage and time.

Calibrated burette rates can also be set using a roller clamp rather than a controller or volumetric pump. It will then be necessary to calculate the flow rate.

EXAMPLE 3   An antibiotic dosage of 50 mg has been ordered diluted in 10 mL of D5W to infuse over 20 min. A 15 mL flush of D5W is to follow. A microdrip will be used, but an infusion control device will not be used.

STEP 1   Read the medication label to determine what volume contains 50 mg. You determine that 50 mg is contained in 2 mL.

STEP 2   Run 8 mL of D5W into the burette and add the 2 mL containing 50 mg of drug. Roll between hands to mix thoroughly.

STEP 3   Determine the flow rate necessary to deliver the medication plus the flush in the 20 minute time period ordered. Either the Formula or the Division Factor method may be used for flow rate calculation.

FORMULA METHOD

$$\text{Flow Rate} = \frac{\text{Total Volume} \times \text{Set Calibration}}{\text{Time in Minutes}}$$

$$\frac{10 \text{ mL (medication)} + 15 \text{ mL (flush)} \times 60 \text{ (gtt/mL)}}{20 \text{ min}}$$

$$\frac{25 \times 60}{20} = \textbf{75 gtt/min}$$

DIVISION FACTOR METHOD

Flow Rate = mL/hr ÷ Division Factor

To use the division factor method you must express the volume in mL/hr (mL/60 min).

25 mL in 20 min = 75 mL in 60 min

or use ratio and proportion to determine this

25 mL : 20 min = X mL : 60 min

= 75 mL in 60 min

A 60 gtt/mL microdrip set has a division factor of 1 (60 ÷ 60).

75 (mL/hr) ÷ 1 (division factor) = **75 gtt/min**

 The flow rate in gtt/min is the same as the volume in mL/hr for microdrip sets calibrated at 60 gtt/mL.

STEP 4   Adjust the flow rate to deliver 75 gtt/min.

STEP 5   Label the burette with drug name and dosage, and "medication infusing" label.

STEP 6   When the medication has cleared the burette add the 15 mL of D5W flush. Continue to run at 75 gtt/min. Remove the "medication infusing" label and replace with a "flush infusing" label.

STEP 7   When the burette empties for the second time restart the primary IV, or disconnect from the saline lock. Remove the "flush infusing" label. Chart the dosage and time administered.

Problem

Determine the volume of solution which must be added to the burette to mix the following IV drugs. Then calculate the flow rate in gtt/min for each administration using a microdrip. Indicate the mL/hr setting for a controller.

1.   An IV medication of 75 mg in 3 mL is ordered diluted to 55 mL to infuse over 45 min. A 15 mL flush is to follow.

     Dilution volume ＿＿＿＿＿＿ gtt/min ＿＿＿＿＿＿ mL/hr ＿＿＿＿＿＿

2.   A dosage of 100 mg in 2 mL is diluted to 30 mL D5W to infuse in 20 min. A 15 mL flush is to follow.

     Dilution volume ＿＿＿＿＿＿ gtt/min ＿＿＿＿＿＿ mL/hr ＿＿＿＿＿＿

3.   The volume of a 10 mg dosage of medication is 1 cc. Dilute to 15 mL and administer over 30 min, with a flush of 15 mL to follow.

     Dilution volume ＿＿＿＿＿＿ gtt/min ＿＿＿＿＿＿ mL/hr ＿＿＿＿＿＿

4. A dosage of 15 mg with a volume of 3 mL is to be diluted to 25 mL and administered in 20 min. A 15 mL flush is to follow.

    Dilution volume _____ gtt/min _____ mL/hr _____

5. A medication of 1 g in 4 mL is to be diluted to 30 mL to infuse over 60 min. A 15 mL flush is to follow.

    Dilution volume _____ gtt/min _____ mL/hr _____

ANSWERS **1.** 52 mL; 93 gtt/min; 93 mL/hr **2.** 28 mL; 135 gtt/min; 135 mL/hr **3.** 14 mL; 60 gtt/min; 60 mL/hr **4.** 22 mL; 120 gtt/min; 120 mL/hr **5.** 26 mL; 45 gtt/min; 45 mL/hr

Comparing IV Dosages Ordered with Protocols

Knowing how to compare dosages ordered with the dosage protocols for a particular medication is a nursing responsibility.

 Dosages of IV medications are calculated on the basis of body weight, or BSA

Protocols may list dosages in terms of mg, mcg or U per day, or per hour. BSA in M^2 is most often used to calculate chemotherapeutic drugs, which are administered only by certified nursing staff. The following examples will demonstrate how to use protocols to check dosages ordered.

EXAMPLE 1 A child weighing 22.6 kg has an order for 500 mg of medication in 100 mL D5W q.12.h. The normal dosage range is 40–50 mg/kg/day. Determine if the dosage ordered is within the normal range.

STEP 1 **Calculate the normal daily range for this child.**

40 mg/day × 22.6 kg = **904 mg**

50 mg/day × 22.6 kg = **1130 mg**

STEP 2 **Assess the accuracy of the dosage ordered.**

The normal dosage range is 452–565 mg/dose. The bag contains 500 mg. The dosage is within normal range.

EXAMPLE 2 A child with a body weight of 18.4 kg is to receive a medication with a dosage range of 100–150 mg/kg/day. The order is for 600 mg in 75 mL D5W q.6.h. Determine if the dosage is within normal range.

STEP 1 **Calculate the normal daily dosage range.**

100 mg/kg × 18.4 kg = **1840 mg/day**

150 mg/kg × 18.4 kg = **2760 mg/day**

STEP 2 **Calculate the daily dosage ordered.**

The dosage ordered is 600 mg q.6.h. (4 doses).

600 mg × 4 = **2400 mg/day**

STEP 3   **Assess the accuracy of the dosage ordered.**

The dosage ordered, 2400 mg/day, is within the normal range of 1840–2760 mg/day.

EXAMPLE 3   A child weighing 17.7 kg is receiving an IV of 250 mL D5W containing 2000 U heparin, which is to infuse at 50 mL/hr. The dosage range of heparin is 10–25 U/kg/hr. Assess the accuracy of this dosage.

STEP 1   **Calculate the normal daily dosage range per hour.**

10 U/kg/hr $\times$ 17.7 kg = **177 U/hr**

25 U/kg/hr $\times$ 17.7 kg = **442.5 U/hr**

STEP 2   **Calculate the dosage infusing per hr.**

250 mL : 2000 U = 50 mL : X U

50 mL = **400 U/hr**

STEP 3   **Assess the accuracy of the dosage ordered.**

The IV is infusing at a rate of 50 mL per hour, which is 400 U. The normal dosage range is 177–442.5 U/hr. The dosage is within normal range.

EXAMPLE 4   A child weighing 32.7 kg has an IV of 250 mL D5 ¼S containing 400 mcg of medication to infuse over 5 hours. The normal range for this drug is 1–3 mcg/kg/hr. Determine if this dosage is within the normal dosage range.

STEP 1   **Calculate the hourly dosage range.**

1 mcg/kg/hr $\times$ 32.7 kg = **32.7 mcg/hr**

3 mcg/kg/hr $\times$ 32.7 kg = **98.1 mcg/hr**

STEP 2   **Calculate the dosage infusing per hour.**

250 mL $\div$ 5 hr = **50 mL/hr**

250 mL : 400 mcg = 50 mL : X mcg

= **80 mcg/hr**

STEP 3   **Assess the accuracy of the dosage ordered**

The dosage of 80 mcg/hr infusing is within the normal range of 32.7–98.1 mcg/hr.

Problem

Calculate the normal dosage range to the nearest tenth, and the dosage being administered for the following medications. Assess the dosages ordered.

1.   A child weighing 24.4 kg has an IV of 250 mL D5W containing 2500 U of a drug. The dosage range for this drug is 15–25 U/kg/hr. The infusion

controller is set to deliver 50 mL/hr. Dosage range per hr _____

Dosage infusing per hr _____ Assessment _____

2. A solution of D5W containing 25 mg of a drug is to infuse in 30 min. The dosage range is 4–8 mg/kg/day, q.6.h. The child weighs 18.7 kg.

   Dosage range per day _____ Daily dosage ordered _____

   Assessment _____

3. An IV solution containing 125 mg of medication is infusing. The dosage range is 5–10 mg/kg/dose, and the child weighs 14.2 kg. Dosage range

   per dose _____ Assessment _____

4. A child weighing 14.3 kg is to receive an IV drug with a dosage range of 50–100 mcg/kg/day in two divided doses. An infusion of 50 mL D5W containing 400 mcg to run 30 min has been ordered. Daily dosage range

   _____ Daily dosage ordered _____ Assessment _____

5. A dosage of 4 mg (4000 mcg) of drug in 500 mL of D5 ½S is to infuse over 4 hours. The dosage range of the drug is 24–120 mcg/kg/hr, and the child

   weighs 16.1 kg. Dosage range per hr _____

   Dosage infusing per hr _____ Assessment _____

6. A child weighing 20.9 kg is to receive a medication with a normal dosage range of 80–160 mg/kg/day, in divided doses q.6.h. The IV ordered contains

   500 mg. Dosage range per day _____ Daily dosage ordered _____

   Assessment _____

7. A child weighing 22.3 kg is to receive 750 mL of D5 ¼S containing 6 g of a drug, which is to run over 24 hours. The dosage range of the drug is

   200–300 mg/kg/day. Dosage range per day _____

   Assessment _____

8. An IV of 50 mL D5W containing 55 mcg of a drug is infusing over a 30 min period. The child weighs 14.9 kg and the dosage range is 6–8 mcg/kg/day,

   q.12.h. Dosage range per day _____ Daily dosage ordered _____

   Assessment _____

9. A child weighing 27.1 kg is to receive a medication with a normal range of 0.5–1 mg/kg/dose. An IV containing 20 mg of medication has been ordered.

   Dosage per dose _____ Assessment _____

10. An IV medication of 60 mcg in 200 mL is ordered to infuse over 2 hr. The normal dosage range is 1.5–3 mcg/kg/hr. The child weighs 16.7 kg. Dosage

range per hr _____ Dosage infusing per hr _____

Assessment _____

> **ANSWERS 1.** 366–610 U/hr; 500 U/hr; normal range   **2.** 74.8–149.6 mg/day; 100 mg/day; normal range
> **3.** 71–142 mg/dose; normal range   **4.** 715–1430 mcg/day; 800 mg; normal range   **5.** 386.4–1932 mcg/hr;
> 1000 mcg; normal range   **6.** 1672–3344 mg/day; 2000 mg; normal range   **7.** 4460–6690 mg/day; normal
> range   **8.** 89.4–119.2 mcg/day; 110 mcg; normal range   **9.** 13.6–27.1 mg/dose; normal range
> **10.** 25.1–50.1 mcg/hr; 30 mcg; normal range

Summary

This concludes the chapter on administration of IV drugs to infants and children. The important points to remember from this chapter are:

IV medications may be ordered to infuse over a period of several hours, or minutes

medications to infuse over several hours are usually added to IV solution bags

medications to infuse in less than an hour are often prepared by staff nurses using a calibrated burette

IV medications are diluted for administration, and it is important to determine hospital policy on inclusion of the medication volume as part of the total dilution volume

a flush is used following medication administration to make sure the medication has cleared the tubing and the total dosage has been administered

a 15 mL flush is used for peripheral lines and a 20 mL flush for central lines

the flow rate for IV medication administration is calculated for the total volume of medication including the flush

drug protocols are used to calculate normal dosage ranges, and to assess dosages ordered

pediatric IV medication administration requires constant assessment of the child's ability to tolerate dosage, dilution and rate of administration

children's veins are very fragile, and intravenous sites must be checked for inflammation and infiltration immediately before, during and following each medication administration

Summary Self Test

Directions: Determine the volume of solution which must be added to a calibrated burette to mix the following IV drugs. The medication volume is included in the total dilution volume. Calculate the flow rate in gtt/min for each infusion. A microdrip with a calibration of 60 gtt/mL is used.

1. An IV antibiotic of 750 mg in 3 mL has been ordered diluted to a total of 25 mL D5W to infuse over 40 minutes. A flush of 15 mL is to follow. _____

_____

2. A dosage of 500,000 U of a penicillin preparation with a volume of 4 mL has been ordered diluted to 50 mL D5 ½NS to infuse in 60 min. A 15 mL flush has been ordered. _____ _____

3. A dosage of 1.5 g/2 mL of an antibiotic is to be diluted to a total of 40 mL D5W and administered over 40 min. A 15 mL flush has been ordered.
_____ _____

4. An antibiotic dosage of 200 mg in 4 mL is to be diluted in 50 mL and administered over 60 min. A 20 mL flush has been ordered. _____
_____

5. A dosage of 20 mg in 2 mL has been ordered diluted to 30 mL, to be infused over 30 min. A flush of 15 mL has been ordered. _____ _____

6. A dosage of 25 mg in 5 mL has been ordered diluted to 40 mL and administered in 40 min. A 15 mL flush is to follow. _____ _____

7. A 10 mg in 2 mL dosage has been ordered diluted to 20 mL to infuse over 20 min. A routine 15 mL flush is to follow. _____ _____

8. A medication dosage of 800 mg in 4 mL is to be diluted to 60 mL and infused over 60 min. A 15 mL flush is to follow. _____ _____

9. A dosage of 0.5 g in 2 mL is to be diluted to 40 mL and run in 30 min. A 15 mL flush is ordered. _____ _____

10. A medication of 1000 mg in 1 mL is to be diluted to 15 mL and administered over 20 min. A 15 mL flush is ordered. _____ _____

Directions: The following IV drugs are to be administered using a volumetric pump. Determine the amount of diluent to be added to the burette, and the flow rate in mL/hr to set the pump.

11. A dosage of 40 mg in 4 mL is to be diluted to 50 mL and administered in 90 min. A 20 mL flush is ordered. _____ _____

12. A 2 g in 5 mL dosage has been ordered diluted to a total of 90 mL and administered in 45 min. A 15 mL flush is ordered. _____ _____

13. An 80 mg dosage with a volume of 2 mL is to be diluted to 80 mL and administered in 60 min. A 15 mL flush is to follow. _____ _____

14. A 60 mg dosage with a volume of 4 mL is ordered diluted to 30 mL and run over 20 min. A 15 mL flush is to follow. _____ _____

15. A 5 mg per 2 mL dosage is to be diluted to 10 mL and administered in 10 min. A 15 mL flush follows. _____ _____

16. The dosage ordered is 0.75 g in 3 mL to be diluted to 30 mL. Run in over 30 min with a 15 mL flush. _____ _____

17. A medication of 100 mg in 2 mL is ordered diluted to 20 mL and run in 15 min with a 15 mL flush to follow. _____ _____

18. The dosage ordered is 100 mg in 1 mL to be diluted to 50 mL. Run in over 45 min. Follow with a 15 mL flush. _____ _____

19. A 30 mg dosage in 1 mL has been ordered diluted to 10 mL to infuse in 10 min. A 15 mL flush is ordered. _____ _____

20. A dosage of 250 mg in 5 mL has been ordered diluted to 40 mL and infused in 60 min. A 15 mL flush follows. _____ _____

Directions: Calculate the normal dosage range to the nearest tenth, and the dosage being administered for the following medications. Assess the dosages ordered.

21. A child weighing 15.4 kg is to receive a dosage with a range of 5–7.5 mg/kg/dose. The solution bag is labeled 100 mg. Dosage range _____ Assessment _____

22. The order is for 200 U in 75 mL. The child weighs 13.1 kg and the dosage range is 15–20 U/kg per dose. Dosage range _____ Assessment _____

23. A dosage of 1.5 mg in 20 mL has been ordered. The normal dosage range is 0.1–0.3 mg/kg/day in 2 divided doses. The child's weight is 12.4 kg. Dosage range per day _____ Daily dosage ordered _____ Assessment _____

24. A dosage of 400 mg in 75 mL of medication is to be infused q.8.h. The normal range is 15–45 mg/kg/day, and the child weighs 27.9 kg. Dosage range per day _____ Daily dosage ordered _____ Assessment _____

25. A child weighing 15.7 kg is to receive a medication with a normal hourly range of 3–7 mcg/kg. A 250 mL solution bag containing 350 mcg is infusing

at a rate of 50 mL/hr. Dosage range per hr _____ Dosage infusing

per hour _____ Assessment _____

26. A child weighing 19.6 kg is to receive a medication with a normal dosage range of 60–80 mg/kg/day. A 90 mL infusion containing 375 mg has been

ordered q.6.h. Dosage range per day _____

Daily dosage ordered _____ Assessment _____

27. Two infusions of 250 mL each containing 300 mg of medication are to infuse continuously over a 24 hr period (250 mL q.12.h.). The child receiving the infusion weighs 11.7 kg, and the normal dosage range of the drug is 50–100

mg/kg/day. Dosage range per day _____

Daily dosage ordered _____ Assessment _____

28. The order is for 100 mL D5W containing 150 mg of medication to infuse q.8.h. The normal dosage range is 3–12 mg/kg/day, and the child weighs

40.1 kg. Dosage range per day _____ Daily dosage ordered _____

Assessment _____

29. A child has an infusion of 250 mL containing 500 U of medication to run at 50 mL/hr. The normal dosage range is 10–25 U/hr. The child weighs

10.3 kg. Dosage range per hour _____ Dosage infusing per hour _____

Assessment _____

30. The normal dosage range of a drug is 0.5–1.5 U/hr. A child weighing 10.7 kg has a 150 mL volume of solution containing 45 U infusing at a rate of 20

mL/hr. Normal dosage range per hr _____

Dosage infusing per hour _____ Assessment _____

31. A child weighing 12.5 kg is receiving an IV of 2500 U heparin in 250 mL D5W at 40 mL/hr. The normal dosage range for heparin is 10–25 U/kg/hr. Normal

dosage range per hour _____ Dosage infusing per hour _____

Assessment _____

32. A child with a weight of 10 kg is to receive a medication with a normal dosage range of 60–80 mg/kg/day. The order is for 200 mg q.6.h. Normal dosage

range per day _____ Daily dosage ordered _____

Assessment _____

33. Order: 0.5 g naficillin in 100 mL D5W q.6.h. Normal dosage range is 100–200 mg/kg/day. Child weighs 15 kg. Normal dosage range per day

_____ Daily dosage ordered _____ Assessment

34. A continuous IV of 500 mL with 20 mEq KCl is infusing at 30 mL/hr. The dosage for potassium chloride is not to exceed 40 mEq/day. Dosage infusing

per hour _____ Dosage infusing per day _____

Assessment _____

35. A 24 kg child is receiving 116 mg per hr of rifampin IV for 3 hours. Dosage range for this drug is 10–20 mg/kg/day. Normal dosage range per day

_____ Dosage received after 3 hours _____

Assessment _____

36. A 25% solution of serum Albumin is infusing at 15 mL/hr for a total of 6 hours. Normal dosage for children is 5–25 g/day. Grams infused after

6 hr _____ Assessment _____

37. The usual dosage of chloramphenicol for children is 50 mg/kg/24 hr in equally divided doses. Order: infuse 50 mL with 290 mg chloramphenicol

q.6.h. The child weighs 51 lbs. Normal dosage per day _____

Daily dosage ordered _____ Assessment _____

38. Order: 500 mL D5RL with 30 mEq KCl to infuse at 40 mL/hr. A maximum of 10 mEq/hr of KCl should not be exceeded and the total 24 hr dosage should

not exceed 40 mEq/day. Dosage infusing per hr _____

Dosage infusing per day _____ Assessment _____

39. A child weighing 30 kg has an IV of 100 mL D5W containing 600 mcg of medication to infuse over 2 hours. The normal range for this drug is

2–4 mcg/kg/hr. Normal dosage range per hour _____

Dosage infusing per hour _____ Assessment _____

40. 150 mL with 18 mg of medication is ordered to infuse over 10 hours. The normal range for this drug is 0.2 mg–0.6 mg/kg/hr. Child weighs 9 kg. Normal

dosage range per hr _____ Dosage infusing per hour _____

Assessment _____

ANSWERS **1.** 22 mL; 60 gtt/min **2.** 46 mL; 65 gtt/min **3.** 38 mL; 83 gtt/min **4.** 46 mL; 70 gtt/min **5.** 28 mL; 90 gtt/min **6.** 35 mL; 83 gtt/min **7.** 18 mL; 105 gtt/min **8.** 56 mL; 75 gtt/min **9.** 38 mL; 110 gtt/min **10.** 14 mL; 90 gtt/min **11.** 46 mL; 47 mL/hr **12.** 85 mL; 140 mL/hr **13.** 78 mL; 95 mL/hr **14.** 26 mL; 135 mL/hr **15.** 8 mL; 150 mL/hr **16.** 27 mL; 90 mL/hr **17.** 18 mL; 140 mL/hr **18.** 49 mL; 87 mL/hr **19.** 9 mL; 150 mL/hr **20.** 35 mL; 55 mL/hr **21.** 77–115.5 mg/dose; normal **22.** 196.5–262 U/dose; normal **23.** 1.2–3.7 mg/day; 3 mg; normal **24.** 418.5–1255.5 mg/day; 1200 mg; normal **25.** 47.1–109.9 mcg/hr; 70 mcg; normal **26.** 1176–1568 mg/day; 1500 mg; normal **27.** 585–1170 mg/day; 600 mg; normal **28.** 120.3–481.2 mg/day; 450 mg; normal **29.** 103–257.5 U/hr; 100 U hr; normal **30.** 5.4–16.1 U/hr; 6 U/hr; normal **31.** 125–312.5 U/hr; 400 U/hr; too high **32.** 600–800 mg/day; 800 mg; normal **33.** 1500–3000 mg/day; 2000 mg; normal **34.** 1.2 mEq/hr; 28.8 mEq/day; normal **35.** 240–480 mg/day; 348 mg; normal **36.** 22.5 g/6 hr; normal **37.** 1160 mg/day; 1160 mg; normal **38.** 2.4 mEq/hr; 58 mEq/day; too high **39.** 60–120 mcg/hr; 300 mcg; too high **40.** 1.8–5.4 mg/hr; 1.8 mg; normal

SECTION

NINE

Heparin and Critical Care Calculations

25 Calculating Heparin Infusions

OBJECTIVES

The student will

1. determine the hourly heparin dosage when flow rate set calibrations are known
2. calculate IV flow rates based on Dr. orders of units/hr.
3. determine the safe 24 hr dosage range of IV heparin.

INTRODUCTION

Heparin is classified as an anticoagulant drug which acts to inhibit new clot formation or extension of already existing clots. It is important to remember that heparin does not actually dissolve clots, but retards their growth. Most commonly administered IV, heparin is ordered by the physician in either units per hour or when the IV concentration is known, by mL per hour. In each case it is the nurse's responsibility to first calculate the dosage to determine its safety, and secondly to administer the correct amount.

Heparin therapy is carefully calculated on an individualized basis, and may vary depending on a variety of factors, one of which is a laboratory test frequently ordered daily during heparin administration. This test is called APTT (activated partial thromboplastin time) and is done to determine the current coagulation status. Heparin dosages are always expressed in USP units (U), and it is very important when calculating dosages to remember the normal heparinizing dosage per day, which determines the safety range for administration.

 The normal heparinizing dosage for adults is 20,000–40,000 U every 24 hours.

The action of heparin is short, about 4–6 hours. Actual average half-life is 60 to 90 min. The half-life is prolonged by higher doses and in liver or kidney disease, and shortened in patients with pulmonary embolism.

In this chapter you will learn how to calculate hourly heparin dosages, determine safe parameters, and finally to calculate the IV flow rate to deliver the specified dosage. Two methods of calculating by ratio and proportion are shown. Choose the method easiest for you.

Calculating Hourly Dosage

If a heparin order asks that you infuse an IV at a predetermined flow rate, for example 50 mL per hour, the doctor has already calculated the dosage per hour of heparin the patient is to receive. However, it still remains a nursing responsibility to calculate this dosage for accuracy and to assure the safe administration of the drug. Look closely at the following examples.

EXAMPLE 1 An IV of 1000 mL D5W containing 40,000 U heparin has been ordered to infuse at 30 mL/hr. Calculate the dosage of heparin the patient is receiving per hour.

$$40,000 \text{ U} : 1000 \text{ mL} = \text{X U} : 30 \text{ mL} \quad \text{or} \quad \frac{40,000 \text{ U}}{1000 \text{ mL}} = \frac{\text{X U}}{30 \text{ mL}}$$

$$1000 \text{ X} = 40,000 \times 30 \qquad\qquad 1000 \text{ X} = 40,000 \times 30$$

$$\text{X} = 1,200,000 \div 1000 \qquad\qquad \text{X} = 1,200,000 \div 1,000$$

$$\text{X} = \textbf{1200 U/hr} \qquad\qquad\qquad \text{X} = \textbf{1200 U/hr}$$

The patient is receiving 1200 U of heparin per hour.

Is dosage within the normal heparinizing range?

1200 U/hr $\times$ 24/hr = **28,800 U/24 hr.** This dosage is within the therapeutic range for adults.

EXAMPLE 2 Order: Add 20,000 U heparin to 1 L D5NS and infuse at 80 mL/hr. Calculate the hourly heparin dosage. Is the dose within the normal recommended range?

$$20,000 \text{ U} : 1000 \text{ mL} = \text{X U} : 80 \text{ mL} \quad \text{or} \quad \frac{20,000 \text{ U}}{1000 \text{ mL}} = \frac{\text{X U}}{80 \text{ mL}}$$

$$1000 \text{ X} = 20,000 \times 80 \qquad\qquad 1000 \text{ X} = 20,000 \times 80$$

$$\text{X} = 1,600,000 \div 1000 \qquad\qquad \text{X} = 1,600,000 \div 1,000$$

$$\text{X} = \textbf{1600 U/hr} \qquad\qquad\qquad \text{X} = \textbf{1600 U/hr}$$

1600 U/hr $\times$ 24 hr = **38,400 U/24 hr.** This dose is within the normal therapeutic range.

Refer to the label in figure 103 and determine the number of mL of heparin you will need to add to the D5NS.

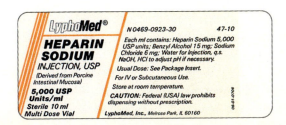

Figure 103

You must add 4 mL of heparin to obtain the 20,000 U dosage.

EXAMPLE 3 An IV of D5W 500 mL with 10,000 U heparin is infusing at 30 mL/hr. Calculate the hourly dosage and determine if the dose is within normal range.

$$10{,}000 \text{ U} : 500 \text{ mL} = \text{X U} : 30 \text{ mL} \quad \text{or} \quad \frac{10{,}000 \text{ U}}{500 \text{ mL}} = \frac{\text{X U}}{30 \text{ mL}}$$

$$500 \text{ X} = 10{,}000 \times 30 \qquad\qquad 500 \text{ X} = 10{,}000 \times 30$$

$$\text{X} = 300{,}000 \div 500 \qquad\qquad \text{X} = 300{,}000 \div 500$$

$$\text{X} = \textbf{600 U/hr} \qquad\qquad\qquad \text{X} = \textbf{600 U/hr}$$

600 U × 24 = **14,400 U/24 hr.** This is less than the recommended dosage and the physician should be notified and the order clarified.

Problem

Calculate the following hourly heparin dosages and determine if they are within the recommended heparinizing range.

1. Order: Add 30,000 U heparin to 750 mL D5W and infuse at 25 mL/hr. _____ Refer to figure 104 and determine the number of mL of this heparin you must add to the D5W. _____

2. A 20,000 U vial of heparin is added to 500 mL D5W and is ordered to infuse at 30 mL/hr. _____ Refer to figure 105 and determine how much heparin you must add to the D5W. _____

3. One liter of D5NS is started with 60,000 U of heparin IV. Doctors orders are to infuse at 40 mL/hr. _____

4. Order: Add 50,000 U heparin to 1 liter D5W and infuse at 75 mL/hr. _____

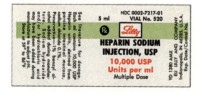

Figure 104

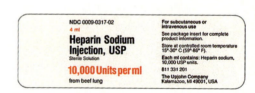

Figure 105

5. A nurse adds 25,000 U heparin to 500 mL D5W and begins the ordered infusion at 30 mL/hr. _____ Refer to figure 106 and determine how many mL of heparin you must add to the D5W. _____

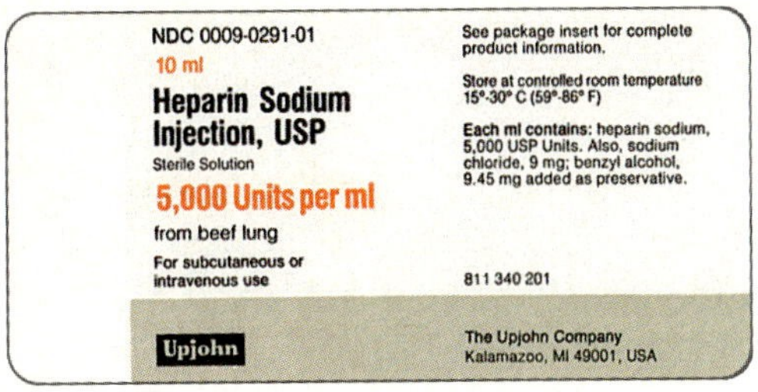

Figure 106

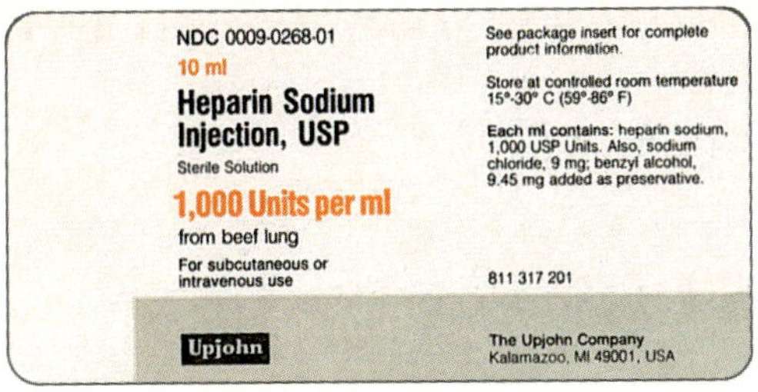

Figure 107

6. Order: Add 10,000 U heparin to 1 liter of D5 ½NS and infuse at 90 mL/hr. _____ Refer to figure 107 and determine how many mL of heparin you must add to the D5 ½NS. _____

7. An IV of 500 mL D5W with 40,000 U heparin is started at 25 mL/hr.
   _____

8. A newly written order is for 1 liter of D5NS with 50,000 U heparin to infuse at 25 mL/hr. _____

ANSWERS 1. 1000 U/hr, within normal range; 3 mL **2.** 1200 U/hr, within normal range; 2 mL
3. 2400 U/hr, above normal range **4.** 3750 U/hr, above normal range **5.** 1500 U/hr, within normal range;
5 mL **6.** 900 U/hr, within normal range; 10 mL **7.** 2000 U/hr, above normal range **8.** 1250 U/hr, within
normal range

Calculating Hourly Dosages from Set Calibration and Flow Rate

Heparin dosages may be calculated hourly from set calibration and flow rate information only. This calculation involves several steps. **First the volume in mL/hr being infused is calculated.** Once this is obtained the same ratio and proportion method is used to determine the heparin dosage being given. Let's look at some examples.

EXAMPLE 1   Calculate the hourly heparin dosage a patient is receiving if the solution contains 25,000 U in 1 L D5W. The set calibration is 15 gtt/mL and the IV flow rate is 30 gtt/min.

■ **Convert gtt/min to mL/min**

$$15 \text{ gtt} : 1 \text{ mL} = 30 \text{ gtt} : X \text{ mL} \quad \text{or} \quad \frac{15 \text{ gtt}}{1 \text{ mL}} = \frac{30 \text{ gtt}}{X \text{ mL}}$$

$$X = \textbf{2 mL/min} \qquad\qquad X = \textbf{2 mL/min}$$

■ **Convert mL/min to mL/hr**

$$2 \text{ mL/min} \times 60 \text{ min} = \textbf{120 mL/hr}$$

■ **Calculate units per hour**

$$25{,}000 \text{ U} : 1000 \text{ mL} = \text{X U} : 120 \text{ mL} \quad \text{or} \quad \frac{25{,}000 \text{ U}}{1{,}000 \text{ mL}} = \frac{\text{X U}}{120 \text{ mL}}$$

$$\text{X} = \textbf{3000 U/hr} \qquad\qquad \text{X} = \textbf{3000 U/hr}$$

The patient is receiving 3000 U of heparin per hour.

EXAMPLE 2 A new IV of 1000 mL D5W with 20,000 U of heparin is infusing at 12 gtt/min. The set calibration is 10 gtt/mL. Calculate the hourly dosage of heparin.

■ **Convert gtt/min to mL/min**

$$10 \text{ gtt} : 1 \text{ mL} = 12 \text{ gtt} : \text{X mL} \quad \text{or} \quad \frac{10 \text{ gtt}}{1 \text{ mL}} = \frac{12 \text{ gtt}}{\text{X mL}}$$

$$\text{X} = \textbf{1.2 mL/min} \qquad\qquad \text{X} = \textbf{1.2 mL/min}$$

■ **Convert mL/min to mL/hr**

$$1.2 \text{ mL/min} \times 60 \text{ min} = \textbf{72 mL/hr}$$

■ **Calculate units per hour**

$$20{,}000 \text{ U} : 1000 \text{ mL} = \text{X U} : 72 \text{ mL} \quad \text{or} \quad \frac{20{,}000 \text{ U}}{1000 \text{ mL}} = \frac{\text{X U}}{72 \text{ mL}}$$

$$\text{X} = \textbf{1440 U/hr} \qquad\qquad \text{X} = \textbf{1440 U/hr}$$

The patient is receiving 1440 U/hr.

EXAMPLE 3 The patient has an IV of 25,000 U of heparin in 1 L D5W infusing at 10 gtt/min. Using a set calibration of 15 gtt/mL determine the hourly heparin dosage. Round off to the nearest hundredth.

■ **Convert gtt/min to mL/min**

$$15 \text{ gtt} : 1 \text{ mL} = 10 \text{ gtt} : \text{X mL} \quad \text{or} \quad \frac{15 \text{ gtt}}{1 \text{ mL}} = \frac{10 \text{ gtt}}{\text{X mL}}$$

$$\text{X} = \textbf{0.67 mL/min} \qquad\qquad \text{X} = \textbf{0.67 mL/min}$$

■ **Convert mL/min to mL/hr**

$$0.67 \text{ mL/min} \times 60 \text{ min} = 40.2 = \textbf{40 mL/hr}$$

■ **Calculate units per hour**

$$25{,}000 \text{ U} : 1000 \text{ mL} = \text{X U} : 40 \text{ mL} \quad \text{or} \quad \frac{25{,}000 \text{ U}}{1{,}000 \text{ mL}} = \frac{\text{X U}}{40 \text{ mL}}$$

$$\text{X} = \textbf{1000 U/hr} \qquad\qquad \text{X} = \textbf{1000 U/hr}$$

The patient is receiving 1000 U/hr.

EXAMPLE 4 Calculate the hourly heparin dosage of a patient who has an IV of 1000 mL D5 ¼NS with 60,000 U heparin that is infusing at 30 gtt/min and has a set calibration of 60 gtt/mL.

■ **Convert gtt/min to mL/min**

$$60 \text{ gtt} : 1 \text{ mL} = 30 \text{ gtt} : X \text{ mL} \quad \text{or} \quad \frac{60 \text{ gtt}}{1 \text{ mL}} = \frac{30 \text{ gtt}}{X \text{ mL}}$$

$$X = \textbf{0.5 mL/min} \qquad\qquad X = \textbf{0.5 mL/min}$$

■ **Convert mL/min to mL/hr**

$$0.5 \text{ mL/min} \times 60 \text{ min} = \textbf{30 mL/hr}$$

■ **Calculate units per hour.**

$$60,000 \text{ U} : 1000 \text{ mL} = X \text{ U} : 30 \text{ mL} \quad \text{or} \quad \frac{60,000 \text{ U}}{1,000 \text{ mL}} = \frac{X \text{ U}}{30 \text{ mL}}$$

$$X = \textbf{1800 U/hr} \qquad\qquad X = \textbf{1800 U/hr}$$

The patient is receiving 1800 U/hr

Problem

Calculate the dosage of heparin each patient is receiving hourly in the following problems.

1. A liter of D5NS with 40,000 U of heparin is infusing IV at 12 gtt/min. The set calibration is 20 gtt/mL. _____

2. A patient is receiving an IV of 500 mL D5W with 25,000 U heparin which is infusing at 10 gtt/min. The tubing administers 10 gtt/mL. _____

3. Orders are to infuse 1 liter of IV solution containing 10,000 U heparin at 20 gtt/min using a set calibration of 15 gtt/mL. _____

4. Your patient has a new IV of 1 L D5W with 30,000 U of heparin infusing at 8 gtt/min. The set calibration is 15 gtt/mL. _____

5. 500 mL of D5W with 25,000 U of heparin is infusing at 25 gtt/min using a set calibration of 60 gtt/mL. _____

ANSWERS   **1.** 1440 U/hr   **2.** 3000 U/hr   **3.** 800 U/hr   **4.** 960 U/hr   **5.** 1250 U/hr

Calculating Heparin Flow Rates

Heparin is frequently ordered in **units per hour** to be administered. In this situation you must **first calculate how many mL/hr will contain the units ordered, then determine the flow rate necessary to deliver this amount.**

EXAMPLE 1 Order: Infuse 1000 U/hr of heparin IV from a solution of 20,000 U in 500 mL D5W. The administration set is a microdrip. Calculate the flow rate.

■ **Calculate mL/hr to be administered**

$$20,000 \text{ U} : 500 \text{ mL} = 1000 \text{ U} : X \text{ mL} \quad \text{or} \quad \frac{20,000 \text{ U}}{500 \text{ mL}} = \frac{1000 \text{ U}}{X \text{ mL}}$$

$$20,000 \text{ X} = 500 \times 1000 \qquad\qquad 20,000 \text{ X} = 500 \times 1000$$

$$X = \textbf{25 mL/hr} \qquad\qquad\qquad X = \textbf{25 mL/hr}$$

■ **Calculate the flow rate in gtt/min**
The set available is a microdrip

$$25 \text{ mL/hr} \div 1 \text{ (division factor)} = \textbf{25 gtt/min}$$

EXAMPLE 2 The doctor orders heparin 800 U/hr IV. Solution available is 40,000 U in 1000 mL D5W. Set calibration is 15 gtt/mL. Calculate the flow rate.

■ **Calculate mL/hr**

$$40,000 \text{ U} : 1000 \text{ mL} = 800 \text{ U} : X \text{ mL} \quad \text{or} \quad \frac{40,000 \text{ U}}{1000 \text{ mL}} = \frac{800 \text{ U}}{X \text{ mL}}$$

$$40,000 \text{ X} = 1000 \times 800 \qquad\qquad 40,000 \text{ X} = 1000 \times 800$$

$$X = \textbf{20 mL/hr} \qquad\qquad\qquad X = \textbf{20 mL/hr}$$

■ **Calculate the flow rate in gtt/min**

$$20 \text{ mL/hr} \div 4 \text{ (division factor)} = \textbf{5 gtt/min}$$

EXAMPLE 3 Order: Infuse 1200 U/hr of heparin IV. Solution available is 60,000 U in 1 L D5W. Set calibration is 20 gtt/mL.

■ **Calculate mL/hr**

$$60,000 \text{ U} : 1000 \text{ mL} = 1200 \text{ U} : X \text{ mL} \quad \text{or} \quad \frac{60,000 \text{ U}}{1000 \text{ mL}} = \frac{1200 \text{ U}}{X \text{ mL}}$$

$$60,000 \text{ X} = 1000 \times 1200 \qquad\qquad 60,000 \text{ X} = 1000 \times 1200$$

$$X = \textbf{20 mL/hr} \qquad\qquad\qquad X = \textbf{20 mL/hr}$$

■ **Calculate the flow rate in gtt/min**

$$20 \text{ mL/hr} \div 3 \text{ (division factor)} = \textbf{6.6} = \textbf{7 gtt/min}$$

Problem

Calculate the flow rates in gtt/min of the following.

1. Administer 1000 U heparin IV every hour. Solution available is 25,000 U in 500 mL of D5W. Set calibration is a microdrip. _____

2. A patient with deep vein thrombosis has orders for heparin 10,000 U every 4 hours IV continuously. Solution available is 50,000 U in 1000 mL D5W. The set calibration is 20 gtt/mL. _____

3. Order: Give 1100 U/hr of heparin IV. Solution 15,000 U in 1 L D5NS. Set calibration is 10 gtt/mL. _____

4. Your newly admitted patient has orders for 50,000 U of heparin in 1 L D5W and infuse 2000 U/hr continuously. Set calibration is 15 gtt/mL. _____

5. Administer 1500 U/hr of heparin IV using a solution of 40,000 U in 750 mL D5 ½NS. Set calibration is 60 gtt/mL. _____

ANSWERS 1. 20 gtt/min **2.** 17 gtt/min **3.** 12 gtt/min **4.** 10 gtt/min **5.** 28 gtt/min

Although we have focused only on the administration of heparin in this chapter, it is intended that the information and calculations learned here be applied to other IV medications you will be administering in the future.

Summary

This ends the chapter on IV heparin calculations. The important points to remember are:

heparin dosages are highly individualized and may be ordered by flow rate, or units per hour

the normal heparinizing dosage for adults is between 20,000–40,000 U every 24 hours

hourly heparin dosages may be calculated from the set calibration of the tubing and the flow rate

when heparin is ordered in units per hour, first determine the number of mL/hr the patient should receive, then determine the actual flow rate

Summary Self Test

Directions: Calculate the following heparin dosages and flow rates.

1. The doctor orders a patient to receive 6000 U of heparin every 6 hours continuously IV. The solution available is 25,000 U in 1 L of D5W. The set calibration is 60 gtt/mL. Calculate the correct flow rate. _____

2. A solution of 25,000 U heparin in 1 L D5 ¼NS is infusing at 15 gtt/min. The tubing set delivers 10 gtt/mL. Calculate the hourly heparin dosage.

   _____

3. A doctor orders a patient to receive 1200 U of heparin every hour IV continuously. The solution is 35,000 U heparin in 1 L D5 ½NS. Calculate the mL/hr the patient will receive. _____

4. There is 20,000 U of heparin in 500 mL D5W infusing at 40 mL per hour. Calculate the hourly unit dosage. _____

5. A newly admitted patient is to receive 1250 U of heparin per hour continuously. The solution available is 1 L D5 ¼NS with 50,000 U heparin. Set calibration is 15 gtt/mL. Calculate the hourly flow rate and gtt/min. _____

6. To help prevent further pulmonary emboli a physician orders 5000 U of heparin IV every 2 hours continuously. The available solution is 40,000 U in 1 L D5RL. Calculate the flow rate if the set calibration is 10 gtt/mL.

   _____

7. Order: Infuse a solution of 25,000 U heparin in 1 L D5W over 24 hours. Calculate the hourly unit dosage, then the flow rate using a set calibration of 10 gtt/mL. _____

8. Calculate the hourly unit dosage of heparin and determine if it is within normal range for a patient receiving 35 gtt/min of an IV containing 40,000 U heparin in 1 L D5W. The set calibration is a microdrip. _____

9. An IV of 35,000 U of heparin in 1 L D5W is ordered to infuse at 50 mL per hour. Calculate the hourly unit dosage. _____

10. A recent open heart patient has 500 mL D5W with 20,000 U of heparin infusing at 20 microdrips/min. Calculate the hourly unit dosage. _____

11. A physician orders a patient to receive 2000 U heparin IV hourly from a solution containing 50,000 U in 1000 mL D5NS. Determine the flow rate if the set calibration is 10 gtt/mL. _____

12. Order: Infuse a solution of 15,000 U heparin in 250 mL NS over 6 hours. Calculate the rate of flow if the set calibration is 20 gtt/mL. _____

13. A patient with a fractured pelvis has orders for an IV solution of 1 L D5 ½NS with 60,000 U of heparin. This is to infuse at 30 mL/hr. Calculate the hourly heparin dosage and determine if it is within normal range. _____

14. A physician orders a patient to receive 1000 U heparin IV hourly from a solution containing 20,000 U in 500 mL D5NS. Determine the flow rate if the set calibration is 60 gtt/mL. _____

15. A newly admitted patient has an order for IV heparin to infuse at 1500 U/hr continuously. The solution available is 20,000 U in 1 L D5W. The set calibration is 20 gtt/mL. Calculate the flow rate. _____

16. Calculate the hourly dosage of 1 L D5 ¼NS with 45,000 U heparin ordered to infuse at 25 mL/hr. _____

17. Calculate the hourly heparin dosage a patient with an IV of 40,000 U heparin in 1 L D5W infusing at 30 mL/hr is receiving. _____

18. A liter of solution containing 15,000 U of heparin is infusing IV at 20 gtt/min. Calculate the hourly unit dosage if the set calibration is 10 gtt/mL. _____

19. During morning rounds you time a patient's IV at 20 gtt/min. The solution infusing is 25,000 U heparin in 1 L D5W. The administration set delivers 10 gtt/mL. The doctor has ordered 1500 U of heparin per hour. Is the patient receiving the ordered dosage? _____

20. Order: Infuse 1 liter of D5RL with 25,000 U heparin over 24 hours. Using a set calibrated at 15 gtt/mL calculate first the hourly unit dosage then calculate the flow rate. Lastly determine if the dosage is within normal limits.

    _____

21. A solution of 500 mL D5NS with 30,000 U heparin is infusing IV at 25 mL/hr. Calculate the hourly unit dosage and determine if it is within normal limits.

    _____

22. For a patient with multiple fractures the doctor has ordered 2 liters D5 ½NS each with 20,000 U heparin to infuse at 50 mL per hour. Calculate the hourly unit dosage. The set calibration is a microdrip. What will the flow rate be?

    _____

23. Calculate the mL/hr and hourly unit dosage for a patient receiving 500 mL D5W with 10,000 heparin IV infusing at 20 gtt/min. Set calibration is 10 gtt/mL. _____

24. Order: Infuse 1 liter D5W with 15,000 U heparin over 10 hours. Calculate mL/hr and U/hr being administered. _____

25. A patient is receiving 20 mL/hr of 1 liter D5W with 35,000 U of heparin. Calculate the hourly unit dosage and flow rate using a set calibration of 20 gtt/mL. _____

26. Order: Infuse 500 mL/D5 ¼NS with 25,000 U heparin at 1500 U/hr. Calculate the flow rate. _____

27. A liter of D5W with 40,000 U heparin is infusing at 25 mL/hr. What is the hourly heparin dosage? _____

28. A 500 mL IV bag with 25,000 U of heparin is infusing at 30 mL per hour. Calculate the hourly dosage of heparin. _____

29. 1000 mL D5W with 55,000 U of heparin is infusing at 20 gtt/min. The set calibration is a microdrip. Calculate hourly dosage. _____

30. Order: Infuse 1 L D5 ½NS with 45,000 U of heparin over 20 hours. Calculate mL/hr and U/hr being administered. _____

31. Order: Infuse 1400 U/hr of heparin. Solution available is 35,000 U of heparin in 1 L D5W. Calculate flow rate to deliver the desired dosage. _____

32. During your initial shift assessment you time a patient's IV at 20 gtt/min. The set calibration is 10 gtt/mL. The order is to administer 1000 U heparin per hour continuously. The IV solution is labeled 20,000 U in 500 mL D5 ½NS. How many mL/hr should the patient be receiving? _____

33. How many mL/hr is the above patient actually receiving? _____

34. Is the dosage this patient is receiving correct? _____

35. There is 250 mL of D5W left in an IV bag. The doctor writes on order to add 10,000 U heparin and infuse at 15 mL/hr. What dosage will the patient be receiving? Is this within the normal heparinizing range? _____

ANSWERS 1. 40 gtt/min **2.** 2250 U/hr **3.** 34 mL/hr **4.** 1600 U/hr **5.** 25 mL/hr; 6 gtt/min **6.** 11 gtt/min
7. 1042 U/hr; 7 gtt/min **8.** 1400 U/hr; Yes, within normal limits **9.** 1750 U/hr **10.** 800 U/hr **11.** 7 gtt/min
12. 14 gtt/min **13.** 1800 U/hr; No, dosage exceeds the normal range **14.** 25 gtt/min **15.** 25 gtt/min **16.** 1125 U/hr
17. 1200 U/hr **18.** 1800 U/hr **19.** No, double the dose is infusing **20.** 1042 U/hr; 11 gtt/min; Yes, dosage within
normal limits. **21.** 1500 U/hr; Yes, within normal limits **22.** 1000 U/hr; 50 gtt/min **23.** 120 mL/hr;
2400 U/hr **24.** 100 mL/hr; 1500 U/hr **25.** 700 U/hr; 7 gtt/min **26.** 30 mL/hr **27.** 1000 U/hr **28.** 1500 U/hr
29. 1100 U/hr **30.** 50 mL/hr; 2250 U/hr **31.** 40 mL/hr **32.** 25 mL/hr **33.** 120 mL/hr **34.** No, too high
35. 600 U/hr; below heparinizing range

Critical Care IV Calculations

26

OBJECTIVES

The student will calculate
1. dosages in mcg/kg per min/hr
2. dosages in mg per min/hr
3. IV flow rates in mL/hr (gtt/min)
4. titrations within an ordered dosage range

INTRODUCTION

A critical care drug is one which maintains or alters a vital physiological function such as heart rate, cardiac output, blood pressure, respirations, or renal function. In general they have a very rapid action and short duration. In emergency situations critical care drugs are administered by IV push or bolus, but once an initial emergency is over the action is sustained by infusion of a smaller concentration of the drug in an IV solution, most commonly D5W.

Physicians ordering critical care IV drugs generally order them by flow rate (mL/hr, gtt/min) or by dosage (mcg/min, or mcg, mg or U/ kg/min or hr). Medications are sometimes ordered to infuse within a dosage range, for example 1– 3 mcg/min, to elicit a specific physiologic response. An example would be to maintain a systolic BP of 100 mm Hg. This adjustment of rate is called titration, and dosage increments are made within the ordered range until the desired response has been established.

Most critical care drugs require close and continuous monitoring. When available an electronic infusion device (EID) should be utilized; if one is not available a microdrip set calibrated at 60 gtt/mL must be used. All calculations in this chapter are for an EID or microdrip, therefore the mL/hr and gtt/min rates are interchangeable and identical.

Critical care calculations will include converting dosages to flow rates, and flow rates to dosage being infused per min, per hr, per mL and per gtt. Since the patient's weight is a critical factor in the ordered dosage, it too is an important component of calculations. Dosage ranges and flow rates for titrated solutions, and calculations of dosage changes during titration are also included.

Remember, accuracy is imperative in calculating and administering critical care drugs because all have narrow margins of safety.

Double checking math is both mandatory and routine.

Read each example and problem through first. Then go back and work through each step slowly and methodically. If you find yourself forgetting the steps you are moving too quickly.

 All calculations in this chapter are for EID or microdrip sets, therefore mL/hr and gtt/min are identical.

Calculating Flow Rate from Dosage Ordered

When a critical care drug is ordered by dosage per minute the flow rate can be quickly calculated.

EXAMPLE 1 A maternity patient has an order for ritodrine HCl 150 mg in 500 mL D5W to infuse at 0.1 mg per min. Calculate the flow rate to deliver this dosage by volumetric pump.

- **Determine the dosage per hour**

  0.1 mg/min × 60 min = **6 mg/hr**

- **Calculate flow rate (mL/hr, gtt/min)**

  150 mg : 500 mL = 6 mg : X mL

  = **20 mL/hr**

To infuse 0.1 mg/min set the flow rate at 20 mL/hr (gtt/min).

EXAMPLE 2 A dosage of 400 mg of dopamine HCl is added to 500 mL D5NS. The order is to infuse 400 mcg/min IV. Calculate the flow rate. This calculation requires one additional step because the solution dosage is in mg, and the order specifies mcg.

- **Determine the dosage per hour**

  400 mcg/min × 60 min = **24000 mcg/hr**

- **Convert to like units (mcg/mg)**

  24000 mcg/hr = **24 mg/hr**

- **Calculate mL/hr flow rate**

  400 mg : 500 mL = 24 mg : X mL

  X = **30 mL/hr**

To deliver 400 mcg/min set the flow rate at 30 mL/hr (gtt/min).

EXAMPLE 3 A patient in CHF has orders for Nitrostat 5 mcg/min IV. Solution available is 8 mg Nitrostat in 250 mL D5W. Calculate the flow rate.

■ **Determine the dosage per hour**

5 mcg/min × 60 min = **300 mcg/hr**

■ **Convert to like units**

300 mcg = **0.3 mg**

■ **Calculate mL/hr**

8 mg : 250 mL = 0.3 mg : X mL

X = 9.4 or **9 mL/hr**

To deliver 5 mcg/min set the flow rate at 9 mL/hr (gtt/min).

Problem

Calculate the following flow rates in mL/hr (gtt/min)

1. For a patient experiencing an acute MI with symptoms of shock, the doctor orders an infusion of Isuprel at 3 mcg/min. Isuprel 2 mg is added to 500 mL D5W. _____

2. Trandate 200 mg has been added to 250 mL D5W and ordered to infuse at 2 mg/min. _____

3. A patient with ventricular irritability has orders to receive Pronestyl at 4 mg/min. Solution available is 500 mg Pronestyl in 250 mL D5W. _____

4. Procanamide 1 g in 250 mL has been ordered to infuse at 2 mg/min. _____

5. A patient with angina has orders for a continuous IV infusion of Nitrostat. Solution available is 8 mg in 250 mL D5W. Orders are to infuse at 10 mcg/min. _____

ANSWERS **1.** 45 mL/hr **2.** 150 mL/hr **3.** 120 mL/hr **4.** 30 mL/hr **5.** 19 mL/hr

Calculating Flow Rate from Dosage per kg

When drugs are ordered on the basis of dosage per kg per min or per hour one additional calculation is necessary.

EXAMPLE 1 Infuse 2 mcg/kg/min of a Nipride solution with a concentration of 50 mg Nipride in 500 mL D5W. The patient weighs 58 kg.

■ **Calculate dosage per minute for this patient**

58 kg × 2 mcg/min = **116 mcg/min**

- **Determine dosage per hour**

  116 mcg/min $\times$ 60 min = **6960 mcg/hr**

- **Convert to like units**

  6960 mcg = 6.96 mg = **7 mg/hr**

- **Calculate mL/hr flow rate**

  50 mg : 500 mL = 7 mg : X mL

  X = **70 mL/hr**

To deliver 2 mcg/kg/min set the flow rate at 70 mL/hr (gtt/min).

EXAMPLE 2 The order is to infuse 10 mcg/kg/min of dobutamine. The solution has a concentration of 500 mg dobutamine in 250 mL D5W. The patient weighs 90 kg.

- **Calculate dosage per min for this patient**

  90 kg $\times$ 10 mcg = **900 mcg/min**

- **Determine dosage per hour**

  900 mcg/min $\times$ 60 min = **54,000 mcg/hr**

- **Convert to like units**

  54000 mcg = **54 mg/hr**

- **Calculate mL/hr flow rate**

  500 mg : 250 mL = 54 mg : X mL

  X = **27 mL/hr**

To deliver a dosage of 10 mcg/kg/min set the flow rate at 27 mL/hr (gtt/min).

EXAMPLE 3 A narcotic overdose patient has an order for a Narcan drip. The IV has 2 mg Narcan in 250 mL D5W, to infuse at a rate of 0.01 mg/kg/hr. The patient weighs 70 kg.

- **Calculate dosage per hr for this patient**

  70 kg $\times$ 0.01 mg/kg = **0.7 mg/hr**

- **Calculate mL/hr flow rate**

  2 mg : 250 mL = 0.7 mg : X mL

  X = 87.5 = **88 mL/hr**

To deliver a dosage of 0.01 mg/kg/hr set the flow rate at 88 mL/hr (gtt/min).

Problem

Calculate flow rates in mL/hr (gtt/min) for the following dosages.

1. A patient with severe chest pain has an order for a Nipride infusion. The order reads to add 50 mg Nipride to 500 mL D5W and infuse at 2 mcg/kg/min.

    The patient weighs 70 kg. _____

2. A patient weighing 83 kg is to receive Lidocaine at the rate of 25 mcg/kg/min. The solution has a concentration of 500 mg Lidocaine in 250 mL D5W.

    _____

3. A post kidney transplant patient weighing 60 kg has orders for cytomegalo-virus immune globulin by constant syringe infusion pump at a rate of 15 mg/kg/hr. A 2500 mg vial of cmv is diluted in 50 mL sterile water.

    _____

4. Esmolol 50 mcg/kg/min has been ordered for a patient who weighs 109 kg.

    The solution ordered is 500 mL D5RL containing 5 g of Esmolol. _____

5. A patient weighing 97 kg has an order for Inocor 7 mcg/kg/min. The solution ordered to infuse is 50 mL NS containing 250 mg of Inocor. _____

ANSWERS 1. 84 mL/hr **2.** 62 mL/hr **3.** 18 mL/hr **4.** 33 mL/hr **5.** 8 mL/hr

Calculating Dosage from Flow Rate

In critical care drugs it may be necessary to know the exact dosage being administered per hr or per min. This can be calculated from the flow rate by using the following steps.

EXAMPLE 1 Order: Infuse dopamine 800 mg in 500 mL D5W at 25 mL/hr. Calculate the dosage in mg/hr and mcg/min infusing.

- **Determine the dosage per hour infusing**

    800 mg : 500 mL = X mg : 25 mL

    X = **40 mg/hr**

- **Convert milligrams to micrograms**

    40 mg = **40,000 mcg/hr**

- **Convert mcg/hr to mcg/min**

    40,000 mcg/hr ÷ 60 min = **666.6 or 667 mcg/min**

    A 25 mL/hr infusion is equal to a dosage of 40 mg/hr, or 667 mcg/min.

EXAMPLE 2 A post-op cardiac bypass patient has orders to infuse Nipride at 30 gtt/min. The solution available is 100 mg Nipride in 500 mL D5W. Calculate the mg/min and mg/hr the patient is receiving.

■ **Convert gtt/min to mL/min**

60 gtt : 1 mL = 30 gtt : X mL

X = **0.5 mL/min**

■ **Determine mg/min**

100 mg : 500 mL = X mg : 0.5 mL

X = **0.1 mg/min**

■ **Calculate mg/hr**

0.1 mg/min × 60 min = **6 mg/hr**

At 30 gtt/min infusing the patient is receiving a dosage of 0.1 mg/min, or 6 mg/hr.

EXAMPLE 3 A patient with ventricular ectopi has stat orders for continuous Lidocaine infusion at a flow rate of 30 mL/hr. The solution available is 1 g Lidocaine in 500 mL D5W. Calculate first the mg/hr then the mg/min the patient will receive.

■ **Convert g to mg**

The answer is in mg so convert g to mg

1 g = 1000 mg

■ **Calculate mg/hr**

1000 mg : 500 mL = X mg : 30 mL

X = **60 mg/hr**

■ **Convert mg/hr to mg/min**

60 mg/hr ÷ 60 min = **1 mg/min**

At the rate of 30 mL/hr this patient is receiving a dosage of 60 mg/hr or 1 mg/min.

The average dosage of Lidocaine is 1–4 mg/min. From the answers you obtained you can quickly ascertain that the dosage is within a safe range.

EXAMPLE 4 0.5 g of Aminophylline is added to 500 mL D5 ¼NS. The order is to infuse IV over 6 hours. Calculate the mg/hr the patient will receive.

■ **Convert g to mg**

0.5 g = **500 mg**

■ **Calculate mg/hr**

500 mg ÷ 6 hours = **83 mg/hr**

The patient is receiving 83 mg/hr of aminophylline.

Problem

Calculate the dosages indicated in the following problems. Express answers to the nearest hundredth.

1. A continuous infusion of Isuprel is ordered for a newly admitted patient in cardiogenic shock at 40 mL/hr. Solution available is 2 mg in 500 mL D5W.

   Calculate the mg/hr and mcg/hr the patient will be receiving. _____

   _____

2. Order: Infuse dobutamine 500 mg in 500 mL D5W at 15 mL/hr. Calculate

   the mg/hr, mg/min, and mcg/min the patient is receiving. _____

   _____   _____

3. Pronestyl 1 g in 250 mL D5W is ordered for a patient with frequent PVC's to run at 1 mL/min. Calculate the number of mg/min the patient is receiving. The normal dosage is between 2–6 mg/min. Is this dosage within normal

   limits? _____   _____

4. A patient in CHF following an MI has an order for Nitrol IV 3 mL/hr by volumetric pump. The IV solution has a dilution of 200 mcg/mL of Nitrol. How

   many mcg/hr and mcg/min is the patient receiving? _____

   _____

5. Esmolol IV is ordered to control the ventricular rate of a patient during surgery. Solution available is 5 g in 500 mL D5W. The doctor orders the infusion to start at 50 mL/hr. Calculate the dosage in mg/hr and mg/min.

   _____   _____

ANSWERS   1. 0.16 mg/hr; 160 mcg/hr   **2.** 15 mg/hr; 0.25 mg/min; 250 mcg/min   **3.** 4 mg/min; Yes   **4.** 600 mcg/hr; 10 mcg/min   **5.** 500 mg/hr; 8 mg/min

Titration of Infusions

Critical care IV medications are often ordered by dosage parameters to obtain a measurable response, for example Isuprel 1–3 mcg/min to maintain heart rate above 64/min. **Adjustment of dosage** in this manner is called **titration.** Dosage will be increased or decreased within the range ordered until the desired response is obtained. **The lowest dosage will be set first,** and adjusted upwards and downwards as necessary. **The upper dosage is never exceeded** unless a new order is obtained.

An electronic infusion device is used for administration of the IV solution. Because these are set in mL/hr the concentration of the IV solution must be calculated in mL, and flow rates must also be calculated in mL/hr. The calculations are similar to those you have already done earlier. Let's look at some examples.

EXAMPLE 1 Levophed 2–6 mcg/min has been ordered to maintain systolic BP > 100. The solution being titrated has 4 mg Levophed in 1 L D5W.

- **Convert to like units**

  4 mg = **4000 mcg**   1 L = **1000 mL**

- **Calculate concentration of solution in mcg/mL**

  4000 mcg : 1000 mL = X mcg : 1 mL

  = **4 mcg/mL**

Concentration of the solution is 4 mcg/mL

- **Convert dosage range to mL/min**

  Use the solution concentration to calculate the lower and upper dosage range.

  Lower dose: 4 mcg : 1 mL = 2 mcg : X mL

  X = **0.5 mL/min**

  Upper dose: 4 mcg : 1 mL = 6 mcg : X mL

  X = **1.5 mL/min**

- **Convert mL/min to mL/hr (gtt/min)**

  The flow rate is set in mL/hr so multiply by 60 min to calculate mL/hr.

  Lower dose: 0.5 mL × 60 min = **30 mL/hr (gtt/min)**

  Upper dose: 1.5 mL × 60 min = **90 mL/hr (gtt/min)**

A dosage of 2–6 mcg/min is equal to a flow rate of 30–90 mL/hr (gtt/min).

Several changes in mL/hr (gtt/min) rate may be made within this range to sustain the blood pressure. At any time the actual dosage titrating can easily be calculated. For example **after several adjustments** the IV is now infusing at **42 mL/hr.**

The **solution concentration** is used again for this calculation.

4 mcg : 1 mL = X mcg : 42 mL

X = **168 mcg/hr**

This gives the mcg/hr infusing. Divide by 60 min to obtain the dosage per min.

168 mcg/hr ÷ 60 min = **2.8 mcg/min**

EXAMPLE 2 Inocor is to be titrated between 415–830 mcg/min to maintain diastolic BP < 90 mm. The solution has a concentration of 250 mg in 50 mL NS.

- **Convert to like units**

    250 mg = 250,000 mcg in 50 mL

- **Calculate concentration of solution in mcg/mL**

    250,000 mcg : 50 mL = X mcg : 1 mL

    = **5000 mcg/mL**

Concentration of the solution is 5000 mcg/mL

- **Convert dosage range to mL/min**

    Lower dose: 5000 mcg : 1 mL = 415 mcg : X mL

    = **0.083 mL/min**

    Upper dose: 5000 mcg : 1 mL = 830 mcg : X mL

    = **0.166 mL/min**

- **Convert mL/min to mL/hr (gtt/min)**

    Lower dose: 0.083 mL × 60 min = 4.98 = **5 mL/hr (gtt/min)**

    Upper dose: 0.166 mL × 60 min = 9.96 = **10 mL/hr (gtt/min)**

A dosage of 415–830 mcg/min is equal to a flow rate of 5–10 mL/hr (gtt/min)

If the rate has been titrated several times and is now infusing at **8 mL/hr** how many mcg/min are infusing?

    5000 mcg : 1 mL = X mcg : 8 mL

    X = **40,000 mcg/hr**

    40,000 mcg/hr ÷ 60 min = **666.7 mcg/min**

EXAMPLE 3 Nitroprusside is to be titrated between 0.5–1.5 mcg/kg/min to maintain systolic BP at > 100 mm. The patient weighs 103 kg, and the solution concentration is 50 mg in 250 mL D5W. Calculate the flow rate to deliver this titration.

This calculation will have one additional step because the dosage is based on body weight.

- **Calculate the dosage range**

    Lower dose: 0.5 mcg × 103 kg = **51.5 mcg/min**

    Upper dose: 1.5 mcg × 103 kg = **154.4 mcg/min**

- **Convert to like units**

    50 mg in 250 mL = 50,000 mcg in 250 mL

- **Calculate concentration of solution**

    50,000 mcg : 250 mL = X mcg : 1 mL

    $$X = \textbf{200 mcg/mL}$$

Concentration of the solution is 200 mcg/mL

- **Convert dosage range to mL/min**

    Lower dose: 200 mcg : 1 mL = 51.5 mcg : X mL

    $$X = \textbf{0.258 mL/min}$$

    Upper dose: 200 mcg : 1 mL = 154.4 mcg : X mL

    $$X = \textbf{0.772 mL/min}$$

- **Convert mL/min to mL/hr (gtt/min)**

    Lower dose: 0.258 mL × 60 min = 15.48 = **15 mL/hr (gtt/min)**

    Upper dose: 0.772 mL × 60 min = 46.32 = **46 mL/hr (gtt/min)**

A dosage of 0.5–1.5 mcg/kg/min is equal to a flow rate of 15–46 mL/hr (gtt/min)

If after several increases and decreases the patient stabilizes at a titrated rate of **22 mL/hr,** what is the dosage of nitroprusside infusing per min?

$$200 \text{ mcg} : 1 \text{ mL} = X \text{ mcg} : 22 \text{ mL}$$

$$X = \textbf{4400 mcg/hr}$$

$$4400 \text{ mcg} \div 60 \text{ min} = \textbf{73.3 mcg/min}$$

EXAMPLE 4 Nipride has been ordered to titrate at 3–6 mcg/kg/min. The solution contains 50 mg Nipride in 250 mL D5W. The patient weighs 72 kg. Determine the flow rate setting for a volumetric pump.

- **Convert to like units**

    50 mg = 50,000 mcg

■ **Calculate concentration of solution**

50,000 mcg : 250 mL = X mcg : 1 mL

X = **200 mcg/mL**

Concentration of the solution is 200 mcg/mL

■ **Calculate the dosage range**

Lower dose: 3 mcg $\times$ 72 kg = **216 mcg/min**

Upper dose: 6 mcg $\times$ 72 kg = **432 mcg/min**

■ **Convert dosage range to mL/min**

Lower dose: 200 mcg : 1 mL = 216 mcg : X mL

X = **1.08 mL/min**

Upper dose: 200 mcg : 1 mL = 432 mcg : X mL

X = **2.16 mL/min**

■ **Convert mL/min to mL/hr**

Lower dose: 1.08 mL $\times$ 60 min = 64.8 = **65 mL/hr (gtt/min)**

Upper dose: 2.16 mL $\times$ 60 min = 129.6 = **130 mL/hr (gtt/min)**

A dosage range of 3–6 mcg/kg/min is equal to a flow rate of 65–130 mL/hr (gtt/min)

If after several adjustments upwards the rate is titrated lower and maintained at **75 mL/hr** what dosage will be infusing per minute?

200 mcg : 1 mL = X mcg : 75 mL

X = **15,000 mcg/hr**

15,000 mcg $\div$ 60 min = **250 mcg/min**

Problem

In each of the following problems calculate the lower and upper dosage range in mL/hr (gtt/min). Use the titrated rate changes provided to calculate current dosages infusing.

1. A patient has a 2 g in 250 mL solution of Bretylium ordered to titrate at 1–2 mg/min for ventricular arrhythmias. _____ After several titrations upward the patient stabilizes at a rate of 12 mL/hr. The dosage infusing per min is _____ .

2.   Isuprel is ordered to titrate between 1–3 mcg/min to sustain heart rate at a minimum of 64/min. The solution infusing has a strength of 2 mg per 500 mL. _____ The IV is currently titrating at 35 mL/hr. What dosage is infusing per min? _____

3.   A titration of 0.15–0.35 mg/min of ritodrine is ordered for a patient in premature labor. The solution infusing has a strength of 150 mg in 500 mL D5W. _____ . At 40 mL/hr contractions stop and the titration is maintained at this rate. What dosage is infusing per min? _____

4.   Esmolol is to titrate between 50–75 mcg/kg/min. The patient weighs 78 kg and the solution strength is 5000 mg in 500 mL D5W. _____ After several titrations the rate is at 30 mL/hr. What dosage is infusing per min? _____

5.   A patient weighing 70 kg has a Dobutrex solution of 250 mg in 500 mL D5W ordered to titrate between 2.5–5 mcg/kg/min. _____ After many adjustments the titrated rate is now 27 mL/hr. What dosage is infusing per min? _____

ANSWERS 1. 8–15 mL/hr; 1.6 mg/min **2.** 15–45 mL/hr; 2.33 mcg/min **3.** 30–70 mL/hr; 0.2 mg/min **4.** 23–35 mL/hr; 5 mg/min **5.** 21–42 mL/hr; 0.23 mg/min

Summary

This concludes the chapter on critical care calculations most commonly encountered. The important points to remember from this chapter are:

critical care drugs have a rapid action and short duration, and alter or maintain vital body functions

all dosages and flow rates must be routinely double checked as critical care drugs have a narrow margin of safety

critical care drugs are infused by electronic infusion device or a 60 gtt/mL microdrip set

when an electronic infusion device or microdrip set is used the flow rate in mL/hr and gtt/min are identical

titration is the adjustment of dosage within a specific range to obtain a measurable change in a vital physiologic function

titrations are initiated at the lowest range ordered, and increased or decreased very slowly to obtain the desired response

all patients receiving critical care drugs must be monitored continuously

Summary Self Test

Directions: Read each question thoroughly then calculate only the dosages and flow rates indicated.

1. Dobutrex 6 mcg/kg/min is ordered to infuse IV to sustain the blood pressure of a patient weighing 75 kg. The solution available is 250 mg in 1 L of D5W. Calculate the mL/hr a volumetric pump will deliver. _____

2. Order: Infuse a Nipride solution of 50 mg in 500 mL D5W at 0.8 mcg/kg/min. Calculate the flow rate in mL/hr a 65 kg patient will receive. _____

3. A patient with aspiration pneumonia has an order for Aminophylline 1 g in 1000 mL D5W to infuse at 75 mL/hr. Calculate the dosage in mg/hr the patient will receive. _____

4. A solution of 400 mg dopamine HCl in 500 mL D5NS is infusing at 20 microdrops per min. Calculate the mg/hr the patient is receiving. _____

5. A doctor orders a pitocin drip by continuous IV infusion at 40 microdrops per min. The solution contains 20 U of pitocin in 1000 mL D5W. Calculate the U/hr dosage. _____

6. A patient with bigeminy has orders for an infusion of 500 mg Lidocaine in 250 mL D5W at 45 mL/hr. Calculate the mg/min and mg/hr this patient will receive. Is this within the normal range of 1–4 mg/min? _____

7. A terminal cancer patient has orders for continuous morphine sulfate IV. The solution available provides 0.5 mg/mL. The order is to infuse the drug at 8 mg/hr. Calculate the flow rate in mL/hr for a volumetric pump. _____

8. Order: Give 500 mg Aldomet in 150 mL D5W and infuse over 60 minutes. At what rate will you set the volumetric pump. _____

9. A patient in heart block has an Isuprel infusion ordered at 4 mcg/min. Solution available is 1 mg in 250 mL D5W. Calculate the flow rate in gtt/min for an IVAC controller. _____

10. For treatment of severe hypercalcemia a doctor orders Didronel 7.5 mg/kg diluted in 250 mL of NS to infuse over 3 hours. The patient weighs 46 kg. Calculate the dosage you would prepare, then determine the flow rate in mL/hr. Lastly, how many mg/hr would the patient receive? _____

11. 200 mg of dopamine is added to 250 mL D5W and an infusion is started at 45 gtt/min. Calculate the mcg/min and mg/hr the patient is receiving.

    _____

12. A patient with tetanus weighing 54 kg has orders for Thorazine 0.5 mg/kg in 500 mL NS. The infusion is run over 8 hours. First calculate the dosage, then the number of mL/hr at which you will infuse the drug. _____

13. A patient with chronic bronchitis and a severe respiratory infection is receiving 75 mL/hr of Aminophylline 1 g in 1 liter D5 ½NS. Determine the number of mg/hr the patient is receiving. _____

14. A physician orders 6 mg morphine sulfate every 30 minutes via a continuous IV drip. The available solution is 1 g in 1 liter D5NS. Calculate the flow rate in gtt/min using a microdrip. _____

15. A doctor orders 2 ampules of dopamine HCl to be added to 500 mL D5W to infuse at 25 mL/hr. Each ampule contains 200 mg. Calculate the mg/hr and mcg/min the patient is receiving. _____

16. A patient in CHF has orders to infuse 0.25 mg Lanoxin in 50 mL D5W over 15 min. Calculate the mg/min the patient will receive during the infusion.

    _____

17. Order: dopamine HCl 5 mcg/kg/min IV continuous. Solution available: 250 mL D5W with 400 mg dopamine. Patient weight 70 kg. Calculate the flow rate in mL/hr for a volumetric pump. _____

18. The doctor orders Pronestyl 3 mg/min IV. Solution available 500 mg in 250 mL D5 ¼NS. Calculate the flow rate in mL/hr. _____

19. A nitroglycerin solution of 25 mcg/mL is infusing at 30 gtt/min. Calculate the mcg/min the patient is receiving. _____

20. A patient with aplastic anemia has orders for 5 g Amicar to be added to 250 mL NS and infused over 90 min. Calculate the mg/hr and flow rate in gtt/min using a microdrip set. _____

21. Order: give 7 mg/kg of Amikin IV in 250 mL D5W over 2 hours. Patient weighs 82 kg. Calculate the dosage you would prepare then the mL/hr to deliver the drug on time. _____

22. For treatment of a gram negative infection the doctor has ordered polymyxin B 12,000 U in 500 mL D5W at 200 mL/hr. Calculate the U/hr the patient is receiving. _____

23. A patient with severe hypotension is receiving 3 mL/min of a solution of Levophed that contains 4 mg in 500 mL D5W. Calculate the mcg/min the patient is receiving. _____

24. A continuous infusion of Aminophylline at 0.7 mg/kg/hr is ordered for a patient weighing 45 kg. Solution available is 1 g in 1 liter D5W. Calculate mL/hr for delivery on a volumetric pump. _____

25. A patient in hypertensive crisis has orders for Arfonad 1.5 mg/min IV. Solution available is 500 mg in 500 mL D5W. Calculate gtt/min using an IVAC controller. _____

26. Calculate the flow rate for 100 mcg/min of dobutamine from a solution of 500 mg in 250 mL. _____

27. Amrinone 5–10 mcg/kg/min is to be titrated for a patient weighing 79 kg. The solution available is 250 mg in 50 mL NS. Determine the range in mL/hr flow rate. _____ After several titrations the IV is now infusing at 7 mL/hr. What dosage per min is this rate delivering? _____

28. Order: Dopamine 200 mg in 500 mL D5W. Titrate at 2–5 mcg/kg/min to maintain systolic BP > 110. The patient weighs 62 kg. Calculate the flow rate range for this titration in mL/hr. _____ After several adjustments the IV is now infusing at 32 mL/hr. What dosage is infusing per hr, and per min? _____ _____

29. Dobutamine has been ordered for a patient weighing 84 kg to titrate at 2.5–10 mcg/kg/min. The solution strength is 250 mg of dobutamine in 500 mL D5W. Calculate the mL/hr to deliver this dosage range. _____ After numberous adjustments the patient has finally stabilized at 78 mL/hr. What dosage per hr and per min is infusing? _____ _____

30. An 80 kg patient with multiple PVC's has a titration of Pronestyl 1–6 mg/min ordered. The solution available is 1 g in 250 mL D5W. Calculate the lower and upper flow rates to deliver. This dosage. _____ After 30 min the doctor orders the dosage increased to 3 mg/min. What flow rate will be set to titrate to this new dosage? _____

ANSWERS **1.** 108 mL/hr **2.** 31 mL/hr **3.** 75 mg/hr **4.** 16 mg/hr **5.** 0.8 U/hr **6.** 1.5 mg/min; 90 mg/hr; Yes **7.** 16 mL/hr **8.** 150 mL/hr **9.** 60 gtt/min **10.** 345 mg; 83 mL/hr; 115 mg/hr **11.** 36 mg/hr; 600 mcg/min **12.** 27 mg; 63 mL/hr **13.** 75 mg/hr **14.** 12 gtt/min **15.** 20 mg/hr; 333 mcg/min **16.** 0.017 mg/min **17.** 13 mL/hr **18.** 90 mL/hr **19.** 13 mcg/min **20.** 3,333 mg/hr; 167 gtt/min **21.** 574 mg; 125 mL/hr **22.** 4800 U/hr **23.** 24 mcg/min **24.** 32 mL/hr **25.** 90 gtt/min **26.** 3 mL/hr **27.** 5–10 mL/hr; 0.58 mg or 583 mcg/min **28.** 19–47 mL/hr; 12.8 mg/hr; 21.3 mg or 213 mcg/min **29.** 25–101 mL/hr; 39 mg/hr; 0.650 mg or 650 mcg/min **30.** 15–90 mL/hr; 45 mL/hr

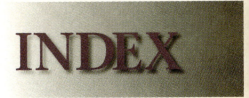